THE NATIONAL ACADEMIES PRESS   500 Fifth Street, N.W.   Washington, DC 20001

NOTICE: The project that is the subject of this report was approved by the Governing Board of the National Research Council, whose members are drawn from the councils of the National Academy of Sciences, the National Academy of Engineering, and the Institute of Medicine. The members of the committee responsible for the report were chosen for their special competences and with regard for appropriate balance.

This study was supported by Contract 200-2005-13434, TO#16, between the National Academy of Sciences and the Department of Health and Human Services (with support from the Centers for Disease Control and Prevention, the Office of Minority Health, and the Department of Veterans Affairs) and by the Task Force for Child Survival and Development on behalf of the National Viral Hepatitis Roundtable. Any opinions, findings, conclusions, or recommendations expressed in this publication are those of the author(s) and do not necessarily reflect the view of the organizations or agencies that provided support for this project.

Library of Congress Cataloging-in-Publication Data

Hepatitis and liver cancer : a national strategy for prevention and control of hepatitis B and C / Heather M. Colvin and Abigail E. Mitchell, editors ; Committee on the Prevention and Control of Viral Hepatitis Infections, Board on Population Health and Public Health Practice.
   p. ; cm.
  Includes bibliographical references and index.
  ISBN 978-0-309-14628-9
  1. Hepatitis B—United States. 2. Hepatitis C—United States. 3. Liver—Cancer—United States. I. Colvin, Heather M. II. Mitchell, Abigail E. III. Institute of Medicine (U.S.). Committee on the Prevention and Control of Viral Hepatitis Infections. IV. Institute of Medicine (U.S.). Board on Population Health and Public Health Practice. V. National Academies Press (U.S.).
  [DNLM: 1. Hepatitis B—complications—United States. 2. Hepatitis B—prevention & control—United States. 3. Hepatitis C—complications—United States. 4. Hepatitis C—prevention & control—United States. 5. Liver Neoplasms—prevention & control—United States. 6. Viral Hepatitis Vaccines—therapeutic use—United States. WC 536 H5322 2010]
  RA644.H4H37 2010
  616.99'436—dc22
                                 2010003194

Additional copies of this report are available from the National Academies Press, 500 Fifth Street, N.W., Lockbox 285, Washington, DC 20055; (800) 624-6242 or (202) 334-3313 (in the Washington metropolitan area); Internet, http://www.nap.edu.

For more information about the Institute of Medicine, visit the IOM home page at **www.iom.edu**.

Copyright 2010 by the National Academy of Sciences. All rights reserved.

Printed in the United States of America

The serpent has been a symbol of long life, healing, and knowledge among almost all cultures and religions since the beginning of recorded history. The serpent adopted as a logotype by the Institute of Medicine is a relief carving from ancient Greece, now held by the Staatliche Museen in Berlin.

Suggested citation: IOM (Institute of Medicine). 2010. *Hepatitis and Liver Cancer: A National Strategy for Prevention and Control of Hepatitis B and C.* Washington, DC: The National Academies Press.

HEPATITIS AND LIVER CANCER

A National Strategy for Prevention and Control of Hepatitis B and C

Heather M. Colvin and Abigail E. Mitchell, *Editors*

Committee on the Prevention and Control of Viral Hepatitis Infections

Board on Population Health and Public Health Practice

INSTITUTE OF MEDICINE
OF THE NATIONAL ACADEMIES

THE NATIONAL ACADEMIES PRESS
Washington, D.C.
www.nap.edu

"Knowing is not enough; we must apply.
Willing is not enough; we must do."
—Goethe

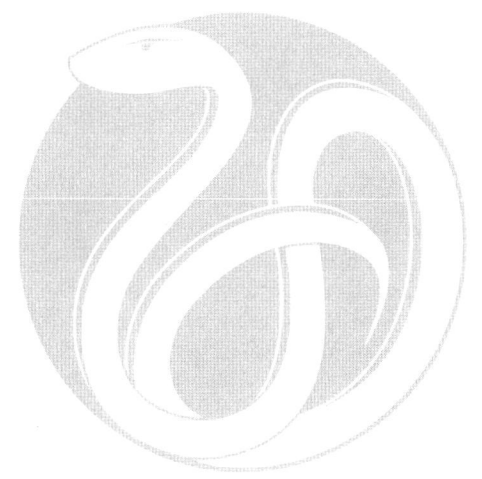

INSTITUTE OF MEDICINE
OF THE NATIONAL ACADEMIES

Advising the Nation. Improving Health.

THE NATIONAL ACADEMIES
Advisers to the Nation on Science, Engineering, and Medicine

The **National Academy of Sciences** is a private, nonprofit, self-perpetuating society of distinguished scholars engaged in scientific and engineering research, dedicated to the furtherance of science and technology and to their use for the general welfare. Upon the authority of the charter granted to it by the Congress in 1863, the Academy has a mandate that requires it to advise the federal government on scientific and technical matters. Dr. Ralph J. Cicerone is president of the National Academy of Sciences.

The **National Academy of Engineering** was established in 1964, under the charter of the National Academy of Sciences, as a parallel organization of outstanding engineers. It is autonomous in its administration and in the selection of its members, sharing with the National Academy of Sciences the responsibility for advising the federal government. The National Academy of Engineering also sponsors engineering programs aimed at meeting national needs, encourages education and research, and recognizes the superior achievements of engineers. Dr. Charles M. Vest is president of the National Academy of Engineering.

The **Institute of Medicine** was established in 1970 by the National Academy of Sciences to secure the services of eminent members of appropriate professions in the examination of policy matters pertaining to the health of the public. The Institute acts under the responsibility given to the National Academy of Sciences by its congressional charter to be an adviser to the federal government and, upon its own initiative, to identify issues of medical care, research, and education. Dr. Harvey V. Fineberg is president of the Institute of Medicine.

The **National Research Council** was organized by the National Academy of Sciences in 1916 to associate the broad community of science and technology with the Academy's purposes of furthering knowledge and advising the federal government. Functioning in accordance with general policies determined by the Academy, the Council has become the principal operating agency of both the National Academy of Sciences and the National Academy of Engineering in providing services to the government, the public, and the scientific and engineering communities. The Council is administered jointly by both Academies and the Institute of Medicine. Dr. Ralph J. Cicerone and Dr. Charles M. Vest are chair and vice chair, respectively, of the National Research Council.

www.national-academies.org

COMMITTEE ON THE PREVENTION AND CONTROL OF VIRAL HEPATITIS INFECTIONS

R. Palmer Beasley (*Chair*), Ashbel Smith Professor and Dean Emeritus, University of Texas, School of Public Health, Houston, Texas
Harvey J. Alter, Chief, Infectious Diseases Section, Department of Transfusion Medicine, National Institutes of Health, Bethesda, Maryland
Margaret L. Brandeau, Professor, Department of Management Science and Engineering, Stanford University, Stanford, California
Daniel R. Church, Epidemiologist and Adult Viral Hepatitis Coordinator, Bureau of Infectious Disease Prevention, Response, and Services, Massachusetts Department of Health, Jamaica Plain, Massachusetts
Alison A. Evans, Assistant Professor, Department of Epidemiology and Biostatistics, Drexel University School of Public Health, Drexel Institute of Biotechnology and Viral Research, Doylestown, Pennsylvania
Holly Hagan, Senior Research Scientist, College of Nursing, New York University, New York
Sandral Hullett, CEO and Medical Director, Cooper Green Hospital, Birmingham, Alabama
Stacene R. Maroushek, Staff Pediatrician, Department of Pediatrics, Hennepin County Medical Center, Minneapolis, Minnesota
Randall R. Mayer, Chief, Bureau of HIV, STD, and Hepatitis, Iowa Department of Public Health, Des Moines, Iowa
Brian J. McMahon, Medical Director, Liver Disease and Hepatitis Program, Alaska Native Tribal Health Consortium, Anchorage, Alaska
Martín Jose Sepúlveda, Vice President, Integrated Health Services, International Business Machines Corporation, Somers, New York
Samuel So, Lui Hac Minh Professor, Asian Liver Center, Stanford University School of Medicine, Stanford, California
David L. Thomas, Chief, Division of Infectious Diseases, Department of Medicine, Johns Hopkins School of Medicine, Baltimore, Maryland
Lester N. Wright, Deputy Commissioner and Chief Medical Officer, New York Department of Correctional Services, Albany, New York

Study Staff

Abigail E. Mitchell, Study Director
Heather M. Colvin, Program Officer
Kathleen M. McGraw, Senior Program Assistant
Norman Grossblatt, Senior Editor
Rose Marie Martinez, Director, Board on Population Health and Public Health Practice

Reviewers

This report has been reviewed in draft form by persons chosen for their diverse perspectives and technical expertise, in accordance with procedures approved by the National Research Council's (NRC's) Report Review Committee. The purpose of this independent review is to provide candid and critical comments that will assist the institution in making its published report as sound as possible and to ensure that the report meets institutional standards for objectivity, evidence, and responsiveness to the study charge. The review comments and draft manuscript remain confidential to protect the integrity of the deliberative process. We wish to thank the following individuals for their review of this report:

Scott Allen, Brown University Medical School
Jeffrey Caballero, Association of Asian Pacific Community Health Organizations
Colleen Flanigan, New York State Department of Health
James Jerry Gibson, South Carolina Department of Health and Environmental Control
Fernando A. Guerra, San Antonio Metropolitan Health District
Theodore Hammett, Abt Associates Inc.
Jay Hoofnagle, National Institute of Diabetes and Digestive and Kidney Diseases
Charles D. Howell, University of Maryland School of Medicine
Walter A. Orenstein, Bill & Melinda Gates Foundation
Philip E. Reichert, Florida Department of Health
Charles M. Rice III, The Rockefeller University

Tracy Swan, Treatment Action Group
Su Wang, Charles B. Wang Community Health Center
John B. Wong, Tufts Medical Center

Although the reviewers listed above have provided many constructive comments and suggestions, they were not asked to endorse the conclusions or recommendations, nor did they see the final draft of the report before its release. The review of the report was overseen by **Bradford H. Gray,** Senior Fellow, The Urban Institute, and **Elena O. Nightingale,** Scholar-in-Residence, Institute of Medicine. Appointed by the Institute of Medicine and the National Research Council, they were responsible for making certain that an independent examination of the report was carried out in accordance with institutional procedures and that all review comments were carefully considered. Responsibility for the final content of the report rests entirely with the author committee and the institution.

Acknowledgments

The committee acknowledges the valuable contributions made by the many persons who shared their experience and knowledge with the committee. The committee appreciates the time and insight of the presenters during the public sessions: **John Ward, Dale Hu, Cindy Weinbaum,** and **David Bell,** Centers for Disease Control and Prevention; **Chris Taylor** and **Martha Saly,** National Viral Hepatitis Roundtable; **Lorren Sandt,** Caring Ambassadors Program; **Joan Block,** Hepatitis B Foundation; **Gary Heseltine,** Council of State and Territorial Epidemiologists; **William Rogers,** Centers for Medicare and Medicaid Services; **Tanya Pagán Raggio Ashley,** Health Resources Services Administration; **Carol Craig,** National Association of Community Health Centers; **Daniel Raymond,** Harm Reduction Coalition; and **Mark Kane,** formerly of the Children's Vaccine Program, PATH. We are also grateful for the thoughtful written and verbal testimony provided by members of the public affected by hepatitis B or hepatitis C.

Several persons contributed their expertise for this report. The committee thanks **David Hutton,** of the Department of Management Science and Engineering at Stanford University; **Victor Toy, Beverly David,** and **Kathleen Tarleton,** of IBM; **Shiela Strauss,** of the New York University College of Nursing; **Ellen Chang** and **Stephanie Chao,** of the Asian Liver Center at Stanford University; **Gillian Haney,** of the Massachusetts Department of Public Health; and all the State Adult Viral Hepatitis Prevention Coordinators that provided information to the committee.

This report would not have been possible without the diligent assistance of **Jeffrey Efird** and **Daniel Riedford,** of the Centers for Disease Control and

Prevention. We appreciate the assistance of **Ronald Valdiserri,** of the Department of Veterans Affairs, for providing literature for the report.

The committee thanks the staff members of the Institute of Medicine, the National Research Council, and the National Academies Press who contributed to the development, production, and dissemination of this report. The committee thanks the study director, Abigail Mitchell, and program officer Heather Colvin for their work in navigating this complex topic and Kathleen McGraw for her diligent management of the committee logistics.

This report was made possible by the support of the Division of Viral Hepatitis and Division of Cancer Prevention and Control of the Centers for Disease Control and Prevention, the Department of Health and Human Services Office of Minority Health, the Department of Veterans Affairs, and the National Viral Hepatitis Roundtable.

Contents

ACRONYMS AND ABBREVIATIONS   xvii

SUMMARY   1
    The Charge to the Committee, 2
    Findings and Recommendations, 2
        Surveillance, 3
        Knowledge and Awareness, 8
        Immunization, 9
        Viral Hepatitis Services, 12
    Recommendation Outcomes, 17

1   INTRODUCTION   19
    Prevalence and Incidence of Hepatitis B and Hepatitis C
    Worldwide, 22
    Prevalence and Incidence of Hepatitis B and Hepatitis C
    in the United States, 25
        Hepatitis B, 25
        Hepatitis C, 28
    Liver Cancer and Liver Disease from Chronic Hepatitis B Virus and
    Hepatitis C Virus Infections, 29
    The Committee's Task, 30
    The Committee's Approach to Its Task, 32
    References, 35

2 SURVEILLANCE   41
   Applications of Surveillance Data, 43
      Outbreak Detection and Control, 44
      Resource Allocation, 45
      Programmatic Design and Evaluation, 45
      Linking Patients to Care, 45
   Disease-Specific Issues Related to Viral-Hepatitis Surveillance, 46
      Identifying Acute Infections, 47
      Identifying Chronic Infections, 51
      Identifying Perinatal Hepatitis B, 54
      Other Challenges for Hepatitis B and Hepatitis C Surveillance Systems, 56
   Infrastructure and Process-Specific Issues with Surveillance, 57
      Funding Sources, 58
      Program Design, 59
      Reporting Systems and Requirements, 59
      Capturing Data on At-Risk Populations, 61
      Case Evaluation, Followup, and Partner Services, 62
      Recommendations, 63
   Model for Surveillance, 66
      Core Surveillance, 67
      Targeted Surveillance, 71
   References, 72

3 KNOWLEDGE AND AWARENESS ABOUT CHRONIC
   HEPATITIS B AND HEPATITIS C   79
   Knowledge and Awareness Among Health-Care and Social-Service Providers, 80
      Hepatitis B, 81
      Hepatitis C, 83
      Recommendation, 85
   Community Knowledge and Awareness, 89
      Hepatitis B, 89
      Hepatitis C, 93
      Recommendation, 96
   References, 101

4 IMMUNIZATION   109
   Hepatitis B Vaccine, 109
      Current Vaccination Recommendations, Requirements, and Rates, 110
      Immunization-Information Systems, 126

CONTENTS xiii

        Barriers to Hepatitis B Vaccination, 127
    Hepatitis C Vaccine, 136
        Feasibility of Preventing Chronic Hepatitis C, 136
        Need for a Vaccine to Prevent Chronic Hepatitis C, 137
        Cost Effectiveness of a Hepatitis C Vaccine, 137
    References, 138

5   VIRAL HEPATITIS SERVICES   147
    Current Status, 148
    Components of Viral Hepatitis Services, 154
        Identification of Infected Persons, 154
        Prevention, 166
        Medical Management, 166
    Major Gaps in Services, 170
        General Population, 170
        Foreign-Born People, 173
        Illicit-Drug Users, 175
        Pregnant Women, 181
        Correctional Settings, 184
        Community Health Facilities, 186
        Targeting Settings That Serve At-Risk Populations, 189
    References, 192

A   COMMITTEE BIOGRAPHIES   209
B   PUBLIC MEETING AGENDAS   215

BOXES, FIGURES, AND TABLES

Boxes

S-1   Recommendations, 4

2-1   Role of Disease Surveillance, 42
2-2   CDC Acute Hepatitis B Case Definition, 48
2-3   CDC Acute Hepatitis C Case Definition, 49
2-4   CDC Chronic Hepatitis B Case Definition, 52
2-5   CDC Hepatitis C Virus Infection Case Definition (Past or Present), 53
2-6   CDC Perinatal Hepatitis B Virus Infection Case Definition, 55

3-1   Geographic Regions That Have Intermediate and High Hepatitis B Virus Endemicity, 81

4-1 Summary of ACIP Hepatitis B Vaccination Recommendations, 112

5-1 Summary of Recommendations Regarding Viral Hepatitis Services, 148
5-2 Mission Statement of Centers for Disease Control and Prevention Division of Viral Hepatitis, 150
5-3 Components of Comprehensive Viral Hepatitis Services, 155
5-4 Summary of CDC At-Risk Populations for Hepatitis B Virus Infection, 156
5-5 Summary of CDC At-Risk Populations for Hepatitis C Virus Infection, 158
5-6 Hepatitis B Virus-Specific Antigens and Antibodies Used for Testing, 160

Figures

1-1 Approximate global preventable death rate from selected infectious diseases and other causes, 2003, 20
1-2 The committee's approach to its task, 34

2-1 Natural progression of hepatitis B infection, 46
2-2 Natural progression of hepatitis C infection, 47

4-1 Estimated cost of adult hepatitis B vaccination per quality adjusted life year (QALY) gained for different age groups and different rates of acute hepatitis B virus (HBV) infection incidence, 119
4-2 Trends in private health-insurance coverage, 133

5-1 Hepatitis B services model, 157
5-2 Essential viral hepatitis services for illicit-drug users, 180

Tables

1-1 Key Characteristics of Hepatitis B and Hepatitis C, 21
1-2 Burden of Selected Serious Chronic Viral Infections in the United States, 26

4-1 Hepatitis B Vaccine Schedules for Newborns, by Maternal HBsAg Status—ACIP Recommendations, 114
4-2 Hepatitis B Immunization Management of Preterm Infants Who Weigh Less Than 2,000 g, by Maternal HBsAg Status—ACIP Recommendations, 115

4-3 Estimated Chance That an Acute Hepatitis B Infection Becomes Chronic with Age, 118
4-4 Studies of Hepatitis B Vaccination Rates in Injection-Drug Users, 122
4-5 Public Health-Insurance Plans, 130

5-1 Summary of Adult Viral Hepatitis Prevention Coordinators Survey, 153
5-2 Interpretation of Hepatitis B Serologic Diagnostic Test Results, 161
5-3 Interpretation of Hepatitis C Virus Diagnostic Test Results, 164
5-4 Studies of Association Between Opiate Substitution Treatment and Hepatitis C Virus Seroconversion, 178

Acronyms and Abbreviations

AASLD	American Association for the Study of Liver Diseases
ACIP	Advisory Committee on Immunization Practices
ACOG	American College of Obstetricians and Gynecologists
AHRQ	Agency for Healthcare Research and Quality
AIDS	acquired immunodeficiency syndrome
ALT	alanine aminotransferase
anti-HBc	Hepatitis B core antibody
anti-HBs	Hepatitis B surface antibody
anti-HCV	Hepatitis C antibody
API	Asian and Pacific Islander
AST	aspartate transaminase
AVHPC	adult viral hepatitis prevention coordinators
CDC	Centers for Disease Control and Prevention
CHIP	Children's Health Insurance Program
CI	confidence interval
CIA	enhanced chemiluminescence
CMS	Centers for Medicare and Medicaid Services
DIS	disease intervention specialist
DTaP	diptheria and tetanus toxoids and acellular pertussis adsorbed vaccine
DUIT	drug user intervention trial
DVH	Division of Viral Hepatitis

EIA	enzyme immunoassay
EIP	Emerging Infections Program
EPSDT	early periodic screening diagnosis and treatment program
FDA	Food and Drug Administration
FEHBP	Federal Employee Health Benefit Program
FQHC	federally qualified health center
HAV	Hepatitis A virus
HBIG	Hepatitis B immunoglobulin
HBsAg	Hepatitis B surface antigen
HBV	Hepatitis B virus
HCC	hepatocellular carcinoma
HCV	Hepatitis C virus
HCW	health-care workers
HDHP	high deductable health plan
HIAA	Health Insurance Association of America
HIB	haemophilus influenzae type B
HIV	human immunodeficiency virus
HMO	health maintenance organization
HPV	human papilloma virus
HRSA	Health Resources and Services Administration
IDU	injection-drug user
IIS	immunization information systems
IOM	Institute of Medicine
IPV	inactivated polio virus
MMTP	methadone maintenance treatment program
NASTAD	National Alliance of State and Territorial AIDS Directors
NAT	nucleic acid test
NCHHSTP	National Center for HIV/AIDS, Viral Hepatitis, Sexually Transmitted Diseases, and Tuberculosis Prevention
NEDSS	National Electronic Disease Surveillance System
NETSS	National Electronic Telecommunications System for Surveillance
NGO	nongovernmental organization
NHANES	National Health and Nutrition Examination Survey
NIDU	non-injection-drug user
NVAC	National Vaccine Advisory Committee

OB/GYN	obstetrician/gynecologist
OMH	Office of Minority Health
OR	odds ratio
PEI	peer education intervention
PHIN	Public Health Information Network
POS	point of service
PPO	preferred provider organization
PY	person year
QALY	quality adjusted life year
RCT	randomized clinical trial
RIBA	recombinant immunoblot assay
RNA	ribonucleic acid
RSV	respiratory syncytial virus
SAMHSA	Substance Abuse and Mental Health Services Administration
SARS	severe acute respiratory syndrome
SEP	syringe exchange program
STD	sexually transmitted disease
STRIVE	Study To Reduce Intravenous Exposures
TB	tuberculosis
TCM	traditional Chinese medicine
USPHS	US Public Health Service
USPSTF	US Preventive Services Task Force
VA	Department of Veterans Affairs
vCJD	variant Creutzfeldt-Jakob disease
VFC	Vaccines for Children
WHO	World Health Organization

Summary

In the next 10 years, about 150,000 people in the United States will die from liver cancer and end-stage liver disease associated with chronic hepatitis B and hepatitis C. It is estimated that 3.5–5.3 million people—1–2% of the US population—are living with chronic hepatitis B virus (HBV) or hepatitis C virus (HCV) infections. Of those, 800,000 to 1.4 million have chronic HBV infections, and 2.7–3.9 million have chronic HCV infections. Chronic viral hepatitis infections are 3–5 times more frequent than HIV in the United States.

Because of the asymptomatic nature of chronic hepatitis B and hepatitis C, most people infected with HBV and HCV are not aware that they have been infected until they have symptoms of cirrhosis or a type of liver cancer, hepatocellular carcinoma (HCC), many years later. About 65% and 75% of the infected population are unaware that they are infected with HBV and HCV, respectively. Importantly, the prevention of chronic hepatitis B and chronic hepatitis C prevents the majority of HCC cases because HBV and HCV are the leading causes of this type of cancer.

Although the incidence of acute HBV infection is declining in the United States, due to the availability of hepatitis B vaccines, about 43,000 new acute HBV infections still occur each year. Of those new infections, about 1,000 infants acquire the infection during birth from their HBV-positive mothers. HBV is also transmitted by sexual contact with an infected person, sharing injection drug equipment, and needlestick injuries. African American adults have the highest rate of acute HBV infection in the United States and the highest rates of acute HBV infection occur in the southern region. People from Asia and the Pacific Islands comprise the largest foreign-born population that is at risk for chronic HBV infection. The number of people in the United States who are living with chronic HBV infection may be increasing as a result of immigration from highly endemic countries. On the basis of immigration patterns in the last decade, it is estimated that every year 40,000–45,000 people from HBV-endemic countries enter the United States legally.

There is no vaccine for hepatitis C. HCV is efficiently transmitted by direct percutaneous exposure to infectious blood. Persons likely to have chronic HCV infection include those who received a blood transfusion before 1992 and past or current injection-drug users (IDUs). Most IDUs in the United States have serologic evidence of HCV infection (that is, they have been exposed to HCV at some time). While HCV incidence appears to have declined over the last decade, a large portion of IDUs, who often do not have access to health-care services, are not identified by current surveillance systems making interpretation of that trend complicated. African Americans and Hispanics have a higher rate of HCV infection than whites.

THE CHARGE TO THE COMMITTEE

Despite federal, state, and local public health efforts to prevent and control hepatitis B and hepatitis C, these diseases remain serious health problems in the United States. Therefore, the Centers for Disease Control and Prevention (CDC) in conjunction with the Department of Health and Human Services Office of Minority Health, the Department of Veterans Affairs, and the National Viral Hepatitis Roundtable sought guidance from the Institute of Medicine (IOM) in identifying missed opportunities related to the prevention and control of HBV and HCV infections. IOM was asked to focus on hepatitis B and hepatitis C because they are common in the United States and can lead to chronic disease. The charge to the committee follows.

> The IOM will form a committee to determine ways to reduce new HBV and HCV infections and the morbidity and mortality related to chronic viral hepatitis. The committee will assess current prevention and control activities and identify priorities for research, policy, and action. The committee will highlight issues that warrant further investigations and opportunities for collaboration between private and public sectors.

FINDINGS AND RECOMMENDATIONS

Upon reviewing evidence on the prevention and control of hepatitis B and hepatitis C, the committee identified the underlying factors that impede current efforts to prevent and control these diseases. Three major factors were found:

1. There is a lack of knowledge and awareness about chronic viral hepatitis on the part of health-care and social-service providers.
2. There is a lack of knowledge and awareness about chronic viral hepatitis among at-risk populations, members of the public, and policy-makers.
3. There is insufficient understanding about the extent and seriousness of this public-health problem, so inadequate public resources are being allocated to prevention, control, and surveillance programs.

That situation has created several consequences:

- Inadequate disease surveillance systems underreport acute and chronic infections, so the full extent of the problem is unknown.
- At-risk people do not know that they are at risk or how to prevent becoming infected.
- At-risk people may not have access to preventive services.
- Chronically infected people do not know that they are infected.
- Many health-care providers do not screen people for risk factors or do not know how to manage infected people.
- Infected people often have inadequate access to testing, social support, and medical management services.

To address those consequences, the committee offers recommendations in four categories: surveillance, knowledge and awareness, immunization, and services for viral hepatitis. The recommendations are discussed below, and listed in Box S-1.

Surveillance

The viral hepatitis surveillance system in the United States is highly fragmented and poorly developed. As a result, surveillance data do not provide accurate estimates of the current burden of disease, are insufficient for program planning and evaluation, and do not provide the information that would allow policy-makers to allocate sufficient resources to viral hepatitis prevention and control programs. The federal government has provided few resources—in the form of guidance, funding, and oversight—to local and state health departments to perform surveillance for viral hepatitis. Additional funding sources for surveillance, such as funding from states and cities, vary among jurisdictions. The committee found little published information on or systematic review of viral hepatitis surveillance in the United States and offers the following recommendation to determine the current status of the surveillance system:

**BOX S-1
Recommendations**

Chapter 2: Surveillance
- 2-1. The Centers for Disease Control and Prevention should conduct a comprehensive evaluation of the national hepatitis B and hepatitis C public-health surveillance system.
- 2-2. The Centers for Disease Control and Prevention should develop specific cooperative viral-hepatitis agreements with all state and territorial health departments to support core surveillance for acute and chronic hepatitis B and hepatitis C.
- 2-3. The Centers for Disease Control and Prevention should support and conduct targeted active surveillance, including serologic testing, to monitor incidence and prevalence of hepatitis B virus and hepatitis C virus infections in populations not fully captured by core surveillance.

Chapter 3: Knowledge and Awareness about Chronic Hepatitis B and Hepatitis C
- 3-1. The Centers for Disease Control and Prevention should work with key stakeholders (other federal agencies, state and local governments, professional organizations, health-care organizations, and educational institutions) to develop hepatitis B and hepatitis C educational programs for health-care and social-service providers.
- 3-2. The Centers for Disease Control and Prevention should work with key stakeholders to develop, coordinate, and evaluate innovative and effective outreach and education programs to target at-risk populations and to increase awareness in the general population about hepatitis B and hepatitis C.

Chapter 4: Immunization
- 4-1. All infants weighing at least 2,000 grams and born to hepatitis B surface antigen-positive women should receive single-antigen hepatitis B vaccine and hepatitis B immune globulin in the delivery room as soon as they are stable and washed. The recommendations of the Advisory Committee on Immunization Practices should remain in effect for all other infants.
- 4-2. All states should mandate that the hepatitis B vaccine series be completed or in progress as a requirement for school attendance.
- 4-3. Additional federal and state resources should be devoted to increasing hepatitis B vaccination of at-risk adults.

- 4-4. States should be encouraged to expand immunization-information systems to include adolescents and adults.
- 4-5. Private and public insurance coverage for hepatitis B vaccination should be expanded.
- 4-6. The federal government should work to ensure an adequate, accessible, and sustainable hepatitis B vaccine supply.
- 4-7. Studies to develop a vaccine to prevent chronic hepatitis C virus infection should continue.

Chapter 5: Viral Hepatitis Services
- 5-1. Federally funded health-insurance programs—such as Medicare, Medicaid, and the Federal Employees Health Benefits Program—should incorporate guidelines for risk-factor screening for hepatitis B and hepatitis C as a required core component of preventive care so that at-risk people receive serologic testing for hepatitis B virus and hepatitis C virus and chronically infected patients receive appropriate medical management.
- 5-2. The Centers for Disease Control and Prevention, in conjunction with other federal agencies and state agencies, should provide resources for the expansion of community-based programs that provide hepatitis B screening, testing, and vaccination services that target foreign-born populations.
- 5-3. Federal, state, and local agencies should expand programs to reduce the risk of hepatitis C virus infection through injection-drug use by providing comprehensive hepatitis C virus prevention programs. At a minimum, the programs should include access to sterile needle syringes and drug-preparation equipment because the shared use of these materials has been shown to lead to transmission of hepatitis C virus.
- 5-4. Federal and state governments should expand services to reduce the harm caused by chronic hepatitis B and hepatitis C. The services should include testing to detect infection, counseling to reduce alcohol use and secondary transmission, hepatitis B vaccination, and referral for or provision of medical management.
- 5-5. Innovative, effective, multicomponent hepatitis C virus prevention strategies for injection-drug users and non-injection-drug users should be developed and evaluated to achieve greater control of hepatitis C virus transmission.
- 5-6. The Centers for Disease Control and Prevention should provide additional resources and guidance to perinatal hepatitis B

continued

> **BOX S-1 Continued**
>
> prevention program coordinators to expand and enhance the capacity to identify chronically infected pregnant women and provide case-management services, including referral for appropriate medical management.
> - 5-7. The National Institutes of Health should support a study of he effectiveness and safety of peripartum antiviral therapy to reduce and possibly eliminate perinatal hepatitis B virus transmission from women at high risk for perinatal transmission.
> - 5-8. The Centers for Disease Control and Prevention and the Department of Justice should create an initiative to foster partnerships between health departments and corrections systems to ensure the availability of comprehensive viral hepatitis services for incarcerated people.
> - 5-9. The Health Resources and Services Administration should provide adequate resources to federally funded community health facilities for provision of comprehensive viral-hepatitis services.
> - 5-10. The Health Resources and Services Administration and the Centers for Disease Control and Prevention should provide resources and guidance to integrate comprehensive viral hepatitis services into settings that serve high-risk populations such as STD clinics, sites for HIV services and care, homeless shelters, and mobile health units.

Recommendation 2-1. The Centers for Disease Control and Prevention should conduct a comprehensive evaluation of the national hepatitis B and hepatitis C public-health surveillance system.

The evaluation should, at a minimum,

- Include assessment of the system's attributes, including completeness, data quality and accuracy, timeliness, sensitivity, specificity, predictive value positive, representativeness, and stability.
- Be consistent with CDC's Updated Guidelines for Evaluating Public Health Surveillance Systems.
- Be used to guide the development of detailed technical guidance and standards for viral hepatitis surveillance.
- Be published in a report.

The committee offers the following recommendations aimed at making viral hepatitis surveillance systems more consistent among jurisdictions and improving their ability to collect and report data on acute and chronic hepatitis B and hepatitis C more accurately:

Recommendation 2-2. The Centers for Disease Control and Prevention should develop specific cooperative viral-hepatitis agreements with all state and territorial health departments to support core surveillance for acute and chronic hepatitis B and hepatitis C.

The agreements should include

- A funding mechanism and guidance for core surveillance activities.
- Implementation of performance standards regarding revised and standardized case definitions, specifically through the use of
  o Revised case-reporting forms with required, standardized components.
  o Case evaluation and followup.
- Support for developing and implementing automated data-collection systems, including
  o Electronic laboratory reporting.
  o Electronic medical-record extraction systems.
  o Web-based, Public Health Information Network-compliant reporting systems.

Recommendation 2-3. The Centers for Disease Control and Prevention should support and conduct targeted active surveillance, including serologic testing, to monitor incidence and prevalence[1] of hepatitis B virus and hepatitis C virus infections in populations not fully captured by core surveillance.

- Active surveillance should be conducted in specific (sentinel) geographic regions and populations.
- Appropriate serology, molecular biology, and followup will allow for distinction between acute and chronic hepatitis B and hepatitis C.

---

[1] Incidence refers to the number of new cases within a specified period of time. Prevalence refers to the number of existing cases in a specified population at a designated time.

Knowledge and Awareness

The committee found that there is relatively poor awareness about hepatitis B and hepatitis C among health-care providers, social-service providers (such as staff of drug-treatment facilities and immigrant-services centers), and the public, especially important, among members of specific at-risk populations. Lack of awareness about the prevalence of chronic viral hepatitis in the United States and the target populations and appropriate methodology for screening, testing, and medical management of chronic hepatitis B and hepatitis C probably contributes to continuing transmission; missing of opportunities for prevention, including vaccination; missing of opportunities for early diagnosis and medical care; and poor health outcomes in infected people.

To improve knowledge and awareness among health-care providers and social-service providers, the committee offers the following recommendation:

Recommendation 3-1. The Centers for Disease Control and Prevention should work with key stakeholders (other federal agencies, state and local governments, professional organizations, health-care organizations, and educational institutions) to develop hepatitis B and hepatitis C educational programs for health-care and social-service providers.

The educational programs should include at least the following components:

- Information about the prevalence and incidence of acute and chronic hepatitis B and hepatitis C both in the general US population and in at-risk populations, particularly foreign-born populations in the case of hepatitis B, and IDUs and incarcerated populations in the case of hepatitis C.
- Guidance on screening for risk factors associated with hepatitis B and hepatitis C.
- Information about hepatitis B and hepatitis C prevention, hepatitis B immunization, and medical monitoring of chronically infected patients.
- Information about prevention of HBV and HCV transmission in hospital and nonhospital health-care settings.
- Information about discrimination and stigma associated with hepatitis B and hepatitis C and guidance on reducing them.
- Information about health disparities related to hepatitis B and hepatitis C.

To increase knowledge and awareness about hepatitis B and hepatitis C in at-risk populations and the general population, the committee offers the following recommendation:

Recommendation 3-2. The Centers for Disease Control and Prevention should work with key stakeholders to develop, coordinate, and evaluate innovative and effective outreach and education programs to target at-risk populations and to increase awareness in the general population about hepatitis B and hepatitis C.

The programs should be linguistically and culturally appropriate and should advance integration of viral hepatitis and liver-health education into other health programs that serve at-risk populations. They should incorporate interventions that meet the following goals:

- Promote better understanding of HBV and HCV infections, transmission, prevention, and treatment in the at-risk and general populations.
- Promote increased hepatitis B vaccination rates among children and at-risk adults.
- Educate pregnant women and women of childbearing age about hepatitis B prevention.
- Reduce perinatal HBV infections and improve at-birth immunization rates.
- Increase testing rates in at-risk populations.
- Reduce stigmatization of chronically infected people.
- Promote safe injections among IDUs and safe drug use among non-injection-drug users (NIDUs).
- Provide culturally and linguistically appropriate educational information for all persons who have tested positive for chronic HBV or HCV infections and those who are receiving treatment.
- Encourage notification of close household and sexual contacts of infected people to be tested for HBV and HCV and encourage hepatitis B vaccination of close contacts.

Immunization

The longstanding availability of effective hepatitis B vaccines makes the elimination of new HBV infections possible, particularly in children. As noted above, about 1,000 newborns are infected by their HBV-positive mothers at birth each year in the United States, and that number has not declined in the last decade. To prevent transmission of HBV from mothers to their newborns, the Advisory Committee on Immunization Practices

(ACIP) recommends that infants born to mothers who are positive for hepatitis B surface antigen (HBsAg) receive hepatitis B immune globulin and a first dose of the hepatitis B vaccine within 12 hours of birth. To improve adherence to that guideline, the committee offers the following recommendation:

> **Recommendation 4-1. All infants weighing at least 2,000 grams and born to hepatitis B surface antigen-positive women should receive single-antigen hepatitis B vaccine and hepatitis B immune globulin in the delivery room as soon as they are stable and washed. The recommendations of the Advisory Committee on Immunization Practices should remain in effect for all other infants.**

The ACIP recommends administration of the hepatitis B vaccine series to unvaccinated children and young adults under 19 years old. School-entry mandates have been shown to increase hepatitis B vaccination rates and to reduce disparities in vaccination rates. Overall, hepatitis B vaccination rates in school-age children are high (for example, about 80% of states reported at least 95% hepatitis B vaccine coverage of children in kindergarten in 2006–2007), but there is variability in coverage among states. Additionally, there are racial and ethnic disparities in childhood vaccination rates—Asian and Pacific Islander (API), Hispanic, and African American children have lower vaccination rates than non-Hispanic white children. Regarding vaccination of children and adults under 19 years old, the committee offers the following recommendation:

> **Recommendation 4-2. All states should mandate that the hepatitis B vaccine series be completed or in progress as a requirement for school attendance.**

Hepatitis B vaccination for adults is directed at high-risk groups—people at risk for HBV infection from infected household contact and sex partners, from injection-drug use, from occupational exposure to infected blood or body fluids, and from travel to regions that have high or intermediate HBV endemicity. Only about half the adults who are at high risk for HBV infection receive the hepatitis B vaccine. Low coverage of high-risk adults is attributed to the lack of dedicated vaccine programs; limitations of funding, insurance coverage, and cost-sharing; and noncompliance of the involved populations. To increase the rate of hepatitis B vaccination of at-risk adults, the committee offers the following recommendation:

> **Recommendation 4-3. Additional federal and state resources should be devoted to increasing hepatitis B vaccination of at-risk adults.**

- Correctional institutions should offer hepatitis B vaccination to all incarcerated persons. Accelerated schedules for vaccine administration should be considered for jail inmates.
- Organizations that serve high-risk populations should offer the hepatitis B vaccination series.
- Efforts should be made to improve identification of at-risk adults. Health-care providers should routinely seek risk behavior histories from adult patients through direct questioning and self-assessment.
- Efforts should be made to increase rates of completion of the vaccine series in adults.
- Federal and state agencies should annually determine gaps in hepatitis B vaccine coverage among at-risk adults and estimate the resources needed to fill those gaps.

Immunization-information systems are used for collection and consolidation of vaccination data from multiple health-care providers, vaccine management, adverse-event reporting, and tracking lifespan vaccination histories. States have made progress on developing and implementing immunization-information systems, particularly with regard to collecting vaccination data on children. The committee believes that it is also important to include vaccination data on adolescents and adults in immunization information systems and offers the following recommendation:

Recommendation 4-4. States should be encouraged to expand immunization-information systems to include adolescents and adults.

Coverage for hepatitis B vaccination is greater for children and youths than for adults. Except for Medicaid's Early Periodic Screening, Diagnosis, and Treatment entitlement, public-health insurance often contains cost-sharing, which may create a barrier to vaccination for some people. Private health insurance has gaps for vaccination coverage because it does not universally cover all ACIP-recommended vaccinations for children and adults. Furthermore, most privately insured persons are required to pay to receive vaccinations. To reduce barriers to children and adults for hepatitis B vaccination, the committee offers the following recommendation:

Recommendation 4-5. Private and public insurance coverage for hepatitis B vaccination should be expanded.

- Public Health Section 317 should be expanded with sufficient funding to become the public safety net for underinsured and uninsured adults to receive the hepatitis B vaccination.

- All private insurance plans should include coverage for all ACIP-recommended vaccinations. Hepatitis B vaccination should be free of any deductible so that first-dollar coverage exists for this preventive service.

There has not been a national shortage of the hepatitis B vaccine, however, temporary supply problems occurred with this vaccine in 2008 (adult and dialysis formulations of Recombivax HB) and 2009 (pediatric formulations of Recombivax HB and Pediatric Engerix-B). A shortage was avoided because other manufacturers were able to provide an adequate supply of the vaccine in adult and dialysis formulations, and CDC released doses of pediatric vaccine from its stockpile. To prevent future supply problems of the hepatitis B vaccine, the committee offers the following recommendation:

Recommendation 4-6. The federal government should work to ensure an adequate, accessible, and sustainable hepatitis B vaccine supply.

Efforts are going on to develop a vaccine for hepatitis C, which could substantially enhance hepatitis C prevention efforts. The committee recognizes the need for a safe, effective, and affordable hepatitis C vaccine and offers the following recommendation:

Recommendation 4-7. Studies to develop a vaccine to prevent chronic hepatitis C virus infection should continue.

Viral Hepatitis Services

Health services related to viral hepatitis prevention, risk-factor screening and serologic testing,[2] and medical management are both sparse and fragmented among entities at the federal, state, and local levels. The committee believes that a coordinated approach is necessary to reduce the numbers of new HBV and HCV infections, illnesses, and deaths associated with these infections. Comprehensive viral hepatitis services should have five core components: outreach and awareness, prevention of new infections, identification of infected people, social and peer support, and medical management of infected people.

The committee identified major gaps in viral hepatitis services for the general population and specific groups that are heavily affected by HBV and HCV infections: foreign-born populations, illicit-drug users, and

---

[2] Risk-factor screening is the process of determining whether a person is at risk for being chronically infected or becoming infected with HBV or HCV. Serologic testing is laboratory testing of blood specimens for biomarker confirmation of HBV or HCV infection.

pregnant women. It also examined venues that provide services to at-risk groups: correctional facilities, community health facilities, STD and HIV clinics, shelter-based programs, and mobile health units. The committee offers recommendations to address major deficiencies for each group and health-care venue.

General Population

Most people who are chronically infected with HBV or HCV are unaware of their infection status. As treatments for chronic hepatitis B and C improve, it becomes critical to identify chronically infected people. Therefore, it is important that the general population have access to screening and testing services so that people who are at risk for viral hepatitis can be identified. The federal government is the largest purchaser of health insurance nationally and is well positioned to be the leader in the development and enforcement of guidelines to ensure that the people for whom it provides health care have access to risk-factor screening, serologic testing for HBV and HCV, and appropriate medical management.

Recommendation 5-1. Federally funded health-insurance programs—such as Medicare, Medicaid, and the Federal Employees Health Benefits Program—should incorporate guidelines for risk-factor screening for hepatitis B and hepatitis C as a required core component of preventive care so that at-risk people receive serologic testing for hepatitis B virus and hepatitis C virus and chronically infected patients receive appropriate medical management.

Foreign-Born Populations

Nearly half of US foreign-born people, or 6% of the total US population, originate in HBV-endemic countries. Thus, there is a growing urgency for culturally appropriate programs to provide hepatitis B screening and related services to this high-risk population. There is a pervasive lack of knowledge about hepatitis B among Asians and Pacific Islanders, and this is probably also the case for other foreign-born people in the United States. The lack of awareness in foreign-born populations from HBV-endemic countries is compounded by the gaps in knowledge and preventive practice among health-care and social-service providers, particularly those who serve a large number of foreign-born, high-risk patients. The committee believes that the needs of foreign-born people are best met with the approach outlined in Recommendations 3-1 and 3-2. The community-based approach as outlined in Recommendation 3-2 would be strengthened by additional resources to provide screening, testing, and vaccination services.

Recommendation 5-2. The Centers for Disease Control and Prevention, in conjunction with other federal agencies and state agencies, should provide resources for the expansion of community-based programs that provide hepatitis B screening, testing, and vaccination services that target foreign-born populations.

Illicit-Drug Users

HBV and HCV infection rates in illicit-drug users are high, particularly in IDUs. HCV is easily transmitted among IDUs, and methods to promote safe injection can be considered essential for HCV control. However, safe-injection strategies alone are insufficient to control HCV transmission. Prevention of HCV infection is a function of multiple factors—safe-injection strategies, education, testing, and drug treatment—so an integrated approach that includes all these elements is more likely to be effective in preventing hepatitis C.

Recommendation 5-3. Federal, state, and local agencies should expand programs to reduce the risk of hepatitis C virus infection through injection-drug use by providing comprehensive hepatitis C virus prevention programs. At a minimum, the programs should include access to sterile needle syringes and drug-preparation equipment because the shared use of these materials has been shown to lead to transmission of hepatitis C virus.

Although illicit-drug use is associated with many serious acute and chronic medical conditions, health-care use among drug users is lower than among persons who do not use illicit drugs. Health care for both IDUs and NIDUs is sporadic and typically received in hospital emergency rooms, corrections facilities, and STD clinics. Given that population's poor access to health care and services, it is important to have prevention and care services in settings that IDUs and NIDUs are likely to frequent or to develop programs that will draw them into care.

Recommendation 5-4. Federal and state governments should expand services to reduce the harm caused by chronic hepatitis B and hepatitis C. The services should include testing to detect infection, counseling to reduce alcohol use and secondary transmission, hepatitis B vaccination, and referral for or provision of medical management.

Studies have shown that the first few years after onset of injection-drug use constitute a high-risk period in which the rate of HCV infection can exceed 40%. Preventing the transition from non-injection-drug use to injection-drug use will probably avert many HCV infections. The committee therefore offers the following research recommendation:

> **Recommendation 5-5.** Innovative, effective, multicomponent hepatitis C virus prevention strategies for injection-drug users and non-injection-drug users should be developed and evaluated to achieve greater control of hepatitis C virus transmission. In particular,
> - Hepatitis C prevention programs for persons who smoke or sniff heroin, cocaine, and other drugs should be developed and tested.
> - Programs to prevent the transition from noninjection use of illicit drugs to injection should be developed and implemented.

Pregnant Women

States and large metropolitan areas are eligible to receive federal funding to support perinatal hepatitis B prevention programs through CDC's National Center for Immunization and Respiratory Diseases. Comprehensive programs have been shown to be effective not only in identifying HBV-infected pregnant women but in providing other case-management services (for example, testing of household and sexual contacts and referral to medical care). However, most programs are understaffed and underfunded and cannot offer adequate case-management services.

> **Recommendation 5-6.** The Centers for Disease Control and Prevention should provide additional resources and guidance to perinatal hepatitis B prevention program coordinators to expand and enhance the capacity to identify chronically infected pregnant women and provide case-management services, including referral for appropriate medical management.

Although an increasing number of effective HBV antiviral suppressive medications have become available for the management of chronic HBV infection, very little research has been done on the use of these medications during the last trimester of pregnancy to eliminate the risk of perinatal transmission. The committee believes that there is a need to fund research to guide the effective use of antiviral medications late in pregnancy to prevent maternofetal HBV transmission, and offers the following research recommendation:

> **Recommendation 5-7.** The National Institutes of Health should support a study of the effectiveness and safety of peripartum antiviral therapy to reduce and possibly eliminate perinatal hepatitis B virus transmission from women at high risk for perinatal transmission.

Correctional Facilities

Incarcerated populations have higher rates of HBV and HCV infections than the general population. Screening of all incarcerated people for risk factors can identify those who need blood tests for infection and, if appropriate, treatment.

> **Recommendation 5-8.** The Centers for Disease Control and Prevention and the Department of Justice should create an initiative to foster partnerships between health departments and corrections systems to ensure the availability of comprehensive viral hepatitis services for incarcerated people.

Community Health Centers

The Health Resources and Services Administration administers grant programs across the country to deliver primary care to uninsured and underinsured people in community health centers, migrant health centers, homeless programs, and public-housing primary-care programs. In general, funding of viral hepatitis services at community health centers is inadequate. Because community health centers provide primary health care for many people who are at risk for hepatitis B and hepatitis C, it is important for them to offer comprehensive viral hepatitis services.

> **Recommendation 5-9.** The Health Resources and Services Administration should provide adequate resources to federally funded community health facilities for provision of comprehensive viral-hepatitis services.

Other Settings That Target At-Risk Populations

STD and HIV clinics, shelter-based programs, and mobile health units are settings that serve populations that are at risk for hepatitis B and hepatitis C. The populations that use the settings may not have access to care through traditional health-care venues. Integration of viral hepatitis services into those settings creates opportunities to identify at-risk clients and to get them other services that they need.

> **Recommendation 5-10.** The Health Resources and Services Administration and the Centers for Disease Control and Prevention should provide resources and guidance to integrate comprehensive viral hepatitis services into settings that serve high-risk populations such as STD

clinics, sites for HIV services and care, homeless shelters, and mobile health units.

RECOMMENDATION OUTCOMES

The committee believes that implementation of its recommendations would lead to reductions in new HBV and HCV infections, in medical complications and deaths that result from these viral infections of the liver, and in total health costs. Advances in three major categories will be needed: in knowledge and awareness about chronic viral hepatitis among healthcare and social-service providers, the general public, and policy-makers; in improvement and better integration of viral hepatitis services, including expanded hepatitis B vaccination coverage; and in improvement of estimates of the burden of disease for resource-allocation purposes.

1

Introduction

The global epidemic of hepatitis B and hepatitis C is a serious public-health problem. Using mortality data from 2003, Weiss and McMichael (2004) ranked the public-health importance of various infectious diseases and other conditions (see Figure 1-1). Those data underscore that chronic hepatitis B and hepatitis C are among the leading causes of preventable death worldwide.

Hepatitis B and hepatitis C are contagious liver diseases caused by the hepatitis B virus (HBV) and the hepatitis C virus (HCV), respectively. HBV is a 42-nanometer, partially double-stranded DNA virus classified in the Hepadnaviridae family; there are eight major HBV genotypes. HCV is a 55-nanometer, enveloped, positive-strand RNA virus classified as a separate genus, *Hepacavirus*, in the Flaviviridae family; there are at least six major HCV genotypes.

Hepatitis B and hepatitis C can be either acute or chronic. The acute form is a short-term illness that occurs within the first 6 months after a person is exposed to HBV or HCV. The diseases can become chronic, although this does not always happen and, particularly in the case of hepatitis B, the likelihood of chronicity depends on a person's age at the time of infection. Chronic hepatitis B and chronic hepatitis C are serious and can result in liver cirrhosis and a type of liver cancer, hepatocellular carcinoma (HCC). The prevention of chronic hepatitis B and chronic hepatitis C prevents the majority of HCC cases because HBV and HCV are the leading causes of this type of cancer. Key characteristics of hepatitis B and hepatitis C are summarized in Table 1-1 and discussed below and in later chapters.

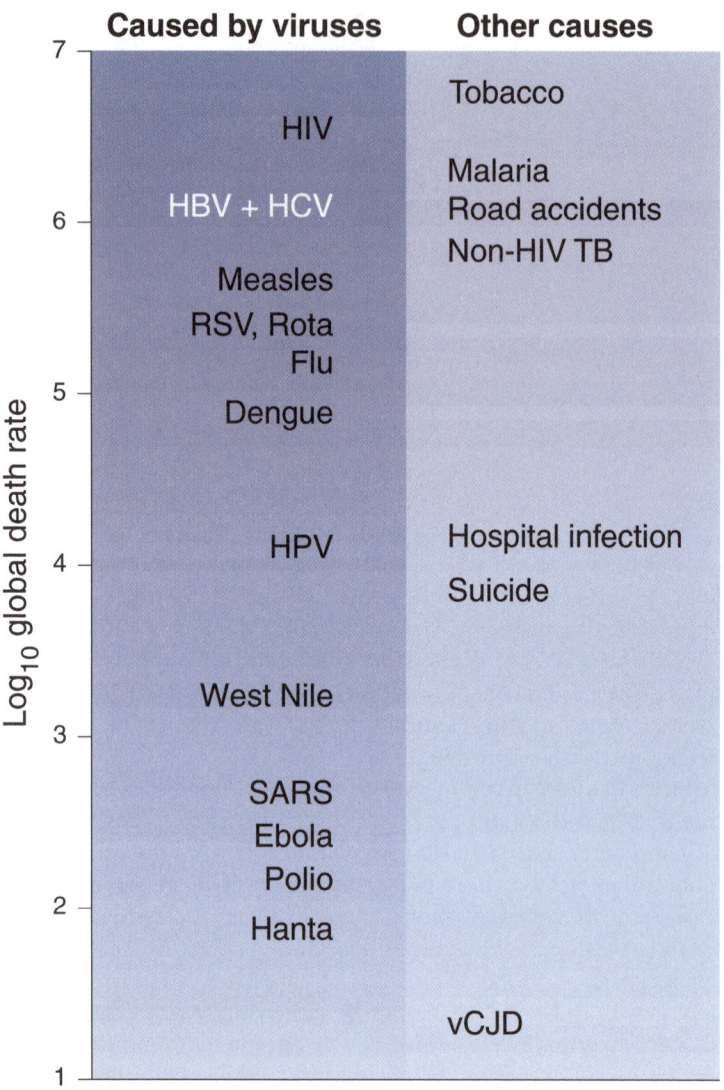

FIGURE 1-1 Approximate global preventable death rate from selected infectious diseases and other causes, 2003.
Abbreviations: HIV, human immunodeficiency virus; HBV, hepatitis B virus; HCV, hepatitis C virus; RSV, respiratory syncytial virus; HPV, human papilloma virus; SARS, severe acute respiratory syndrome; TB, tuberculosis; vCJD, variant Creutzfeldt-Jakob disease.
SOURCE: Weiss and McMichael, 2004. Reprinted with permission from Macmillan Publishers Ltd: *Nature Medicine* 10(12 Suppl):S70-S76, copyright 2004.

TABLE 1-1 Key Characteristics of Hepatitis B and Hepatitis C

	Hepatitis B	Hepatitis C
Causative agent	Partially double-stranded DNA virus Hepadnaviridae family	Enveloped, positive-strand RNA virus *Hepacavirus* genus, Flaviviridae family
Statistics	In the United States, 0.8–1.4 million people are chronically infected with HBV	In the United States, 2.7–3.9 million people are chronically infected with HCV
Routes of transmission	Contact with infectious blood, semen, and other body fluids, primarily through: • Birth to an infected mother • Sexual contact with an infected person • Sharing of contaminated needles, syringes, or other injection-drug equipment Less commonly through: • Contact with infectious blood through medical procedures	Contact with blood of an infected person, primarily through: • Sharing of contaminated needles, syringes, or other injection-drug equipment Less commonly through: • Sexual contact with an infected person • Birth to an infected mother • Contact with infectious blood through medical procedures
Persons at risk	• Persons born in geographic regions that have HBsAg prevalence of at least 2% • Infants born to infected mothers • Household contacts of persons who have chronic HBV infection • Sex partners of infected persons • Injection-drug users • Sexually active persons who are not in long-term, mutually monogamous relationships (for example, more than one sex partner during previous 6 months) • Men who have sex with men	• Persons who have ever injected illegal drugs, including those who injected only once many years ago • Recipients of clotting-factor concentrates made before 1987 • Recipients of blood transfusions or solid-organ transplants before July 1992 • Patients who have ever received long-term hemodialysis treatment • Persons who have known exposures to HCV, such as health-care workers after needlesticks involving HCV-positive blood and recipients of blood or organs from donors who later tested HCV-positive • All persons who have HIV infection

continued

TABLE 1-1 Continued

	Hepatitis B	Hepatitis C
Persons at risk	• Health-care and public-safety workers at risk for occupational exposure to blood or blood-contaminated body fluids • Residents and staff of facilities for developmentally disabled persons • Persons who have chronic liver disease • Hemodialysis patients • Travelers to countries that have intermediate or high prevalence of HBV infection	• Patients who have signs or symptoms of liver disease (for example, abnormal liver-enzyme tests) • Children born to HCV-positive mothers (to avoid detecting maternal antibody, these children should not be tested before the age of 18 months)
Potential for chronic infection	Among newly infected, unimmunized persons, chronic infection occurs in: • >90% of infants • 25–50% of children aged 1–5 years • 6–10% of older children and adults	75–85% of newly infected persons develop chronic infection
Clinical outcomes	• 15–25% of chronically infected persons will die from cirrhosis, liver failure, or hepatocellular carcinoma • 3,000 deaths each year are due to hepatitis B-related liver disease in the United States	• 60–70% of chronically infected persons develop chronic liver disease • 5–20% develop cirrhosis over a period of 20–30 years • 1–5% will die from cirrhosis or hepatocellular carcinoma • 12,000 deaths each year are due to hepatitis C-related liver disease in the United States

Abbreviations: HBV, hepatitis B virus; HCV, hepatitis C virus; HBsAg, hepatitis B surface antigen.
SOURCE: Adapted from CDC, 2009a.

PREVALENCE AND INCIDENCE OF HEPATITIS B AND HEPATITIS C WORLDWIDE

Worldwide, about 1 in 12 persons (480–520 million people) are chronically infected with HBV or HCV (Lavanchy, 2008; WHO, 2009). An estimated 78% of cases of primary liver cancer (HCC) and 57% of cases of liver cirrhosis are caused by chronic HBV or HCV infection (Perz et al., 2006). Chronic liver disease due to coinfection with HBV or HCV has become a major cause of death in persons infected with HIV (Sulkowski, 2008), and coinfection presents additional treatment challenges (Kumar et al., 2008). It is estimated that HBV and HCV infections cause nearly a million deaths each year (Perz et al., 2006).

Chronic viral hepatitis is a silent killer. Without testing for infection, many chronically infected persons are not aware that they have been infected until symptoms of advanced liver disease appear. Advanced liver cancer has a 5-year survival rate of below 5% (American Cancer Society, 2009). Although much progress has been made in reducing the morbidity and mortality through effective treatment of chronic viral hepatitis, there is no global program to provide chronically infected persons with access to affordable treatment.

HBV is 50–100 times more infectious than HIV (WHO, 2009). Acute HBV infection in adults, although often asymptomatic, can cause severe illness and is associated with a 0.5–1% risk of death from liver failure (CDC, 2007). Chronic HBV infection, which occurs when the acute infection is not cleared by the immune system, is associated with a 15–25% risk of premature death from liver cancer or end-stage liver disease (Beasley and Hwang, 1991; WHO, 2009). The World Health Organization (WHO) estimates that up to 2 billion people worldwide have been infected with HBV; about 350 million people live with chronic HBV infection, and about 600,000 people die from HBV-related liver disease or HCC each year (WHO, 2009).

The major transmission routes and prevalence of chronic HBV infection vary by age and geography. Primary HBV infection acquired at an early age (through vertical transmission from an infected mother to her newborn or horizontal transmission during early childhood) is associated with the highest risk of chronic infection and is common in people born in or residing in the highly endemic countries of the western Pacific region, Asia, and sub-Saharan Africa (Shepard et al., 2006). In countries with a low prevalence of HBV carriers, primary infection usually occurs during adolescence or young adulthood as a result of unsafe injections and unprotected sexual activity. An estimated 21 million new HBV infections each year are due to unsafe injections in health-care settings (Hauri et al., 2004). Hepatitis B is also a major basis for social injustice in some endemic countries. For example, myths and misinformation about modes of HBV transmission have resulted in widespread discrimination against chronically infected persons in some endemic countries, such as China, the country with the world's largest population of chronically infected people, who are not allowed to work in the food industry, are often required to undergo routine pre-employment HBV testing, and can be expelled from school or work because of a positive test (*The Economist*, 2006).

An estimated 130–170 million people live with chronic HCV infection worldwide, and an estimated 350,000 die of HCV-related liver disease each year (Perz et al., 2006). There are about 2.3–4.7 million new HCV infections each year from nosocomial transmission alone (Lavanchy, 2009). Unsafe mass immunization has led to exceedingly high HCV prevalence in some areas, such as Egypt, where 14–20% of the population has HCV antibodies (Frank et al., 2000; Lavanchy, 2008). In most populations in Africa, North America, South America, Europe, and Southeast Asia, the prevalence in the general population is less than 3% (Lavanchy, 2008).

HCV is efficiently transmitted via direct percutaneous exposure to infectious blood. Hepatitis C became a global epidemic in the 20th century as blood transfusions, hemodialysis, and the use of injection needles to administer licit and illicit drugs increased throughout the world (Drucker et al., 2001; Pybus et al., 2007). For example, the extremely high prevalence of HCV in Egypt is due to a schistosomiasis-eradication campaign that began in the 1960s, when more than 35 million injections were administered to about 6 million Egyptians (Deuffic-Burban et al., 2006; Frank et al., 2000; Lehman and Wilson, 2009). The identification of the virus in 1989 led to measures to reduce health-care–related exposure to HCV, particularly in industrialized nations. However, more than six billion unsafe injections are given worldwide each year (Hutin et al., 2003).

With the reduction in health-care–related exposures to HCV and the recent introduction of the practice of illicit-drug injection in new regions of the world, HCV infection through injection-drug use has become the major source of exposure to HCV worldwide. Explosive increases in HCV infection have occurred in regions of Asia and central and eastern Europe because of poor access to sterile injection equipment and lack of drug treatment. A recent meta-analysis reported that HCV prevalence was 84% in injection-drug users (IDUs) surveyed in the Guangxi region bordering the Golden Triangle in China (Xia et al., 2008). In that region, drug use is highly stigmatized, which reduces community support for prevention efforts and inhibits IDUs' access to prevention services. Antiviral treatments for chronic HBV and HCV infections can effectively reduce the associated morbidity and mortality from liver disease. However, access to treatment is often limited by high costs of care and by the asymptomatic nature of chronic HBV and HCV infections. Therefore, many infected people are not identified in time to benefit from antiviral treatment.

Global eradication or elimination of new HBV infections is plausible because the infections can be prevented with the hepatitis B vaccine. No vaccine to prevent hepatitis C has been licensed. Given the limitations of the scope of the committee's work, it did not assess global prevention and control efforts for hepatitis B and hepatitis C and did not consider the international effects of its recommendations.

PREVALENCE AND INCIDENCE OF HEPATITIS B AND HEPATITIS C IN THE UNITED STATES

HBV and HCV infections pose a major public-health problem in the United States and are major causes of chronic liver disease. Three to five times more people are living with chronic viral hepatitis infections than with HIV infection. Table 1-2 presents the burden of HBV, HCV, and HIV infections in the United States. The US Centers for Disease Control and Prevention (CDC) estimates that 3.5–5.3 million people in the United States—1–2% of the population—are living with chronic HBV or HCV infection—about 800,000 to 1.4 million people with chronic hepatitis B and an additional 2.7–3.9 million people with chronic hepatitis C (CDC, 2009d). However, an accurate estimate is difficult to obtain because there is no national chronic-hepatitis surveillance program. Each year, about 15,000 deaths are caused by HBV- or HCV-associated liver cancer or end-stage liver disease (CDC, 2009d). Almost half the liver transplantations in the United States are necessitated by end-stage liver disease associated with HBV or HCV infection (Kim et al., 2009).

The annual costs of HBV and HCV infections are difficult to determine. The direct medical cost associated with HBV infection has been estimated at $5.8 million based on the number of new cases in 2000 among persons 5–24 years old (Chesson et al., 2004). An estimated $1.8 billion in medical care costs was associated with HCV infections in 1997 (Leigh et al., 2001). Indirect costs, such as lost productivity, add to the HCV-associated cost burden. Because of the aging of people now infected (including some people with asymptomatic infections who will become symptomatic), HCV-related illnesses, deaths, and costs are all expected to rise substantially during the next two decades (Pyenson et al., 2009; Wong et al., 2000).

Hepatitis B

The national strategy for preventing new HBV infection in infants and children—including routine screening of pregnant women for hepatitis B surface antigen (a blood marker for chronic HBV infection), universal infant hepatitis B immunization, and catchup vaccination of unvaccinated children and adolescents—has resulted in a dramatic reduction in chronic HBV infection in infants and acute HBV infection in children of all ethnicities (CDC, 2004; Mast et al., 2005, 2006). Despite those achievements, the goal of eliminating perinatal HBV transmission has not been achieved, largely because coverage of newborns with a birth dose of hepatitis B vaccine is incomplete (CDC, 2008c). As a result, CDC estimates that each year about 1,000 newborns develop chronic HBV infection, which puts them at risk for premature death from HBV-related liver disease (Ward, 2008b).

TABLE 1-2 Burden of Selected Serious Chronic Viral Infections in the United States

Virus	Prevalence[a,b]	Percentage of Population Unaware of Infection Status[c,d,e]	Deaths in 2006 Related to Infection[a,b]	Vaccine-Preventable	Transmission Routes	Percentage of CDC NCHHSTP FY 2008 Budget[f]
HBV	0.8–1.4 million	About 65%	3,000	Yes	Birth, blood, sex	2% combined
HCV	2.7–3.9 million	About 75%	12,000	No	Birth, blood, sex	
HIV/AIDS	1.1 million	About 21%	14,016	No	Birth, blood, sex	69% (domestic activities)

Abbreviations: CDC NCHHSTP, Centers for Disease Control and Prevention National Center for HIV/AIDS, Viral Hepatitis, Sexually Transmitted Disease, and Tuberculosis Prevention; HBV, hepatitis B virus; HCV, hepatitis C virus; HIV/AIDS, human immunodeficiency virus/acquired immunodeficiency syndrome.

SOURCES: [a]CDC, 2009b; [b]CDC, 2009d; [c]Lin et al., 2007; [d]Hagan et al., 2006; [e]CDC, 2008b; [f]Ward, 2008a.

Based upon surveillance data and modeling, CDC estimates that there has been an 82% decline in incidence of acute HBV infection since 1990 with the total number of new infections in 2007 estimated at 43,000 (Daniels et al., 2009). Because many children have been vaccinated against HBV, most reported cases of acute HBV infection are in adults. The national strategy for preventing HBV transmission in adults—by recommending hepatitis B vaccination selectively for high-risk adults (including men who have sex with men, IDUs, and correctional-facility inmates)—has had only little success in reducing the incidence of acute HBV infection in US adults (Mast et al., 2006). Acute HBV infections are often asymptomatic or have symptoms similar to those of other common illnesses, such as influenza, so there is a high probability of underreporting.

In the United States, data on reported cases of acute HBV infection in 2007 indicate that the highest rate of infection is in non-Hispanic black men: 2.3 per 100,000. The incidence is substantially lower in other populations: 0.9 per 100,000 Asians and Pacific Islanders (APIs) and 1.0 per 100,000 non-Hispanic whites and Hispanics. There also appear to be geographic variations in incidence; the highest rates of acute HBV infection are in the South[1] (Daniels et al., 2009).

Although the incidence of acute HBV infection is declining in the United States, the number of people who are living with chronic HBV infection may be increasing as a result of immigration from highly endemic countries (that is, the hepatitis B surface antigen prevalence is ≥ 2%). On the basis of immigration patterns in the last decade, it is estimated that every year 40,000–45,000 people enter the United States legally from HBV-endemic countries (Mast et al., 2006; U.S. Department of Homeland Security, 2009). Some populations are at higher risk for chronic HBV infection, including API Americans, who make up only 4.5% of the general US population (U.S. Census Bureau, 2008) but account for more than 50% of Americans who are living with chronic HBV infection (CDC, 2009c). The prevalence of chronic HBV infection in API Americans is as high as 15% in some studies and constitutes an important health disparity (CDC, 2006). Having been born in an HBV-endemic country appears to be the major risk factor for chronic HBV infection in the API population (Lin et al., 2007).

Recent studies suggest that routine HBV testing of all adult API Americans is cost-effective (Hutton et al., 2007), but almost two-thirds of chronically infected API Americans are unaware of their infection status because they have not been tested for HBV (CDC, 2006; Lin et al., 2007).

---

[1] CDC's southern region includes Alabama, Arkansas, Delaware, the District of Columbia, Florida, Georgia, Kentucky, Louisiana, Maryland, Mississippi, North Carolina, Oklahoma, South Carolina, Tennessee, Texas, Virginia, and West Virginia.

Hepatitis C

Persons likely to have chronic HCV infection include those who received a blood transfusion before 1992 and past or current IDUs. US veterans who use the Department of Veterans Affairs (VA) health-care system have a higher prevalence of HCV infection (4–35%) than the general population (about 2%) (Cheung, 2000; Dominitz et al., 2005; Groom et al., 2008; Sloan et al., 2004), so VA has established a program to test all VA patients for HCV infection and to manage HCV-positive patients clinically (Kussman, 2007). As is the case with HBV infection, most patients who have acute or chronic HCV infection are asymptomatic, and their disease remains undiagnosed (Kamal, 2008).

In the United States, most IDUs have serologic evidence of HCV infection, but the prevalence is highly variable. For example, in a study of young IDUs in four US cities, the prevalence of HCV antibody was 35% overall but varied from 14% in Chicago and 27% in Los Angeles to 51% in Baltimore and New York City (Amon et al., 2008). Prevalence is strongly associated with time engaged in risky behaviors, rising as the number of years of drug-injecting accumulates and reaching 65–90% in longer-term injectors (Hagan et al., 2008). HCV prevalence in IDUs in industrialized nations has fallen in recent years. For example, in IDUs injecting for less than 1 year, HCV prevalence fell from 46% before 1995 to 32% in a more recent period and in IDUs injecting for 5 years or more, prevalence fell from 67% before 1995 to 53% in the period after 1995 (Hagan et al., 2008). Most of the estimates of HCV incidence rates in IDUs in the United States have been between 15 and 30 per 100 person years at risk, with higher incidence found in recent-onset injectors (Garfein et al., 1998; Hagan et al., 2001, 2008; Hahn et al., 2002; Maher et al., 2006; Smyth et al., 2000; Thorpe et al., 2002).

The prevalence of HCV infection in the incarcerated population has been reported to vary from 12% to 35% (Boutwell et al., 2005; Weinbaum et al., 2003). Although some HCV transmission occurs within correctional settings (Hunt and Saab, 2009; Macalino et al., 2004), the vast majority of HCV-infected inmates became infected by injection-drug use in the community and not while incarcerated (Weinbaum et al., 2003).

Although reporting of acute HCV infection does not accurately reflect the underlying incidence in the United States, the number of acute HCV infections peaked in the late 1980s and declined throughout the 1990s (Armstrong et al., 2006; Shepard et al., 2005). The decline observed in the 1990s may reflect changes in IDUs' behavior and practices, including greater participation in needle-exchange programs (Wasley et al., 2008). It is consistent with results of studies summarized previously that suggest that HCV seroconversion rates in IDUs have declined since 1995 (Armstrong et al., 2006; Shepard et al., 2005). The decline slowed and then leveled off starting in 2003, and there was a slight increase in reported acute cases in 2006 (Wasley et al., 2008). Interpretation of those trends is complicated, however, inasmuch as reporting is related to access to health care and diagnosis of acute infection; many IDUs, who often have limited access to health care and no symptoms from infection, are not included in the trend analysis.

LIVER CANCER AND LIVER DISEASE FROM CHRONIC HEPATITIS B VIRUS AND HEPATITIS C VIRUS INFECTIONS

Both chronic HBV and HCV infections can lead to HCC, a type of liver cancer, and liver disease (But et al., 2008; McMahon, 2004, 2008; Tan et al., 2008). The two most important risk factors for HCC are chronic HBV and HCV infections. As stated above, an estimated 78% of HCC cases and 57% of liver cirrhosis cases are caused by chronic HBV and HCV infections (Perz et al., 2006).

In the United States, an estimated 3,000 people die each year from HCC or chronic liver disease caused by HBV infection (CDC, 2008a). However, risks of those outcomes vary and are higher in men and in people who are older, ingest large amounts of alcohol, and are coinfected with HIV (McMahon, 2004; Pungpapong et al., 2007). Outcomes of HBV infections occur much more often in those with high blood concentrations of HBV DNA, in persons over 40 years old, and in persons infected with HBV genotype C (Chen et al., 2006; Dehesa-Violante and Nuñez-Nateras, 2007; McMahon, 2004; Pungpapong et al., 2007). There are an especially high prevalence of chronic HBV infection and a high risk of HCC in the API American population, who make up the largest pool of chronically infected persons in the United States and are most commonly infected with HBV genotype C (Chang et al., 2007). HCC incidence tripled in the United States from 1975 through 2005, and the highest incidence is in API Americans who immigrated to the United States (Altekruse et al., 2009). American Indian and Alaska Native peoples have been found to have the highest rate of liver-related death of ethnic groups in the United States (Vong and Bell, 2004). The age-specific rate of death in American Indian and Alaska Native peoples due to chronic liver disease is much higher than that in any other population and chronic HBV infection and increasing rates of chronic HCV infection play a large role (Vong and Bell, 2004).

In the United States, about 12,000 people die from complications of chronic hepatitis C each year (CDC, 2008a). Deaths related to hepatitis C have increased; the highest number of deaths are in middle-aged men, non-Hispanic blacks, and American Indians (Wise et al., 2008). As is the case with chronic hepatitis B, complications occur more often in men and in people who are older, have metabolic syndrome secondary to obesity, ingest large amounts of alcohol, and are coinfected with HIV (Ghany et al., 2009; Missiha et al., 2008; Pradat et al., 2007). There are also important ethnic and racial differences in the burden of chronic hepatitis C. The prevalence of HCV infection is higher in blacks than in whites (Armstrong et al., 2006; Thomas et al., 2000). Blacks also are less likely to respond to interferon-alpha-based treatment for chronic hepatitis C; this seems to be explained to a large extent by differences in DNA sequences near the interferon lambda 3 gene (Ge et al., 2009; Jeffers et al., 2004; Muir et al., 2004; Thomas et al., 2009). Likewise, there appears to be a greater burden of chronic hepatitis C and reduced response to treatment in Hispanic whites than in non-Hispanic whites (Armstrong et al., 2006; Bonacini et al., 2001; Rodriguez-Torres et al., 2009). In both Hispanics and blacks, HCC risk is increasing, in large part because of chronic hepatitis C (Altekruse et al., 2009). However, there is less evidence than in the case of HBV infection that different HCV genotypes or higher blood HCV concentrations increase the risk of long-term disease outcomes. Health-care use trends from 1994 to 2001 show a 20–30% yearly increase in HCV-related hospitalizations, length of hospital stays, total hospitalization costs, and hospital deaths (Grant et al., 2005).

THE COMMITTEE'S TASK

CDC has developed recommendations for the prevention and control of hepatitis B (Mast et al., 2005, 2006; Weinbaum et al., 2008) and hepatitis C (CDC, 1998, 2001). The National Institutes of Health (NIH) has developed consensus documents on the management of hepatitis B (NIH, 2008) and hepatitis C (NIH, 2002). WHO has published guidelines related to hepatitis B vaccination of children (WHO, 2001). A number of not-for-profit organizations have also worked to increase awareness of the diseases, educate the public about prevention, and advocate for those chronically infected with HBV and HCV. Although government and nongovernment efforts have led to a decline in the number of cases, chronic hepatitis B and hepatitis C continue to be serious public-health problems in the United States. For that reason, CDC in conjunction with the National Viral Hepatitis Roundtable, a not-for-profit coalition of public, private, and voluntary organizations; the Department of Health and Human Services Office of Minority Health; and VA sought guidance from the Institute of Medicine (IOM) in identifying missed opportunities related to the prevention and control of HBV and HCV infections. IOM was asked to focus on hepatitis B and hepatitis C because they are common in the United States and can lead to chronic disease. This report does not address hepatitis A virus, hepatitis E virus, or hepatitis D virus (also called the hepatitis delta virus) infections.

INTRODUCTION

The specific charge to the committee follows:

The IOM will form a committee to determine ways to reduce new HBV and HCV infections and the morbidity and mortality related to chronic viral hepatitis. The committee will assess current prevention and control activities and identify priorities for research, policy, and action. The committee will highlight issues that warrant further investigations and opportunities for collaboration between private and public sectors. In conducting its work, the committee might want to consider:

Strategies for preventing new HBV and HCV infections:

- Improving vaccine coverage among vulnerable populations to reach national transmission elimination goals.
- Increasing the proportion of persons aware of their chronic infection status.
- Identifying barriers to the identification, counseling, and testing of persons at risk for chronic hepatitis, and ways they can be reduced and eliminated.
- Promoting prevention among adolescents and adults who engage in risky behaviors, particularly those known to have screened positive for HCV and HBV infection.
- Determining optimal ways to identify, develop, and implement prevention programs among at-risk populations.
- Development of an effective HCV vaccine.

Strategies for reducing morbidity and mortality from chronic HBV and HCV infections:

- Providing appropriate medical referral, evaluation, and management of chronically infected persons.
- Assessing health-care utilization and outcomes for persons with chronic infections, and opportunities for prevention and care to reduce health-care-related costs.
- Reducing health disparities in morbidity and mortality from viral hepatitis.
- Improving clinical surveillance of markers of disease progression and stage of hepatocellular carcinoma associated with chronic viral hepatitis and associated cirrhosis.

Assess the type and quality of data needed from state and local viral hepatitis surveillance systems to guide and evaluate prevention services:

- Assess the role of acute disease surveillance in monitoring new infections, detecting outbreaks, identifying vaccine failures and documenting the elimination of HBV transmission.
- Assess the role of state and local chronic disease surveillance in describing the burden of morbidity and mortality related to chronic hepatitis B and hepatitis C and related liver cirrhosis and cancer, the extent of

ongoing risk behaviors, and the impact of HIV co-infection and other cofactors.
- Assess the role of state and local disease registries in the delivery of prevention and care services for persons with chronic hepatitis B and persons with hepatitis C.
- Assess the role of laboratory testing strategies for the identification of markers for acute HCV infection.
- Assess laboratory testing strategies for identification of antiviral resistance for HBV and HCV.

Finally, the committee should pay attention to addressing the special needs of specific subpopulations at high risk, such as Asian Americans, African Americans, and persons born in HBV-endemic countries.

THE COMMITTEE'S APPROACH TO ITS TASK

To address its charge, the committee first reviewed available evidence on a variety of topics related to the prevention of hepatitis B and hepatitis C, management of these diseases, and surveillance activities related to viral hepatitis. The evidence was drawn from the published literature and from open-session presentations by recognized experts in the field (see Appendix B). Oral testimony presented by members of the public during the open sessions was also taken into account. Additional information was obtained from written testimony submitted to the committee (available from the National Academies' Public Access Records Office, publicac@nas.edu).

A comprehensive review and evaluation of treatments for HBV and HCV infections (for example, which medications to use) is beyond the scope of this report. However, treatment information can be found in guidelines published by the American Association for the Study of Liver Diseases (Ghany et al., 2009; Lok and McMahon, 2009) and in NIH consensus statements on the management of hepatitis B (NIH, 2008) and hepatitis C (NIH, 2002).

The committee also has not been tasked with comprehensively reviewing information about the safety of the hepatitis B vaccine. Safety issues surrounding this vaccine were reviewed in the IOM report *Immunization Safety Review: Hepatitis B Vaccine and Demyelinating Neurological Disorders* (IOM, 2002). The committee that wrote that report concluded that the evidence favored rejection of a causal relationship between hepatitis B vaccine administered to adults and incident multiple sclerosis and multiple-sclerosis relapse. It also found the evidence inadequate for accepting or rejecting a causal relationship between hepatitis B vaccine and the first episode of a central nervous system demyelinating disorder, acute disseminated encephalomyelitis, optic neuritis, transverse myelitis, Guillain-Barré syndrome, or brachial neuritis. IOM has undertaken another review of the safety of the hepatitis B vaccine, and the findings are expected to be available in 2011.

The committee that wrote the present report met five times in the period December 2008–August 2009. During the meetings, the committee evaluated the evidence and deliberated on issues relevant to its charge. Types of evidence taken into consideration included international, federal, state, and community guidelines, programs, and other activities aimed at preventing new cases of HBV and HCV infection, identifying chronic cases of hepatitis B and hepatitis C, and managing those cases. It also explored federal and state surveillance mechanisms for identifying and tracking hepatitis B and hepatitis C cases. The committee began by identifying problems with and gaps in the current prevention and control systems. It also examined model programs for other infectious diseases, such as those covered under the Ryan White CARE Act (Health Resources and Services Administration, 2009). The committee developed evidence-based recommendations to address the problems with the current systems to reduce the numbers of new HBV and HCV infections, to manage the care of chronically infected people more effectively by reducing morbidity and mortality, and to improve surveillance of chronic hepatitis B and hepatitis C cases.

The committee focused on making recommendations that could be implemented with existing knowledge and available tools to advance prevention and control of chronic viral hepatitis in a timely manner. Although the committee recognizes the importance of basic research in this field, it believes that given the scope of the problem and the lack of available resources, its focus should be on improving prevention and control services. As a result, the committee did not address basic-research questions in the field extensively. Nor did it conduct cost–benefit analyses of its recommendations.

The committee's general approach is presented in Figure 1-2. After defining the scope of the problem and reviewing the available evidence, the committee identified the primary underlying factors that impede current efforts to prevent and control hepatitis B and hepatitis C. The committee believes that a lack of awareness about viral hepatitis among both the general public and health-care and social-service providers is leading to continued high rates of morbidity and mortality from hepatitis B and hepatitis C. Consistent themes were found in all the materials reviewed by the committee; as a result, this report is organized according to four principal categories:

- Improved disease surveillance (Chapter 2).
- Improved knowledge and awareness on the part of health-care and social-service providers and the public (Chapter 3).

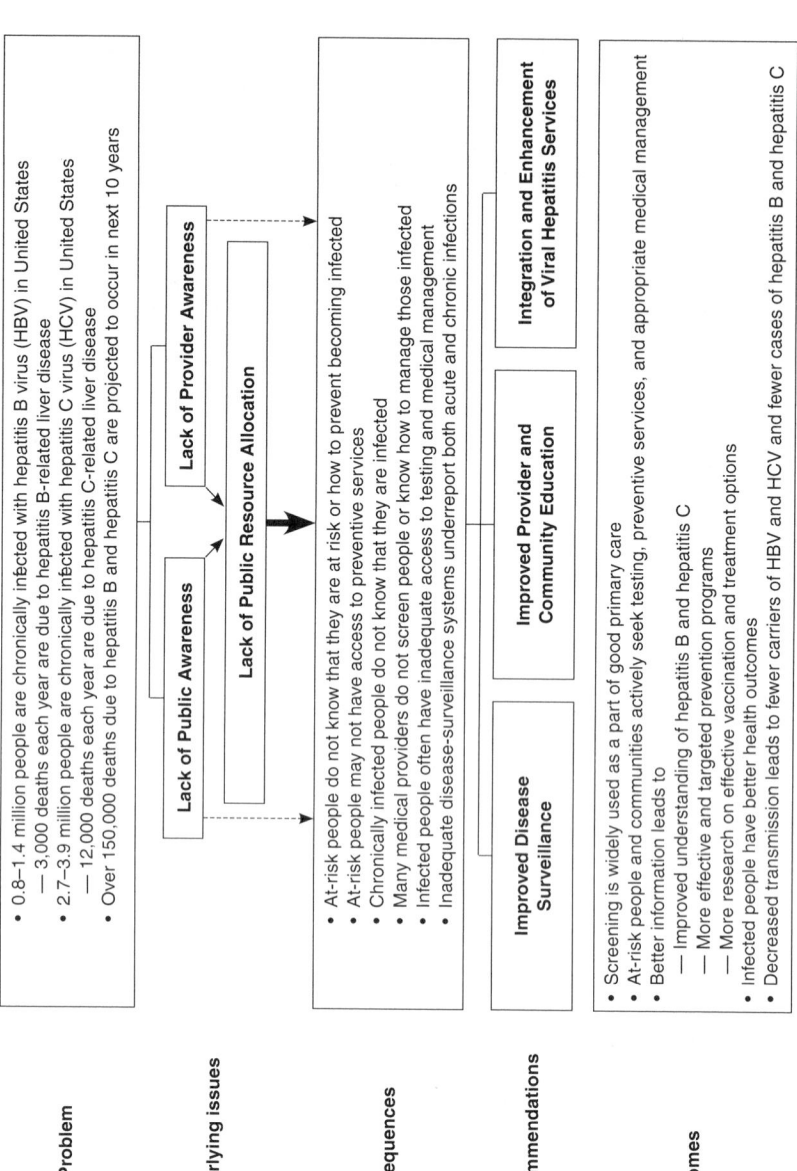

FIGURE 1-2 The committee's approach to its task.

- Increased hepatitis B vaccination rates in various populations (Chapter 4).
- Improved integration and enhancement of viral hepatitis services for specific at-risk populations and in health-care and other settings (Chapter 5).

REFERENCES

Altekruse, S. F., K. A. McGlynn, and M. E. Reichman. 2009. Hepatocellular carcinoma incidence, mortality, and survival trends in the United States from 1975 to 2005. *Journal of Clinical Oncology* 27(9):1485-1491.

American Cancer Society. 2009. *Cancer facts & figures, 2009.* Atlanta, GA.

Amon, J. J., R. S. Garfein, L. Ahdieh-Grant, G. L. Armstrong, L. J. Ouellet, M. H. Latka, D. Vlahov, S. A. Strathdee, S. M. Hudson, P. Kerndt, D. Des Jarlais, and I. T. Williams. 2008. Prevalence of hepatitis C virus infection among injection drug users in the United States, 1994-2004. *Clinical Infectious Diseases* 46(12):1852-1858.

Armstrong, G. L., A. Wasley, E. P. Simard, G. M. McQuillan, W. L. Kuhnert, and M. J. Alter. 2006. The prevalence of hepatitis C virus infection in the United States, 1999 through 2002. *Annals of Internal Medicine* 144(10):705-714.

Beasley, R., and L. Hwang. 1991. Overview of the epidemiology of heptocellular carcinoma. In *Viral hepatitis and liver disease. Proceedings of the 1990 international symposium on viral hepatitis and liver disease*, edited by F. B. Hollinger, S. Lemon, and H. S. Margolis. Baltimore: Williams & Wilkins. Pp. 532-525.

Bonacini, M., M. D. Groshen, M. C. Yu, S. Govindarajan, and K. L. Lindsay. 2001. Chronic hepatitis C in ethnic minority patients evaluated in Los Angeles county. *American Journal of Gastroenterology* 96(8):2438-2441.

Boutwell, A. E., S. A. Allen, and J. D. Rich. 2005. Opportunities to address the hepatitis C epidemic in the correctional setting. *Clinical Infectious Diseases* 40(s5):S367-S372.

But, D. Y., C. L. Lai, and M. F. Yuen. 2008. Natural history of hepatitis-related hepatocellular carcinoma. *World Journal of Gastroenterology* 14(11):1652-1656.

CDC (Centers for Disease Control and Prevention). 1998. Recommendations for prevention and control of hepatitis C virus (HCV) infection and HCV-related chronic disease. *Morbidity and Morality Weekly: Recommendations and Reports* 47(RR-19):1-39.

———. 2001. Updated U.S. Public Health Service guidelines for the management of occupational exposures to HBV, HCV, and HIV and recommendations for postexposure prophylaxis. *Morbidity and Morality Weekly: Recommendations and Reports* 50(RR-11):1-52.

———. 2004. Incidence of acute hepatitis B—United States, 1990-2002. *Morbidity and Mortality Weekly Report* 52(51-52):1252-1254.

———. 2006. Screening for chronic hepatitis B among Asian/Pacific Islander populations—New York City, 2005. *Morbidity and Mortality Weekly Report* 55(18):505-509.

———. 2007. *FAQs for health professionals: Hepatitis B.* http://www.cdc.gov/hepatitis/HBV/HBVfaq.htm#overview (accessed August 21, 2009).

———. 2008a. *Disease burden from hepatitis A, B, and C in the United States.* http://www.cdc.gov/hepatitis/statistics.htm (accessed August 21, 2209)

———. 2008b. HIV prevalence estimates—United States, 2006. *Morbidity and Mortality Weekly Report* 57(39):1073-1076.

———. 2008c. Newborn hepatitis B vaccination coverage among children born January 2003-June 2005—United States. *Morbidity and Mortality Weekly Report* 57(30):825-828.

———. 2009a. *The ABCs of hepatitis*. http://www.cdc.gov/hepatitis/Resources/Professionals/PDFs/ABCTable.pdf (accessed November 6, 2009).

———. 2009b. *HIV/AIDS statistics and surveillance*. http://www.cdc.gov/hiv/topics/surveillance/basic.htm (accessed August 24, 2009).

———. 2009c. Notice to readers: National hepatitis B initiative for Asian Americans/Native Hawaiian and other Pacific Islanders. *Morbidity and Mortality Weekly Report* 58(18):503.

———. 2009d. *Viral hepatitis: Statistics and surveillance*. http://www.cdc.gov/hepatitis/Statistics.htm (accessed August 24, 2009).

Chang, E. T., T. H. M. Keegan, S. L. Gomez, G. M. Le, C. A. Clarke, S. K. So, and S. L. Glaser. 2007. The burden of liver cancer in Asians and Pacific Islanders in the greater San Francisco Bay area, 1990 through 2004. *Cancer* 109(10):2100-2108.

Chen, G., W. Lin, F. Shen, U. H. Iloeje, W. T. London, and A. A. Evans. 2006. Past HBV viral load as predictor of mortality and morbidity from HCC and chronic liver disease in a prospective study. *American Journal of Gastroenterology* 101(8):1797-1803.

Chesson, H. W., J. M. Blandford, T. L. Gift, G. Tao, and K. L. Irwin. 2004. The estimated direct medical cost of sexually transmitted diseases among American youth, 2000. *Perspectives on Sexual and Reproductive Health* 36(1):11-19.

Cheung, R. C. 2000. Epidemiology of hepatitis C virus infection in American veterans. *American Journal of Gastroenterology* 95(3):740-747.

Daniels, D., S. Grytdal, and A. Wasley. 2009. Surveillance for acute viral hepatitis—United States, 2007. *Morbidity and Mortality Weekly Report: Surveillance Summaries* 58(3):1-27.

Dehesa-Violante, M., and R. Nuñez-Nateras. 2007. Epidemiology of hepatitis virus B and C. *Archives of Medical Research* 38(6):606-611.

Deuffic-Burban, S., M. K. Mohamed, B. Larouze, F. Carrat, and A. J. Valleron. 2006. Expected increase in hepatitis C-related mortality in Egypt due to pre-2000 infections. *Journal of Hepatology* 44(3):455-461.

Dominitz, J. A., E. J. Boyko, T. D. Koepsell, P. J. Heagerty, C. Maynard, J. L. Sporleder, A. Stenhouse, M. A. Kling, W. Hrushesky, C. Zeilman, S. Sontag, N. Shah, F. Ona, B. Anand, M. Subik, T. F. Imperiale, S. Nakhle, S. B. Ho, E. J. Bini, B. Lockhart, J. Ahmad, A. Sasaki, B. van der Linden, D. Toro, J. Martinez-Souss, V. Huilgol, S. Eisen, and K. A. Young. 2005. Elevated prevalence of hepatitis C infection in users of United States Veterans Medical Centers. *Hepatology* 41(1):88-96.

Drucker, E., P. G. Alcabes, and P. A. Marx. 2001. The injection century: Massive unsterile injections and the emergence of human pathogens. *Lancet* 358(9297):1989-1992.

The Economist. 2006. Asia: B is for bigotry; hepatitis B in China. November 18, 2006, p. 66.

Frank, C., M. K. Mohamed, G. T. Strickland, D. Lavanchy, R. R. Arthur, L. S. Magder, T. El Khoby, Y. Abdel-Wahab, E. S. Aly Ohn, W. Anwar, and I. Sallam. 2000. The role of parenteral antischistosomal therapy in the spread of hepatitis C virus in Egypt. *Lancet* 355(9207):887-891.

Garfein, R. S., M. C. Doherty, E. R. Monterroso, D. L. Thomas, K. E. Nelson, and D. Vlahov. 1998. Prevalence and incidence of hepatitis C virus infection among young adult injection drug users. *Journal of Acquired Immune Deficiency Syndromes and Human Retrovirology* 18 Suppl 1:S11-19.

Ge, D., J. Fellay, A. J. Thompson, J. S. Simon, K. V. Shianna, T. J. Urban, E. L. Heinzen, P. Qiu, A. H. Bertelsen, A. J. Muir, M. Sulkowski, J. G. McHutchison, and D. B. Goldstein. 2009. Genetic variation in IL28B predicts hepatitis C treatment-induced viral clearance. *Nature* 461(7262):399-401.

Ghany, M. G., D. B. Strader, D. L. Thomas, and L. Seeff. 2009. Diagnosis, management, and treatment of hepatitis C: An update. *Hepatology* 49(4):1335-1374.

Grant, W. C., R. R. Jhaveri, J. G. McHutchison, K. A. Schulman, and T. L. Kauf. 2005. Trends in health care resource use for hepatitis C virus infection in the United States. *Hepatology* 42(6):1406-1413.

Groom, H., E. Dieperink, D. B. Nelson, J. Garrard, J. R. Johnson, S. L. Ewing, H. Stockley, J. Durfee, Y. Jonk, M. L. Willenbring, and S. B. Ho. 2008. Outcomes of a hepatitis C screening program at a large urban VA medical center. *Journal of Clinical Gastroenterology* 42(1):97-106.

Hagan, H., J. Campbell, H. Thiede, S. Strathdee, L. Ouellet, F. Kapadia, S. Hudson, and R. S. Garfein. 2006. Self-reported hepatitis C virus antibody status and risk behavior in young injectors. *Public Health Reports* 121(6):710-719.

Hagan, H., E. R. Pouget, D. C. Des Jarlais, and C. Lelutiu-Weinberger. 2008. Meta-regression of hepatitis C virus infection in relation to time since onset of illicit drug injection: The influence of time and place. *American Journal of Epidemiology* 168(10):1099-1109.

Hagan, H., H. Thiede, N. S. Weiss, S. G. Hopkins, J. S. Duchin, and E. R. Alexander. 2001. Sharing of drug preparation equipment as a risk factor for hepatitis C. *American Journal of Public Health* 91(1):42-46.

Hahn, J. A., K. Page-Shafer, P. J. Lum, P. Bourgois, E. Stein, J. L. Evans, M. P. Busch, L. H. Tobler, B. Phelps, and A. R. Moss. 2002. Hepatitis C virus seroconversion among young injection drug users: Relationships and risks. *Journal of Infectious Diseases* 186(11):1558-1564.

Hauri, A. M., G. L. Armstrong, and Y. J. Hutin. 2004. The global burden of disease attributable to contaminated injections given in health care settings. *International Journal of STD and AIDS* 15(1):7-16.

Health Resources and Services Administration. 2009. *The Ryan White HIV/AIDS program.* http://hab.hrsa.gov/about/ (accessed August 21, 2009).

Hunt, D. R., and S. Saab. 2009. Viral hepatitis in incarcerated adults: A medical and public health concern. *American Journal of Gastroenterology* 104(4):1024-1031.

Hutin, Y. J. F., A. M. Hauri, and G. L. Armstrong. 2003. Use of injections in healthcare settings worldwide, 2000: Literature review and regional estimates. *BMJ* 327(7423):1075-1080.

Hutton, D. W., D. Tan, S. K. So, and M. L. Brandeau. 2007. Cost-effectiveness of screening and vaccinating Asian and Pacific Islander adults for hepatitis B. *Annals of Internal Medicine* 147(7):460-469.

IOM (Institute of Medicine). 2002. *Immunization safety review: Hepatitis B vaccine and demyelinating neurological disorders.* Edited by K. Stratton, D. Almario, and M. C. McCormick. Washington, DC: The National Academies Press.

Jeffers, L. J., W. Cassidy, C. D. Howell, S. Hu, and K. R. Reddy. 2004. Peginterferon alfa-2a (40 kd) and ribavirin for black American patients with chronic HCV genotype 1. *Hepatology* 39(6):1702-1708.

Kamal, S. M. 2008. Acute hepatitis C: A systematic review. *American Journal of Gastroenterology* 103(5):1283-1297; quiz 1298.

Kim, W. R., N. A. Terrault, R. A. Pedersen, T. M. Therneau, E. Edwards, A. A. Hindman, and C. L. Brosgart. 2009. Trends in waitlist registration for liver transplantation for viral hepatitis in the US. *Gastroenterology* 137(5):1608-1686.

Kumar, R., V. Singla, and S. Kacharya. 2008. Impact and management of hepatitis B and hepatitis C virus co-infection in HIV patients. *Tropical Gastroenterology* 29(3):136-147.

Kussman, M. J. 2007. *National hepatitis C program.* VHA Directive 2007-022. Department of Veterans Affairs.

Lavanchy, D. 2008. Chronic viral hepatitis as a public health issue in the world. *Best Practice and Research. Clinical Gastroenterology* 22(6):991-1008.

———. 2009. The global burden of hepatitis C. *Liver International* 29(s1):74-81.

Lehman, E. M., and M. L. Wilson. 2009. Epidemic hepatitis C virus infection in Egypt: Estimates of past incidence and future morbidity and mortality. *Journal of Viral Hepatitis* 16(9):650-658.

Leigh, J. P., C. L. Bowlus, B. N. Leistikow, and M. Schenker. 2001. Costs of hepatitis C. *Archives of Internal Medicine* 161(18):2231-2237.

Lin, S. Y., E. T. Chang, and S. K. So. 2007. Why we should routinely screen Asian American adults for hepatitis B: A cross-sectional study of Asians in California. *Hepatology* 46:1034-1040.

Lok, A. S., and B. J. McMahon. 2009. Chronic hepatitis B: Update 2009. *Hepatology* 50(3):661-662.

Macalino, G. E., J. C. Hou, M. S. Kumar, L. E. Taylor, I. G. Sumantera, and J. D. Rich. 2004. Hepatitis C infection and incarcerated populations. *International Journal of Drug Policy* 15(2):103-114.

Maher, L., B. Jalaludin, K. G. Chant, R. Jayasuriya, T. Sladden, J. M. Kaldor, and P. L. Sargent. 2006. Incidence and risk factors for hepatitis C seroconversion in injecting drug users in Australia. *Addiction* 101(10):1499-1508.

Mast, E. E., H. S. Margolis, A. E. Fiore, E. W. Brink, S. T. Goldstein, S. A. Wang, L. A. Moyer, B. P. Bell, and M. J. Alter. 2005. A comprehensive immunization strategy to eliminate transmission of hepatitis B virus infection in the United States: Recommendations of the advisory committee on immunization practices (ACIP) part 1: Immunization of infants, children, and adolescents. *Morbidity and Morality Weekly: Recommendations and Reports* 54(RR-16):1-31.

Mast, E. E., C. M. Weinbaum, A. E. Fiore, M. J. Alter, B. P. Bell, L. Finelli, L. E. Rodewald, J. M. Douglas, Jr., R. S. Janssen, and J. W. Ward. 2006. A comprehensive immunization strategy to eliminate transmission of hepatitis B virus infection in the United States: Recommendations of the advisory committee on immunization practices (ACIP) part II: Immunization of adults. *Morbidity and Morality Weekly: Recommendations and Reports* 55(RR-16):1-33; quiz CE31-34.

McMahon, B. J. 2004. The natural history of chronic hepatitis B virus infection. *Seminars in Liver Disease* 24(Suppl 1):17-21.

———. 2008. Natural history of chronic hepatitis B—clinical implications. *Medscape Journal of Medicine* 10(4):91.

Missiha, S. B., M. Ostrowski, and E. J. Heathcote. 2008. Disease progression in chronic hepatitis C: Modifiable and nonmodifiable factors. *Gastroenterology* 134(6):1699-1714.

Muir, A. J., J. D. Bornstein, and P. G. Killenberg. 2004. Peginterferon alfa-2b and ribavirin for the treatment of chronic hepatitis C in blacks and non-Hispanic whites. *New England Journal of Medicine* 350(22):2265-2271.

NIH (National Institutes of Health). 2002. NIH consensus statement on management of hepatitis C: 2002. *NIH Consensus and State-of-the-Science Statements* 19(3):1-46.

———. 2008. *NIH consensus development conference statement on the management of Hepatitis B.* http://consensus.nih.gov/2008/hebB%20draft%20statement%20102208_FINAL.pdf (accessed August 21, 2009)

Perz, J. F., G. L. Armstrong, L. A. Farrington, Y. J. Hutin, and B. P. Bell. 2006. The contributions of hepatitis B virus and hepatitis C virus infections to cirrhosis and primary liver cancer worldwide. *Journal of Hepatology* 45(4):529-538.

Pradat, P., N. Voirin, H. L. Tillmann, M. Chevallier, and C. Trepo. 2007. Progression to cirrhosis in hepatitis C patients: An age-dependent process. *Liver International* 27(3):335-339.

Pungpapong, S., W. R. Kim, and J. J. Poterucha. 2007. Natural history of hepatitis B virus infection: An update for clinicians. *Mayo Clinic Proceedings* 82(8):967-975.

Pybus, O. G., P. V. Markov, A. Wu, and A. J. Tatem. 2007. Investigating the endemic transmission of the hepatitis C virus. *International Journal for Parasitology* 37(8-9):839-849.

Pyenson, B., K. Fitch, and K. Iwasaki. 2009. *Consequences of hepatitis C virus (HCV). Costs of a baby boomer epidemic of liver disease.* New York: Vertex Pharmaceuticals Incorporated.

Rodriguez-Torres, M., L. J. Jeffers, M. Y. Sheikh, L. Rossaro, V. Ankoma-Sey, F. M. Hamzeh, and P. Martin. 2009. Peginterferon alfa-2a and ribavirin in Latino and non-Latino whites with hepatitis C. *New England Journal of Medicine* 360(3):257-267.

Shepard, C. W., L. Finelli, and M. J. Alter. 2005. Global epidemiology of hepatitis C virus infection. *The Lancet Infectious Diseases* 5(9):558-567.

Shepard, C. W., E. P. Simard, L. Finelli, A. E. Fiore, and B. P. Bell. 2006. Hepatitis B virus infection: Epidemiology and vaccination. *Epidemiologic Reviews* 28:112-125.

Sloan, K. L., K. A. Straits-Troster, J. A. Dominitz, and D. R. Kivlahan. 2004. Hepatitis C tested prevalence and comorbidities among veterans in the US Northwest. *Journal of Clinical Gastroenterology* 38(3):279-284.

Smyth, B. P., E. Keenan, and J. J. O'Connor. 2000. Assessment of hepatitis C infection in injecting drug users attending an addiction treatment clinic. *Irish Journal of Medical Science* 169(2):129-132.

Sulkowski, M. S. 2008. Viral hepatitis and HIV coinfection. *Journal of Hepatology* 48(2):353-367.

Tan, A., S. H. Yeh, C. J. Liu, C. Cheung, and P. J. Chen. 2008. Viral hepatocarcinogenesis: From infection to cancer. *Liver International* 28(2):175-188.

Thomas, D. L., J. Astemborski, R. M. Rai, F. A. Anania, M. Schaeffer, N. Galai, K. Nolt, K. E. Nelson, S. A. Strathdee, L. Johnson, O. Laeyendecker, J. Boitnott, L. E. Wilson, and D. Vlahov. 2000. The natural history of hepatitis C virus infection: Host, viral, and environmental factors. *Journal of the American Medical Association* 284(4):450-456.

Thomas, D. L., C. L. Thio, M. P. Martin, Y. Qi, D. Ge, C. O'Huigin, J. Kidd, K. Kidd, S. I. Khakoo, G. Alexander, J. J. Goedert, G. D. Kirk, S. M. Donfield, H. R. Rosen, L. H. Tobler, M. P. Busch, J. G. McHutchison, D. B. Goldstein, and M. Carrington. 2009. Genetic variation in IL28B and spontaneous clearance of hepatitis C virus. *Nature* 461(7265):798-801.

Thorpe, L. E., L. J. Ouellet, R. Hershow, S. L. Bailey, I. T. Williams, J. Williamson, E. R. Monterroso, and R. S. Garfein. 2002. Risk of hepatitis C virus infection among young adult injection drug users who share injection equipment. *American Journal of Epidemiology* 155(7):645-653.

U.S. Census Bureau. 2008. *2007 American community survey.* http://factfinder.census.gov/servlet/STTable?_bm=y&-qr_name=ACS_2008_3YR_G00_S0502&-geo_id=01000US&-ds_name=ACS_2008_3YR_G00_&-_lang=en&-format=&-CONTEXT=st (accessed August 20, 2009).

U.S. Department of Homeland Security. 2009. *Yearbook of immigration statistics: 2008. Table 3: Persons obtaining legal permanent resident status by region and country of birth: Fiscal years 1999 to 2008.* http://www.dhs.gov/files/statistics/publications/yearbook.shtm (accessed August 21, 2009).

Vong, S., and B. P. Bell. 2004. Chronic liver disease mortality in the United States, 1990-1998. *Hepatology* 39(2):476-483.

Ward, J. 2008a. FY 2008 domestic enacted funds. Presentation to the committee: December 4, 2008.

Ward, J. W. 2008b. Time for renewed commitment to viral hepatitis prevention. *American Journal of Public Health* 98(5):779-781.

Wasley, A., S. Grytdal, and K. Gallagher. 2008. Surveillance for acute viral hepatitis—United States, 2006. *Morbidity and Mortality Weekly Report: Surveillance Summaries* 57(2):1-24.

Weinbaum, C., R. Lyerla, and H. S. Margolis. 2003. Prevention and control of infections with hepatitis viruses in correctional settings. Centers for Disease Control and Prevention. *Morbidity and Morality Weekly: Recommendations and Reports* 52(RR-1):1-36; quiz CE31-CE34.

Weinbaum, C. M., I. Williams, E. E. Mast, S. A. Wang, L. Finelli, A. Wasley, S. M. Neitzel, and J. W. Ward. 2008. Recommendations for identification and public health management of persons with chronic hepatitis B virus infection. *Morbidity and Morality Weekly: Recommendations and Reports* 57(RR-8):1-20.

Weiss, R. A., and A. J. McMichael. 2004. Social and environmental risk factors in the emergence of infectious diseases. *Nature Medicine* 10(12 Suppl):S70-S76.

WHO (World Health Organization). 2001. *Introduction of hepatitis B vaccine into childhood immunization services: Management guidelines, including information for health workers and parents.* Geneva: World Health Organization.

———. 2009. *Hepatitis B fact sheet no. 204.* http://www.who.int/mediacentre/factsheets/fs204/en/ (accessed October 20, 2008).

Wise, M., S. Bialek, L. Finelli, B. P. Bell, and F. Sorvillo. 2008. Changing trends in hepatitis C-related mortality in the United States, 1995-2004. *Hepatology* 47(4):1128-1135.

Wong, J., G. McQuillan, J. McHutchison, and T. Poynard. 2000. Estimating future hepatitis C morbidity, mortality, and costs in the United States. *American Journal of Public Health* 90(10):1562-1569.

Xia, X., J. Luo, J. Bai, and R. Yu. 2008. Epidemiology of hepatitis C virus infection among injection drug users in China: Systematic review and meta-analysis. *Public Health* 122(10):990-1003.

2

Surveillance

Public-health surveillance is an essential tool in the prevention and control of infectious and chronic diseases and the medical management of people who have the diseases. Surveillance data are used to estimate the magnitude of a health problem, to describe the natural history of a disease, to detect epidemics, to document the distribution and spread of a health event or disease, to evaluate control and prevention measures, and to aid in public-health planning (Thacker, 2000). Public-health surveillance requires standardized, systematic, continuing collection and management of data. In addition, surveillance should encompass timely analysis and dissemination to allow public-health action (CDC, 2001a; Thacker, 2000). Through those steps, federal agencies and state and local health departments are able to inform stakeholders by providing reliable information that can be used to reduce morbidity and mortality through public policy, appropriate resource distribution, and programmatic and educational interventions. The committee has defined (see Box 2-1) the role of surveillance for hepatitis B virus (HBV) and hepatitis C virus (HCV) that is within the scope of its study.

This chapter describes how surveillance data are used or could be used to determine the focus and scope of viral hepatitis prevention and control efforts. The committee reviewed the weaknesses of the current surveillance system for hepatitis B and hepatitis C, including the timeliness, accuracy, and completeness of data collection, analysis, and dissemination. It found that there were few published sources of information about viral hepatitis surveillance. To obtain a clearer picture of the activities that were taking place at state and local levels, the committee gathered information from

> **BOX 2-1**
> **Role of Disease Surveillance**
>
> 1. Identify acute hepatitis B virus (HBV) and hepatitis C virus (HCV) outbreaks and individual acute cases and measure incidence
>   - Respond to outbreaks by
>   o Identifying cases
>   o Mobilizing appropriate resources to provide preventive services to eliminate or minimize further transmission
>   - Develop accurate estimates of the burden of acute hepatitis B and hepatitis C in United States
> 2. Identify chronic cases of hepatitis B and C and measure prevalence
>   - Develop accurate estimates of the burden of chronic disease in United States
>   - Prevent secondary cases
>   o Hepatitis B: Education, vaccination, and screening
>   o Hepatitis C: Education, harm reduction, and screening
> 3. Link cases to appropriate services, including medical management
> 4. Evaluate current practices and prevention efforts

various sources. Its findings are based on its review of the literature and on information gathered through surveys of and direct contact with professionals working in this field.

Much of the information gathered through surveys involved state-level and city-level public-health department staff who were working on programs funded by the Centers for Disease Control and Prevention (CDC). Forty-nine states have a cooperative agreement with CDC that funds a coordinator who conducts viral-hepatitis prevention activities, such as health-care provider and consumer education, integration of viral-hepatitis prevention services into health-care and public-health settings, and development of state viral-hepatitis prevention plans. Although the cooperative agreements do not include funds for viral-hepatitis surveillance, the coordinators are good sources of information about surveillance activities being conducted in each jurisdiction. CDC's Division of Viral Hepatitis (DVH) performed a brief survey of the CDC-funded hepatitis C coordinators in 2006 to gather information about viral-hepatitis surveillance activities. At the request of the committee, CDC again surveyed the coordinators (now called adult viral-hepatitis prevention coordinators, AVHPCs) in April 2009. As part of a national assessment of viral-hepatitis surveillance initiatives, the National

Alliance of State and Territorial AIDS Directors interviewed staff involved in enhanced viral-hepatitis surveillance projects funded through CDC's Emerging Infections Programs early in 2009 (the programs are described in more detail later in this chapter). Committee members also contacted several AVHPCs directly in April and May 2009 to discuss their work.

The recommendations for surveillance based on the committee's findings focus on the development of a model designed to improve the quality and accuracy of information by developing systems to collect, analyze, and disseminate data on acute and chronic HBV and HCV infections. The recommendations call for a two-part system: core surveillance activities, building the capacity of state and local health departments to conduct standard disease surveillance on newly diagnosed acute and chronic HBV and HCV infections, and targeted surveillance to obtain data on specific populations that are not represented fully in the collection of core surveillance data. Core surveillance means those activities in which all jurisdictions must engage to provide accurate, complete, and timely information to monitor incidence, prevalence, and trends in disease diagnoses. Data from other activities, such as targeted surveillance, supplement information from core surveillance, and are necessary to provide accurate incidence estimates, given the challenges of conducting hepatitis B and C surveillance, as detailed in this chapter. The recommendations also include guidance regarding the interpretation and dissemination of surveillance data.

APPLICATIONS OF SURVEILLANCE DATA

Surveillance data are used in a variety of ways by a broad base of state health-department staff, researchers, clinicians, policy-makers, and private industry. Federal and state health-department surveillance systems provide population-based information that can be used to improve the public's health. They also offer an opportunity for public-health intervention at the individual level by linking infected people to appropriate care and support services (Klevens et al., 2009). Overall, surveillance data are critical in estimating incidence and prevalence of HBV and HCV infections (CDC, 2008c), and they provide a basis for studying and understanding the mechanisms of diverse outcomes in the natural history of these infections (Thacker, 2000).

Public health surveillance generally involves name-based reporting of cases of specified diseases to state and local health departments. As such, it requires the gathering of information that some people consider private. Public health officials and state legislatures have weighed the costs and benefits of public health surveillance and have required name-based reporting of specific diseases with confidentiality safeguards in place to protect private information (Fairchild et al., 2008). Confidential name-based reporting is standard practice for infectious diseases surveillance, including HIV surveillance (CDC, 2008d). Acute HBV infections are reportable in all states and acute HCV infections are reportable in all but one state. All states report the cases to CDC. Chronic HBV infections are reportable in all but six states and chronic HCV infections are reportable in all but seven states (CSTE, 2009).

Outbreak Detection and Control

Accurate and timely surveillance data are necessary to identify outbreaks of acute HBV and HCV infection in the health-care and community settings. The data can assist in recognizing and addressing breaches in infection control, and they can help to mitigate the size of outbreaks. There have been several outbreaks of hepatitis B and hepatitis C in health-care settings in recent years (CDC, 2003b, 2003d, 2005b, 2008a, 2009c; Fabrizi et al., 2008; Thompson et al., 2009). Research on those outbreaks has shown that they typically occurred in dialysis units, medical wards, nursing homes, surgery wards, and outpatient clinics and resulted from breaches in infection control (Lanini et al., 2009). In a 2009 study, researchers found evidence of 33 outbreaks in nonhospital health-care settings in the United States in the last 10 years. Transmission was primarily patient to patient and was caused by lapses in infection control and aseptic techniques that allowed contamination of shared medical devices, such as dialysis machines. The authors stated that successful outbreak control depended on systematic case identification and investigation, but most health departments did not have the time, funds, personnel resources, or legal authority to investigate health-care–associated outbreaks (Thompson et al., 2009).

Hepatitis B and hepatitis C surveillance data can be used to identify or quantify new trends in the transmission of HBV and HCV. For example, surveillance data can help epidemiologists to determine whether sexual transmission of HCV reported among some cohorts of HIV-positive men who have sex with men (Matthews et al., 2007; van de Laar et al., 2009) is statistically significant on a population level. Surveillance data have also been used to identify clusters of newly acquired cases of hepatitis C in adolescents and young adults and to direct appropriate interventions to persons in the clusters (CDC, 2008f). Those findings can help public-health officials to target their resources at emerging populations being affected by HBV and HCV, such as racial and ethnic populations or geographically linked active injection-drug users (IDUs).

Resource Allocation

Surveillance data are often used to determine how to use resources most effectively. For example, estimates of disease burden are commonly used to provide guidance to policy-makers on the level of funding required for disease-related programs. If surveillance data are not available or understate the disease burden, legislators and public-health officials will not allocate sufficient resources to mount an appropriate public-health response.

Information on disease burden is only one factor that guides policy-makers in allocating public-health resources. Priorities in public funding are also driven by public awareness and advocacy. Therefore, it is important to communicate surveillance trends and disease burden clearly to policy-makers and community advocates. For example, estimates of trends indicate that mortality from HCV may soon exceed that from HIV (Deuffic-Burban et al., 2007). However, despite the large number of individuals and communities affected by hepatitis B and hepatitis C, the resources available for addressing viral hepatitis are only a small fraction of those available for addressing HIV. CDC's National Center for HIV/AIDS, Viral Hepatitis, Sexually Transmitted Diseases, and Tuberculosis Prevention had a budget of almost $1 billion for 2008, and only 2% of it was allocated to hepatitis B and hepatitis C (Ward, 2008). Sixty-nine percent of the budget was allocated for HIV, 15% for sexually transmitted diseases (STDs), and 14% for tuberculosis.

Programmatic Design and Evaluation

Public-health organizations use surveillance data to design programs that target appropriate populations. For example, CDC requires states to set priorities among populations for HIV prevention according to data generated by HIV/AIDS surveillance programs and community-services assessments (CDC, 2003a). Surveillance data can also be used to evaluate systems for delivery of prevention and care service. A key potential role of hepatitis surveillance programs is to evaluate the effect of HBV vaccination programs (Wasley et al., 2007).

Linking Patients to Care

For some diseases, it is desirable to have a surveillance system closely involved in ensuring the linkage of persons who have new diagnoses to health-care services, often called case management (Fleming et al., 2006). For viral-hepatitis surveillance, linking patients who have recent diagnoses to comprehensive viral-hepatitis programs may be indicated to ensure access to appropriate services, including clinical evaluation, regular followup visits, referral to drug-treatment and harm-reduction programs, education about liver health, and prevention of transmission to others. Chapter 5 will discuss the components of viral-hepatitis services.

DISEASE-SPECIFIC ISSUES RELATED TO VIRAL-HEPATITIS SURVEILLANCE

Many of the difficulties that surveillance systems face in identifying and tracking cases of hepatitis B and hepatitis C are related to the complexity of the infections and their associated progression (see Figures 2-1 and 2-2). This section highlights some of those challenges. Chapter 5 will provide more detail on issues related to screening and identification.

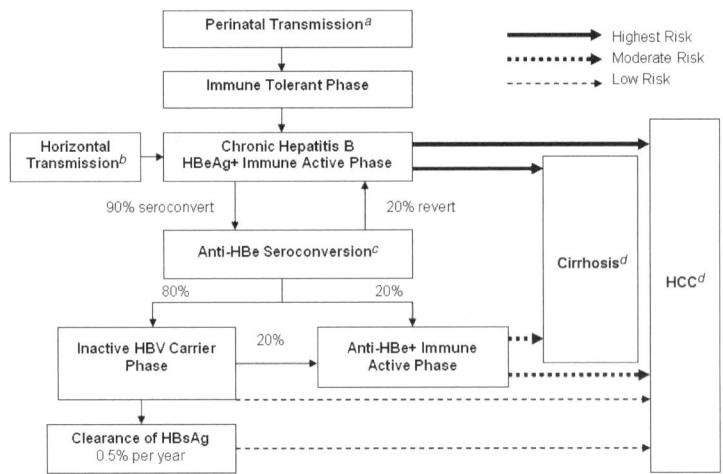

FIGURE 2-1 Natural progression of hepatitis B infection.
Abbreviations: HBeAg, hepatitis B e antigen; anti-HBe, antibody to hepatitis B e antigen; HBsAg, hepatitis B surface antigen; HBV, hepatitis B virus; HCC, hepatocellular carcinoma.
[a]Transmission occurs in 90% of infants of HBsAg+/HBeAg+ mothers and 15% of infants of HBsAg+/anti-HBe+ mothers.
[b]30% of those infected from the age of 1–5 years and under 7% of those infected at the age of 6 years or older.
[c]About 50% of patients by 5 years and 70% of patients by 10 years will seroconvert to anti-HBe.
[d]15-25% risk of premature death from cirrhosis and HCC.

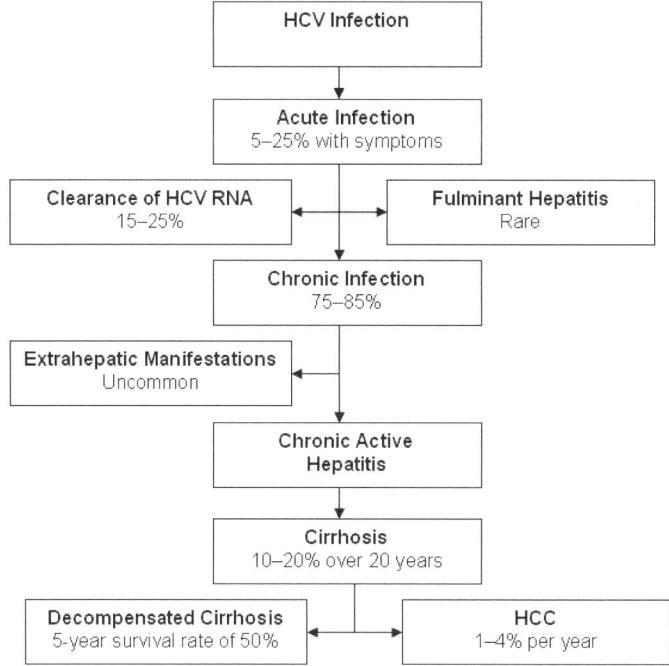

FIGURE 2-2 Natural progression of hepatitis C infection.
Abbreviations: HCV, hepatitis C virus; RNA, ribonucleic acid; HCC, hepatocellular carcinoma.
SOURCE: Adapted from Chen and Morgan, 2006. Reprinted with permission from Ivyspring International Publisher, copyright 2006.

Identifying Acute Infections

Several factors contribute to the difficulty in identifying acute HBV and HCV infections. Many newly acquired cases are asymptomatic, or they may have symptoms similar to those of other common illnesses and so do not prompt health-care providers to conduct serologic testing for HBV and HCV, or the serologic tests that are conducted are inadequate to distinguish between acute and chronic cases. About 90% of acute HBV infections in children under 5 years of age and 70% of HBV infections in adults are asymptomatic (McMahon et al., 1985); 75–95% of acute HCV infections are asymptomatic (Chen and Morgan, 2006; Guerrant et al., 2001), so few infected patients seek care for the acute illness; and there is a very high probability of underreporting even when care is obtained (Chen and Morgan, 2006; Cox et al., 2005; Hagan et al., 2002). Clinicians often are not fully aware of reporting requirements in connection with other reportable diseases and do not initiate reports routinely (Allen and Ferson, 2000). In addition, some persons with chronic HBV infection can experience sudden increases in alanine aminotransferase (ALT) that may be associated with jaundice or liver decompensation. That change may have a variety of causes, including infection with another hepatitis virus; alcohol, drug, or medication use; or sudden hepatitis B disease reactivation that can be associated with the period of seroconversion from a hepatitis B e antigen (HBeAg) state to an antibody to hepatitis B e (anti-HBe) state or reversion from an anti-HBe state back to an HBeAg-positive state (Koff, 2004). Therefore, in investigating acute symptomatic infections, it is important to identify outbreaks so that preventive measures can be undertaken and, in the case of hepatitis B, to identify and screen close contacts who might benefit from the hepatitis B vaccine. Such information is needed if surveillance staff is to determine which cases are newly diagnosed, the result of recent exposure, or chronic (Fleming et al., 2006).

Classifying acute cases of hepatitis B and hepatitis C requires a complex integration of clinical data, positive and negative laboratory data, and prior or repeat testing (see Boxes 2-2 and 2-3). Many of the test results—for

---

BOX 2-2
CDC Acute Hepatitis B Case Definition

Clinical case definition:
An acute illness with
- discrete onset of symptoms

and
- jaundice or elevated serum aminotransferase levels

Laboratory criteria for diagnosis:
- IgM antibody to hepatitis B core antigen (anti-HBc) positive

or
- hepatitis B surface antigen (HBsAg) positive
- IgM anti-HAV negative (if done)

Case classification:
Confirmed: a case that meets the clinical case definition and is laboratory confirmed

---

Abbreviations: CDC, Centers for Disease Control and Prevention; HAV, hepatitis A virus; HBV, hepatitis B virus.
SOURCE: CDC, 2009a.

SURVEILLANCE

> **BOX 2-3**
> **CDC Acute Hepatitis C Case Definition**
>
> **Clinical case definition:**
> An acute illness with a discrete onset of any sign or symptom consistent with acute viral hepatitis (e.g., anorexia, abdominal discomfort, nausea, vomiting), and either jaundice or serum alanine aminotransferase (ALT) levels >400 IU/L.
>
> **Laboratory criteria for diagnosis:**
> **One or more of the following three criteria:**
>   1) Antibodies to hepatitis C virus (anti-HCV) screening test positive with a signal to cut-off ratio predictive of a true positive as determined for the particular assay as defined by CDC, OR
>   2) Hepatitis C Virus Recombinant Immunoblot Assay (HCV RIBA) positive, OR
>   3) Nucleic Acid Test (NAT) for HCV RNA positive
>
> **and, meets the following two criteria:**
>   1) IgM antibody to hepatitis A virus (IgM anti-HAV) negative, AND
>   2) IgM antibody to hepatitis B core antigen (IgM anti-HBc) negative
>
> **Case classification:**
> *Confirmed:* A case that meets the clinical case definition, is laboratory confirmed, and is not known to have chronic hepatitis C.
>
> ---
> Abbreviations: CDC, Centers for Disease Control and Prevention; HAV, hepatitis A virus; HCV, hepatitis C virus; RIBA, recombinant immunoblot assay; RNA, ribonucleic acid.
> NOTE: URL for the signal-to-cutoff ratios: http://www.cdc.gov/ncidod/diseases/hepatitis/c/sc_ratios.htm.
> SOURCE: CDC, 2009a.

example, for ALT, aspartate transaminase, immunoglobulin M (IgM) antibody to the hepatitis A virus, and IgM antibody to the hepatitis B core antigen (HBcAg)—are difficult for health departments to obtain, particularly because negative test results often are not automatically reported to health departments (Fleming et al., 2006). Because auxiliary test results are not systematically reported to health departments, surveillance staff must actively follow up with health-care providers to obtain them and other clinical indicators of acute disease. If the data cannot be obtained, either because the proper tests were not ordered or because there is insufficient staff to conduct followup, cases will be classified ambiguously as nonacute infections.

Furthermore, current CDC case definitions may miss a substantial fraction of clinically apparent acute cases because they lack clinical markers that could improve case identification and help to distinguish between acute and chronic cases. Using data from electronic medical records, Klompas et al. (2008) found that CDC's case definition of acute HBV had a positive predictive value of only 47.2% (that is, out of 1,000 people identified as having acute hepatitis B with the CDC case definition, only 472 of them were found to truly have acute hepatitis B). When patients with prior positive tests for HBV infection (or International Classification of Diseases, revision 9, codes for chronic HBV infection) were excluded, the positive predictive value increased to 68.4%. However, the positive predictive value was raised to above 96% by adding the requirement for peak ALT over 1,000 or total bilirubin over 1.5. Most important, when applying the most sensitive algorithm (the algorithm that detected the greatest number of cases of acute hepatitis B), the study found that only four of the eight cases of acute hepatitis B were in the state's surveillance system and only one of the four was correctly classified as acute; this suggests that 88% of acute hepatitis B cases may be missed if current reporting algorithms are used (Klompas et al., 2008).

Similarly, detection of acute hepatitis C can be challenging because no single case definition is either sensitive or specific for it. HCV seroconversion may be missed, and there is no IgM-based assay that reliably distinguishes acute hepatitis C from chronic hepatitis C, unlike the situation with hepatitis A virus or HBV infection. Relatively low HCV ribonucleic acid (RNA) concentrations and more than one log fluctuation in HCV RNA concentration are features of acute HCV infection that may be useful for the development of more dynamic diagnostic algorithms, but the accuracy of these algorithms has not been validated (Cox et al., 2005; McGovern et al., 2009; Villano et al., 1999).

In summary, the identification of acute hepatitis infection is inherently flawed because the vast majority of cases are asymptomatic and patients do not seek medical care or testing. Such persons would be identified only in prospective studies that include routine serial testing of liver enzyme concentrations, such as those previously conducted to identify the incidence of transfusion-associated hepatitis. Underreporting of diagnosed cases and misclassification of reported cases seriously limit the accuracy of data on cases of acute viral hepatitis collected by state and territorial surveillance programs and transmitted to CDC. Thus, the estimates of the incidence of acute hepatitis in the United States are based solely on symptomatic cases. The majority of those cases may be missing from the surveillance system because of poor access to health care, underreporting, and misclassification. Taken together, published surveillance summaries of reported cases of acute viral hepatitis substantially underestimate the number of cases; these summaries may give misleading impressions of the incidence of disease to policy-makers and program planners.

Identifying Chronic Infections

Given that both hepatitis B and hepatitis C infections are largely asymptomatic, most people do not receive a diagnosis until the infection is chronic. For hepatitis B, the chance of developing a chronic infection varies with age at the time of infection.

In persons over 6 years old, the vast majority of acute HBV infections are self-limited (Hyams, 1995). However, hepatitis B infections become chronic in over 90% of infants who are infected at birth or in the first year of life and in 30% of children who are infected at the age of 1–5 years (Pungpapong et al., 2007). Although hepatitis B surface antigen (HBsAg) is detectable within 4–10 weeks after infection, it is indicative of chronic HBV infection only if it persists for more than 6 months (Koff, 2004). An accurate diagnosis of chronic hepatitis B may therefore require the reporting of multiple serologic markers at more than one time (Koff, 2004).

For disease-surveillance purposes, it can be challenging for health departments to obtain the complete laboratory results that are necessary to classify a chronic hepatitis B case according to CDC's case definitions (see Box 2-4). In general, a full hepatitis B panel (including any negative results for IgM anti-HBc) is required or two HBsAg results at least 6 months apart. Although states govern laboratory-reporting requirements in their jurisdictions, negative test results are generally not reportable and must be actively obtained. CDC's *Guidelines for Viral Hepatitis Surveillance and Case Management* recommend that only positive HBsAg-test results be reported, but this test alone is inadequate to distinguish acute from chronic infection. Automated systems attached to electronic medical records may help to address surveillance for chronic HBV cases in the future, but in the meantime many diagnoses of chronic HBV infection probably will not be correctly captured and classified as confirmed cases (CDC, 2005a).

Surveillance for chronic HCV infection also presents challenges (see Box 2-5). In adults, about 15–25% of acute hepatitis C infections resolve spontaneously (Villano et al., 1999). That may increase to about 45% in children and young adults (Vogt et al., 1999). The presence of HCV RNA is generally detected within 1 week of infection (Mosley et al., 2005), but antibodies to HCV (anti-HCV) can be detected in only 50–70% of infected persons at the onset of symptoms; this increases to more than 90% after 3 months (NIH, 2002). A chronic infection is characterized by the persistent presence of HCV RNA for at least 6 months (NIH, 2002).

Typically, when a patient presents for HCV testing, the first test that is conducted is for the presence of anti-HCV. This test is generally an en-

BOX 2-4
CDC Chronic Hepatitis B Case Definition

Clinical description
Persons with chronic HBV infection may have no evidence of liver disease or may have a spectrum of disease ranging from chronic hepatitis to cirrhosis or liver cancer. Persons with chronic infection may be asymptomatic.

Laboratory criteria
- IgM antibodies to anti-HBc negative
and
- a positive result on one of the following tests: hepatitis B surface antigen HBsAg, HBeAg, or hepatitis B virus (HBV) DNA,
or
- HBsAg positive or HBV DNA positive or HBeAg positive two times at least 6 months apart (Any combination of these tests performed 6 months apart is acceptable.)

Case classification
Confirmed: a case that meets either laboratory criteria for diagnosis
Probable: a case with a single HBsAg positive or HBV DNA positive or HBeAg positive lab result when no IgM anti-HBc results are available

Comment
Multiple laboratory tests indicative of chronic HBV infection may be performed simultaneously on the same patient specimen as part of a "hepatitis panel." Testing performed in this manner may lead to seemingly discordant results, e.g., HBsAg-negative and HBV DNA-positive. For the purposes of this case definition, any positive result among the three laboratory tests mentioned above is acceptable, regardless of other testing results. Negative HBeAg results and HBV DNA levels below positive cutoff level do not confirm the absence of HBV infection.

Abbreviations: CDC, Centers for Disease Control and Prevention; anti-HBc, hepatitis B core antigen; HBsAg, hepatitis B surface antigen; HBeAg, hepatitis B e antigen; HBV, hepatitis B virus; DNA, deoxyribonucleic acid.
SOURCE: CDC, 2009a.

> **BOX 2-5**
> **CDC Hepatitis C Virus Infection Case Definition**
> **(Past or Present)**
>
> **Clinical description:**
> Most HCV-infected persons are asymptomatic. However, many have chronic liver disease, which can range from mild to severe including cirrhosis and liver cancer.
>
> **Laboratory criteria for diagnosis:**
> - Anti-HCV positive (repeat reactive) by EIA, verified by an additional more specific assay (e.g., RIBA for anti-HCV or nucleic acid testing for HCV RNA),
>
> or
> - HCV RIBA positive,
>
> or
> - Nucleic acid test for HCV RNA positive,
>
> or
> - Report of HCV genotype,
>
> or
> - Anti-HCV screening-test-positive with a signal to cut-off ratio predictive of a true positive as determined for the particular assay (e.g., ≥3.8 for the enzyme immunoassays) as determined and posted by CDC.
>
> **Case classification:**
> *Confirmed:* a case that is laboratory confirmed and that does not meet the case definition for acute hepatitis C.
> *Probable:* a case that is anti-HCV positive (repeat reactive) by EIA and has ALT or SGPT values above the upper limit of normal, but the anti-HCV EIA result has not been verified by an additional more specific assay or the signal to cutoff ratio is unknown.
>
> ---
> Abbreviations: CDC, Centers for Disease Control and Prevention; HCV, hepatitis C virus; EIA, enzyme immunoassay; RIBA, recombinant immunoblot assay; RNA, ribonucleic acid; ALT or SGPT, alanine aminotranferase.
> SOURCE: CDC, 2009a.

zyme immunoassay (EIA). A repeatedly reactive EIA is followed by a more specific assay to detect viremia, such as the recombinant immunoblot assay (RIBA) for anti-HCV, or by nucleic acid testing for HCV RNA. In some cases, an EIA with a high signal-to-cutoff ratio predictive of a true positive will be used in the place of a confirmatory RIBA. However, all confirmed anti-HCV test results should be followed by a test for the presence of HCV

RNA (Alter et al., 2003; Ghany et al., 2009). The difficulty in identifying chronic cases often revolves around the need for two separate tests (or other supplemental antibody tests) and the 6-month timeframe required for a diagnosis of chronic HCV infection. Many infected people are tested at public or nonclinical testing sites—such as drug-treatment facilities, sites for testing for HIV or STDs, or community-based organizations—that conduct only the less expensive anti-HCV tests. Persons tested at those sites might not have access to an HCV RNA test, or the laboratory conducting the initial EIA test might not routinely test for HCV RNA when an EIA has been positive. The process leads to incomplete diagnoses and inaccurate reporting of the number of chronic cases.

The CDC-recommended case definition of nonacute HCV infection also poses some problems in interpreting the collected data. Although it is assumed that the majority of nonacute hepatitis C cases represent chronic infections, this case definition also includes acute cases that do not meet the confirmed acute case classification (CDC, 2005a). However, a case defined only by the presence of anti-HCV could be a late acute infection, a chronic infection, a resolved infection, or a false-positive assay result. It is therefore essential that anti-HCV testing be supplemented by testing for HCV RNA and by followup samples to classify cases correctly and to use the data for program-planning purposes.

Identifying Perinatal Hepatitis B

Since 1992, CDC has awarded funds to 64 grantees to support perinatal hepatitis B prevention programs through its Immunization Services Division's cooperative agreements with health departments. The funds support perinatal hepatitis B coordinators, who are charged with identifying all HBsAg-positive pregnant women, ensuring the administration of appropriate immunoprophylaxis to all infants born to these women, ensuring the completion of postvaccination serologic testing of the infants, and ensuring the completion of the hepatitis B vaccine series. Most coordinator programs also include ensuring vaccination of household contacts and sexual partners of HBsAg-positive women in their mission (CDC, 2009g).

In an economic analysis of immunization strategies to prevent hepatitis B transmission in the United States, Margolis et al. (1995) found that prevention of perinatal infection and routine infant vaccination would reduce the lifetime risk of HBV infection by at least 68%. They estimated that prevention of perinatal HBV infections would save $41.8 million in medical and work-loss costs. Routine hepatitis B vaccination of infants would provide additional savings of $19.7 million. Both strategies were found to be cost-effective, with estimated costs per year of life saved of $164 for preventing perinatal HBV infection and of $1,522 for infant vaccination.

In 1992, the Connecticut Department of Public Health found that hiring a state-level perinatal coordinator led to significantly better compliance with the recommendation to administer hepatitis B immune globulin (HBIG) than followup by local health departments. They also found that completion of the three-dose vaccination series was higher in cases followed by the state coordinator than in those followed by local public-health officials (CDC, 1996).

Two major problems occur in the identification and management of possible cases (see Box 2-6). The first involves linking pregnancy status with positive HBsAg laboratory reports on females of child-bearing age in a timely manner. In 2005, the Advisory Committee on Immunization Practices called for improving prevention of perinatal and early childhood HBV transmission by improving laws and regulations to improve identification of HBsAg-positive and HBsAg-undetermined mothers (Mast et al., 2005).

BOX 2-6
CDC Perinatal Hepatitis B Virus Infection Case Definition

Clinical description
Perinatal hepatitis B in the newborn may range from asymptomatic to fulminant hepatitis.

Laboratory criteria
HBsAg positive

Case classification
HBsAg positivity in any infant aged >1–24 months who was born in the United States or in US territories to an HBsAg-positive mother

Comment: Infants born to HBsAg-positive mothers should receive hepatitis B immune globulin (HBIG) and the first dose of hepatitis B vaccine within 12 hours of birth, followed by the second and third doses of vaccine at 1 and 6 months of age, respectively. Postvaccination testing for HBsAg and anti-HBs (antibody to HBsAg) is recommended from 3 to 6 months following completion of the vaccine series. If HBIG and the initial dose of vaccine are delayed for >1 month after birth, testing for HBsAg may determine if the infant is already infected.

Abbreviations: CDC, Centers for Disease Control and Prevention; HBsAg, hepatitis B surface antigen; anti-HBs, antibody to HBsAg; HBIG, hepatitis B immune globulin.
SOURCE: CDC, 2009a.

Implementation of automated electronic systems can greatly increase the speed with which cases can be identified (LaPorte et al., 2008), but they are not available in most states. The second problem involves a lack of resources to follow up on all potential and known cases and their contacts in a timely manner. Followup of an infant can take up to 2 years. In addition, a substantial number of HBsAg-positive mothers are not identified in time to ensure the required followup of the mothers and their infants (see Chapter 4).

Other Challenges for Hepatitis B and Hepatitis C Surveillance Systems

Repeat testing in high-risk populations can confuse the number of suspected acute versus chronic infections. Members of some populations, such as IDUs, may repeatedly incur HCV infection that resolves spontaneously without ever becoming chronic (Mehta et al., 2002). Those cases could mistakenly be classified as chronic infections based on antibody results alone.

Many of the people affected by hepatitis B and hepatitis C have limited access to health care (for example, active IDUs, homeless people, some Pacific Islanders, legal immigrants living in poverty, and undocumented immigrants) and are less likely to be diagnosed appropriately, to provide complete and accurate demographic and behavioral information, or to access followup care. Structural and political barriers, stigma, and fear of legal repercussions contribute to the limitations on their access. Each HBV-infected or HCV-infected person who does not enter into appropriate medical care represents a missed opportunity for secondary prevention and may contribute to the collection of inaccurate and less detailed surveillance data. Finding ways to ensure that patients receive comprehensive and culturally appropriate care and referrals not only would increase the likelihood of improving their health outcomes but is likely to affect surveillance-data collection favorably.

Finally, because of the chronic nature of viral hepatitis, it is important that surveillance staff communicate well between jurisdictions. Persons with chronic disease can be misclassified as having acute cases if earlier diagnoses made in other jurisdictions are not identified. Not infrequently, a previous diagnosis has been reported in another state or jurisdiction. The ability of state and local surveillance-program staff to track cases across jurisdictions is hampered by various factors, including inadequacy of staff resources, nonstandardized surveillance software systems, and the lack of a national database that could be used to identify potential matches in other jurisdictions.

INFRASTRUCTURE AND PROCESS-SPECIFIC ISSUES WITH SURVEILLANCE

Current public-health surveillance systems for hepatitis B and hepatitis C are poorly developed and are inconsistent among jurisdictions. As a result, surveillance data do not provide accurate estimates of the current burden of disease, are insufficient for program planning and evaluation, and do not provide the information that would allow policy-makers to allocate sufficient resources to address the problem. The AVHPCs, funded by CDC in state and territorial health departments, are tasked with identifying mechanisms for educating the public, at-risk populations, and medical-service and social-service providers about viral hepatitis; for managing and coordinating viral-hepatitis prevention activities; and for integrating viral-hepatitis screening programs and related services into health-care settings and public-health programs that serve at-risk adults. In most cases, however, CDC funding covers only the AVHPC's salary. No funding is provided for viral-hepatitis testing, hepatitis B immunizations, or other services. Most important, AVHPCs are not funded to conduct surveillance activities, although many of them provide technical assistance for such programs.

In addition, CDC's DVH has scant resources for providing funding and guidance to local and state health departments to perform surveillance for viral hepatitis. The resources provided for viral-hepatitis surveillance contrast sharply with the resources that CDC provides for HIV surveillance. For example, CDC has specific cooperative agreements with the states and territories to conduct core HIV/AIDS surveillance activities. The cooperative agreements are accompanied by dedicated funding, specific CDC project officers and epidemiologists, regular technical-assistance meetings and training, and a help desk that has trained staff to answer database-related questions. The guidance for HIV/AIDS surveillance is a three-volume set containing more than 500 pages of detailed instructions, standards, and guidelines. In contrast, CDC's cooperative agreements with state and territorial health departments for viral hepatitis do not include surveillance activities. In addition, although CDC's DVH has produced guidelines for viral-hepatitis surveillance for state and territorial health departments, they are presented in fewer than 50 pages (CDC, 2005a). Given that the guidelines cover three distinct and complex diseases (hepatitis A, hepatitis B, and hepatitis C), they lack the detail necessary to create surveillance practices that are consistent among jurisdictions. As a result of the deficiency of resources dedicated to hepatitis surveillance, data are incomplete, variable, and inaccurate. Inconsistency between jurisdictions seriously undermines the validity of the data provided at the state, regional, and national levels.

The inability of health departments to track all diagnosed cases also seriously undermines case-management and prevention efforts. For example, studies have shown that vaccinating close contacts of persons chronically infected with HBV (that is, ring vaccination) is cost-effective (Hutton et al., 2007). The strategy remains cost-effective even in populations in which the prevalence of chronic HBV infection is as low as 2%. However, without funding and staffing for surveillance and identification of new cases of HBV, ring vaccination is not a public-health activity that is typically supported by most health departments.

CDC has funded seven enhanced projects through the Viral Hepatitis Surveillance Emerging Infections Programs (EIPs). The projects began in 2004 and were scheduled to end in 2009. CDC plans to extend the program for 2 more years (personal communication, J. Efird, CDC, May 18, 2009). They are in Colorado, Connecticut, Minnesota, New York state, New York City, Oregon, and San Francisco. Although the projects focus on surveillance for hepatitis A, hepatitis B, and hepatitis C, they all take different approaches, including multiple approaches in individual jurisdictions. Project funding supports epidemiologic and data-entry staffing. Methods used in the seven programs include verification of diagnoses with medical providers, chart review, followup calls to infected persons that focus on education or data collection, educational mailings (for example, letters and booklets), followup with persons that are household or close contacts (especially acute HBV cases), sampling for followup of cases of chronic HBV and HCV, review of all data, and matching with HIV and STD programs. There is no uniform evaluation of the projects.

In February and March 2009, staff of the National Alliance of State and Territorial AIDS Directors (NASTAD) interviewed the coordinators of the seven EIPs. From those interviews, staff identified additional programmatic issues that affect reporting. They include resource issues, such as the varied capacity of county and city health departments (which leads to inconsistencies in data collection and data systems, in some instances in the same state); the staffing requirements needed to collect, process, and manage data; and the staff and time needed to investigate health-care–related outbreaks adequately. Other issues are the need to educate medical providers better on which laboratory tests are needed for appropriate diagnosis (also noted by Fleming et al., [2006]), and the difficulty that staff face in obtaining demographic data (including data on race, ethnicity, and country of origin) and data on risk history (Klevens et al., 2009; NASTAD, 2009).

Funding Sources

Funding for hepatitis surveillance is highly fragmented. No federal funds are dedicated to chronic-hepatitis surveillance except for the seven jurisdictions that receive funds from CDC's DVH to perform enhanced surveillance activities. State, territorial, or city health-department viral-hepatitis surveillance units, where they exist, often receive no dedicated federal funding for this activity. Others may receive funding directly from their state or city, or they may be integrated into or receive funding from other programs or units that receive federal funding from CDC programs whose missions are related to epidemiology or viral hepatitis. The CDC programs include the Immunization Services Division (related to perinatal hepatitis B), the Epidemiology and Laboratory Capacity for Infectious Diseases program (acute hepatitis B), EIPs, and the DVH. Funding may also be available through private organizations or foundations. Some surveillance units receive funding from multiple sources. Each funding source may require different activities and may provide varied guidance on the receiving unit's activities. The recent survey of AVHPCs conducted by NASTAD found that fewer than one-fourth of the 43 responding jurisdictions reported receiving funding for surveillance for either chronic HBV or chronic HCV infection (NASTAD, 2009).

Program Design

Variability among jurisdictions is also due to a wide array of program structures. In a 2006 survey, 33% of the 52 hepatitis C coordinators funded by CDC reported being in their jurisdictions' communicable-diseases or epidemiology programs, 25% in HIV–STD programs, 14% in HIV programs, and the remainder in the immunization or STD programs (CDC, 2006). The hepatitis C coordinators' locations within public health departments may or may not correspond with the health department program responsible for conducting surveillance, which can lead to reduced involvement and oversight by the coordinator of viral hepatitis surveillance activities.

In a later survey of the (renamed) AVHPCs by CDC in April 2009, only 32 states reported having state viral-hepatitis plans. Of the 32, 29 included surveillance as a component. However, fewer than two-thirds of the program coordinators reported being able to implement the surveillance components. The reasons listed for not implementing plan components were lack of staff and lack of funding (CDC, 2009h).

Reporting Systems and Requirements

Reporting of surveillance data to CDC by state and territorial health departments is voluntary, and in general little federal funding is provided for HBV and HCV surveillance activities (Klein et al., 2008). Chronic hepatitis B is reportable in 42 states, but only 38 states conduct surveillance and maintain systems, and only 20 report cases to CDC (George, 2004). Chronic hepatitis C is reportable in 40 states, but only 20 report cases to CDC (George, 2004). CDC collects data from states that report chronic HBV and HCV infections (and received data on 133,520 cases of HCV infection in 2007 alone), but these data are not presented routinely in *Morbidity and Mortality Weekly Report,* which is published by CDC, or elsewhere (Klevens et al., 2009). Although all states but one perform some degree of surveillance for acute HBV and HCV (Daniels et al., 2009b), much of this surveillance is passive at best.

There are significant barriers to implementing more comprehensive surveillance activities. In the previously mentioned survey conducted by NASTAD in 2009, it was reported that of the 43 responding jurisdictions, almost half received between 1,000 and 10,000 HBV laboratory results annually, and over 70% reported the same range for the number of HCV laboratory results received annually (NASTAD, 2009). Many states do not have the staffing or systems to keep up with such a high volume of information received and are often unable to follow up with medical providers to address underreporting or to obtain demographic and risk-history information, such as race, ethnicity, and drug-use details (Klein et al., 2008). The lack of funding to hire adequate staff is the fundamental barrier to complete and accurate surveillance.

Although CDC provides case-reporting forms for the collection of viral-hepatitis surveillance data, the forms do not have required elements, and they ask for data that are often difficult to obtain. Moreover, the use of the forms is inconsistent among states and local jurisdictions. Of the 43 health departments that responded to inquiries from the present committee, 26 have developed their own HBV case-reporting form, and 21 have developed an HCV case-reporting form. The forms were created to capture behavioral-risk information not included on CDC's form or to improve data collection and entry into the separate jurisdictions' specific software systems. For example, the CDC case-reporting form does not collect risk-behavior information specific to chronic HBV. Finally, 8 states do not use a case-reporting form at all for reporting HBV, and 12 states do not use one for HCV; these jurisdictions rely solely on the reporting of laboratory-test results.

Paradoxically, efforts to modernize and enhance public-health surveillance systems have led to greater inconsistency in data collection. In 1984, CDC began work on the Epidemiologic Surveillance Project. The goal of the project was to develop computer-based transmission of public-health surveillance data between states and CDC. By 1989, all 50 states were participating in the reporting system for certain acute infectious diseases, and the system was renamed the National Electronic Telecommunications System for Surveillance (NETSS) (CDC, 2009f). Data were transmitted weekly to CDC in a standard record format. However, the system quickly became dated with advances in information and surveillance technology, such as electronic laboratory reporting and electronic medical records.

Moreover, other surveillance systems and software were used for reporting of HIV/AIDS, STDs, tuberculosis, and some vaccine-preventable diseases.

In 1999, CDC developed the concept of the National Electronic Disease Surveillance System (NEDSS), which was designed to promote the development of interoperable surveillance systems (that is, the Public Health Information Network, or PHIN) at federal, state, and local levels (CDC, 2009e). The NEDSS initiative describes information-system standards to which all systems must adhere but does not require use of CDC-produced software. CDC provides the NEDSS Base System, a software system that may be used, but only 16 jurisdictions have opted to use it. Most jurisdictions use PHIN-compliant systems, which are either purchased from a commercial vendor or developed specifically for a particular jurisdiction. A few jurisdictions continue to use the NETSS system while their PHIN-compliant systems are being developed (personal communication, J. Efird, CDC, April 1, 2009). The result is that CDC no longer provides a standardized database for inputting and reporting data on viral hepatitis. Consequently, there is a wide array of state systems with an even wider array of capabilities. The lack of standardization makes it difficult for states to share information efficiently. In addition, creating and modifying their systems can lead to substantial expenses for states and jurisdictions (CDC, 2009i).

Even states and jurisdictions that have PHIN-compliant systems in place may not have the staff to enter the high volume of viral-hepatitis data received. Four of the 43 states that responded to the recent questionnaire for this committee reported not having any staff to enter data. They do not include states that may not be able to enter all received data fully. In the 2009 NASTAD survey of AVHPCs, it was reported that 27 of the 43 reporting jurisdictions had backlogs of HCV data, with an average of 6,200 cases that needed to have data entered (NASTAD, 2009).

Capturing Data on At-Risk Populations

As discussed previously, current surveillance systems do not adequately capture cases of acute and chronic HBV and HCV infections. That is particularly true for members of marginalized populations. IDUs are at high risk for both HBV and HCV infections. The incidence of HCV infection in IDUs ranges from 2% to 40% per year, with most rates in the range of 15–30% per year[1] (Maher et al., 2006; Mathei et al., 2005; van den Berg et al., 2007), and the incidence of HBV infection from 10% to 12% per year (Ruan et al., 2007). A study of IDUs in Seattle looked at those who became infected with HBV or HCV during the 12-month study period. The study matched study participants who had become infected to those identified in

---

[1] HCV prevalence is calculated in percentages from person years.

the health department's surveillance database. Of the 113 study participants who became infected, only two cases of those identified in the study were picked up by the state's surveillance system (Hagan et al., 2002). None of the 65 acute HCV infections in IDUs was reported.

Enhanced sero-surveillance studies, such as the National Health and Nutrition Examination Survey (NHANES), which are often used to provide supplemental data and prevalence estimates when surveillance systems are inadequate or incomplete, have serious limitations when addressing viral hepatitis. For example, NHANES, the study most commonly used to estimate the disease burden of chronic HBV and HCV infections, excludes or underrepresents populations that are most at risk for HBV and HCV infections. Those populations include homeless persons, institutionalized and incarcerated persons, and persons of Asian and Pacific Island descent. About 1.5 million people are in state or federal prisons in the United States (Department of Justice, 2009). CDC estimated chronic HBV prevalence in the adult prison population to be around 1–3.7%, and the prevalence of chronic HCV infection has been reported to vary from 12–35% (CDC, 2003c). Thus, the national estimate of 2.7–3.9 million people chronically infected with HCV (CDC, 2009b; Daniels et al., 2009a) potentially excludes several hundred thousand cases. Similarly, Asians, Pacific Islanders, American Indian, and Alaska Native people are undersampled among NHANES participants (Coleman et al., 1998). Given the higher prevalence of HBV in those populations, NHANES underreports the number of chronic HBV cases in the national estimates (Kim, 2007).

A supplemental HIV surveillance project funded by CDC's Division of HIV/AIDS Prevention is the National HIV Behavioral Surveillance System. The system surveys persons at high risk for HIV infection in cities with high rates of AIDS diagnoses to determine their risk behavior, testing behavior, and use of prevention services. Even though IDUs are one of the targeted populations studied through the system (CDC, 2009d), HCV testing has not been included systematically as part of the study design, and this leads to missed opportunities to define the injection and injection-related behaviors as they apply to HCV and HCV prevention.

Case Evaluation, Followup, and Partner Services

The reporting of a case of hepatitis B or hepatitis C by a public test site or private clinic provides an opportunity for public-health followup. Part of the followup generally involves ensuring that the persons with the reported diagnoses and their partners receive proper medical evaluation, counseling, vaccination, and referrals to support services as needed. (Fleming et al.,

2006). An inability of a health department to identify a case becomes a missed opportunity to prevent future cases and to ensure that HBV-infected and HCV-infected people receive the care that they need.

In 2007, the Massachusetts Department of Public Health piloted the use of STD disease intervention specialists (DISs) to follow up on cases of HCV infection in people 15–25 years old. The DISs were tasked with collecting risk-history data and providing partner-notification services for drug-sharing partners of the infected people. There was some success in reaching a small sample of the high volume of infected people, but no funding was available to support the staff. In addition, the DISs had competing priorities that kept the department from being able to implement its methods fully so that they could be appropriately evaluated (Onofrey et al., 2008).

Given the demands on staff, most state health-department surveillance units indicated that they were barely able to keep up with the basics of data collection. The 2009 NASTAD survey found that only 18 of the 43 jurisdictions conducted any type of followup; in the ones that did conduct followup, there was wide variation in what that comprised (NASTAD, 2009). Followup can consist of making calls to providers or cases to collect demographic, clinical, or risk-history data and contacting infected people by mail, by telephone, or in person to provide education or referral to medical services. For the most part, even the best resourced surveillance units are able to conduct only very limited case management (Fleming et al., 2006).

Furthermore, the utility and cost effectiveness of conducting partner services for persons who test positive for HBV or HCV is yet to be determined. Currently, states conduct partner notification for HIV and some STDs. Services include notifying sex or needle-sharing partners of exposure to disease and testing, counseling, and referrals for other services. Newly revised CDC guidelines on partner services strongly recommend partner services for persons reported to have HIV or early syphilis; services for gonorrhea and chlamydial infection are recommended for high-priority cases as resources allow (CDC, 2008e). Recommendations for persons who have viral hepatitis were not included in the HIV and STD integrated guidelines.

Recommendations

Recommendation 2-1. The Centers for Disease Control and Prevention should conduct a comprehensive evaluation of the national hepatitis B and hepatitis C public-health surveillance system.

The evaluation should, at a minimum,

- Include assessment of the system's attributes, including completeness, data quality and accuracy, timeliness, sensitivity, specificity, predictive value positive, representativeness, and stability.
- Be consistent with CDC's Updated Guidelines for Evaluating Public Health Surveillance Systems.
- Be used to guide the development of detailed technical guidance and standards for viral hepatitis surveillance.
- Be published in a report.

The committee found little published information on or systematic review of viral-hepatitis surveillance in the United States. Specific information was obtained from a series of surveys of the AVHPCs. In contrast, the history and status of national HIV surveillance is well reviewed and documented (CDC, 1999; Glynn et al., 2007; Nakashima and Fleming, 2003).

In July 2001, CDC published updated guidelines for evaluating public-health surveillance systems (CDC, 2001b). According to the guidelines, the evaluation should "involve an assessment of system attributes, including simplicity, flexibility, data quality, acceptability, sensitivity, predictive value positive, representativeness, timeliness, and stability." The lack of sensitivity of state hepatitis-surveillance systems is well documented for acute cases, and many states do not perform surveillance for chronic HBV or chronic HCV infections. Moreover, the movement of CDC away from NETSS, a CDC-provided system, and toward a national network of PHIN-compliant systems has left state and territorial health departments with a wide array of software systems and capabilities (CDC, 2009i). A comprehensive review is needed to document the current systems and capacities of public-health jurisdictions. The evaluation should focus on developing guidance to improve consistency of data, guide the development of detailed technical guidance and standards for hepatitis-surveillance programs, and allow CDC to improve understanding and description of the limitations of the data collected. Completion of this task should not delay the implementation of other components of the surveillance-related recommendations in this report.

Recommendation 2-2. The Centers for Disease Control and Prevention should develop specific cooperative viral-hepatitis agreements with all state and territorial health departments to support core surveillance for acute and chronic hepatitis B and hepatitis C.

The agreements should include

- A funding mechanism and guidance for core surveillance activities.
- Implementation of performance standards regarding revised and standardized case definitions, specifically through the use of
  o Revised case-reporting forms with required, standardized components.
  o Case evaluation and followup.
- Support for developing and implementing automated data-collection systems, including
  o Electronic laboratory reporting.
  o Electronic medical-record extraction systems.
  o Web-based, PHIN-compliant reporting systems.

CDC should provide more comprehensive guidance to states on surveillance for viral hepatitis. The committee suggests that CDC use the HIV surveillance system as a model. The committee focused on that surveillance model as an alternative to the current model because of its organization, availability of technical assistance, and provision of detailed guidelines. The strength of the model is in its centralized guidance, mandatory process and outcome standards, and oversight at a national level, all of which provide consistency in data among jurisdictions (Hall and Mokotoff, 2007).

CDC is able to oversee its national effort through separate cooperative agreements with each state and territory for specific core HIV surveillance activities (CDC, 2007). The agreements not only provide funding for enough dedicated staff to provide followup directly with providers and to conduct active surveillance but commit states and territories to specific methods and performance expectations. States are also provided with detailed guidance on case investigation, classification, and followup requirements (CDC/CSTE, 2006). To ensure consistency, CDC holds required disease-specific technical-assistance meetings for all grantees. Project officers and epidemiologists are assigned to each grantee. As of April 2008, all states and territories had implemented the confidential, name-based reporting method used for all other reportable infectious diseases (CDC, 2008d). The national HIV surveillance system will soon be able to achieve case counts with no duplicates among jurisdictions through an interstate reciprocal notification system wherein CDC provides quarterly reports on cases that might be duplicated between states on the basis of matching soundex codes,[2] dates

---

[2] A soundex code is a coded last name index based on the way a surname sounds rather than the way it is spelled. It is a census coding system developed so you can find a surname even if it may have been recorded under various spellings. A soundex code consists of a letter and three numbers (CDC/CSTE, 2006).

of birth, race, and sex. There is also guidance and sufficient staffing to be able to investigate cases of public-health importance, including clusters of unusual clinical, laboratory, or geographic occurrences; cases with unusual modes of transmission; cases without detectable antibody response; and cases with unusual strains of HIV, such as HIV-2 and non-B subtypes.

Another aspect of the HIV surveillance model is that all jurisdictions use standardized HIV/AIDS case-report forms. Specific information must be completed before the software system will classify an entry as a case; this information includes laboratory or provider diagnosis confirmation, and patient's date of birth, race, ethnicity, and sex. The case-report form includes the collection of behavioral-risk information, measures of immunologic function (CD4+ cell count and percentage), and viral load.

Most important, the HIV model includes process and outcome standards that all jurisdictions must strive to achieve (CDC, 1999). The outcome standards include completeness, timeliness, accuracy, risk ascertainment, and collection of first CD4+ cell count. Because the new software system is document-based, it will enable evaluation of the completeness of national case ascertainment with a capture-recapture method (Hall et al., 2006). The resulting information can be used to determine weaknesses in the reporting system and to help interpret data appropriately.

Finally, the process and outcome standards have been incorporated into CDC's updated framework for evaluating public-health surveillance systems (Hall and Mokotoff, 2007). CDC assesses national HIV surveillance data against the required outcome standards annually. The HIV/AIDS surveillance evaluation framework promotes continuous improvement in the quality of data through technical guidance, measurement of performance, reporting of assessment results to state and local health departments, and adjustments in guidance, training, or technical assistance according to assessment results.

The cooperative agreement and the associated funding have allowed the development of the national HIV surveillance system. Both are imperative for the development of an accurate, timely, and complete hepatitis surveillance system that will provide accurate incidence and prevalence data to inform proper resource allocation, program development and evaluation, and policy-making.

The following section details the committee's recommended model for structuring surveillance for hepatitis B and hepatitis C.

MODEL FOR SURVEILLANCE

The committee recommends that a two-tiered model be developed: core surveillance and targeted surveillance. The initial focus of the program should be the development and implementation of standardized systems among all states to maximize their capacity to perform core surveillance for acute and chronic HBV and HCV infection. Standardization will be accomplished through cooperative agreements, improved guidance, and adequate and consistent funding. Systems should be integrated into existing HIV or other disease surveillance infrastructure where feasible. Complementary efforts need to be made in building enhanced supplemental surveillance systems to describe trends in underrepresented at-risk populations better and to address the gaps identified in the current surveillance system. Both types of surveillance activities will provide better information to policymakers and service-delivery systems to improve care for people who are at risk for or living with HBV or HCV infection. Changes should be phased and prioritized, with the first step focused on the development and funding of core surveillance systems for each state.

Core Surveillance

Core surveillance—including collection, processing, analysis, and dissemination of data on cases of acute and chronic HBV and HCV infection—is needed in all states. Because of the public-health importance of quick identification of outbreaks and nosocomial transmission, acute-disease surveillance has had the highest priority in surveillance programs in the past. However, chronic-disease surveillance is also critical in that, if funded appropriately, it will assist in the recognition of acute cases, aid in moving people with recent diagnoses into appropriate care, contribute to an increased understanding of disease burden, allow evaluation of prevention efforts, and, given appropriate case management, save on costs associated with treatment of patients who have cirrhosis, hepatocellular carcinoma, or liver transplantation. Proper chronic-disease surveillance can also improve acute-disease surveillance by enhancing the accuracy and efficiency of related data collection. Evaluation of the core surveillance system should be ongoing to ensure that it is meeting emerging needs.

Funding Mechanism

In the proposed model, the state would be the primary unit of surveillance. Funding should be earmarked for viral-hepatitis surveillance through cooperative agreements with the states. CDC should ensure that all states have sufficient infrastructure to identify and appropriately investigate all suspected cases of acute and chronic HBV and HCV infection. Cooperative agreements should require reporting of standardized viral-hepatitis surveillance data within 3 years of implementation. The agreements should include funding for states to hire staff to process laboratory results, enter data, and follow up cases of acute and chronic HBV and HCV infections.

Case Definitions

CDC should revise and standardize definitions and methods. Revised case definitions should reflect active and resolved hepatitis C infection (for example, a case should not be confirmed if only antibody test results are available). Recommended testing for hepatitis C should include, where possible, HCV RNA tests to determine whether a person is actively infected. The case definition for acute HBV and HCV infection should be revised to remove the need for symptoms for classification as a confirmed case. Classification as a suspected case of acute HCV infection should be used to encourage active followup of likely recent infections (for example, in adolescents and young adults) (CDC, 2008f).

Case-Reporting Form

The case-reporting form should be standardized, and core components of it should be required of all jurisdictions to permit better capture of information on cases of acute and chronic HCV and HBV infection. The required elements should be such that they could reasonably be found in a patient's medical record. For example, the current CDC form requests the number of sexual partners in a given period. That information is not typically found in a medical record or known by a medical provider. Additional, more comprehensive epidemiologic studies could be funded to provide for patient interviews and a detailed assessment of risk factors (see Recommendation 2-3). Furthermore, the case-reporting form should collect more detailed demographic data on racial and ethnic populations to identify and address disparities among populations. For example, the case-reporting form should include categories for different ethnicities and should disaggregate Asians and Pacific Islanders (for example, Chinese, Vietnamese, Japanese, and Marshallese).

Automated Data-Collection Systems

Automated or passive methods of accessing and processing test results should be supported and improved. Enhancing and expanding automated methods of collecting data (for example, Web-based disease-reporting systems, electronic laboratory reporting, and electronic medical records) reduce staff time, increase timeliness and completeness, and minimize data-entry errors (Klevens et al., 2009; Klompas et al., 2008; Lazarus et al., 2001; Panackal et al., 2002; Vogt et al., 2006; Wurtz and Cameron, 2005). Given the volume of viral-hepatitis data, automated systems clearly are indicated (Hopkins, 2005). However, it has been noted that although electronic laboratory reporting can greatly increase the timeliness and accuracy of reporting, it does not remove the need for health departments to conduct additional followup to obtain information not contained in laboratory reports, such as symptoms, race and ethnicity, and risk history (Hopkins, 2005; Klevens et al., 2009).

A pilot study of a surveillance system based on electronic medical records in Massachusetts found a 39% increase in reported cases of chlamydia and a 53% increase in reported cases of gonorrhea over a 12-month period compared with cases reported through the existing passive surveillance system. The system was also able to identify 81 instances of pregnancy not identified by passive surveillance in patients with chlamydia or gonorrhea (CDC, 2008b). The system was shown to identify cases of acute HBV infection reliably, including cases that had not yet been reported to state authorities (Klompas et al., 2008). Other studies have found a similar benefit of improving surveillance for infectious diseases via automatic notification with electronic medical records (Allen and Ferson, 2000; Hopkins, 2005). CDC should promote the use of surveillance systems based on electronic medical records and open-source platforms that will enable the extraction and transmission of data to state and local health departments.

Standardized Laboratory Reporting It is essential that laboratory data be standardized and that health departments have automated access to them. Automated electronic laboratory reporting improves the completeness and timeliness of disease surveillance (Effler et al., 1999, 2002; Overhage et al., 2008; Panackal et al., 2002; Ward et al., 2005). Currently, many laboratory-data collection systems do not integrate or link the multiple laboratory tests needed to satisfy a case definition (CDC, 2008b). That could be more easily addressed with electronic laboratory reporting. CDC should work with states and laboratories to develop and standardize electronic systems. In addition, it may be useful for CDC to document and monitor which laboratory tests are reportable in each state, as is done for the HIV surveillance system.

Identifying Pregnant Women There is a strong need to identify pregnant women who have chronic HBV to ensure that appropriate followup of the newborn is conducted with regard to receipt of HBIG and hepatitis B vaccine. Currently, most health departments lack an automated means of determining whether the subject of a reported positive HBsAg test was a pregnant woman. Local health departments have to investigate all positive hepatitis B tests in women of childbearing age, and this creates a substantial workload. CDC should work with national laboratory vendors to identify ways of reporting whether positive HBV tests are linked with prenatal panels. Web-based surveillance systems may be useful for improving capture of data on pregnant women who have HBV infection (LaPorte et al., 2008).

PHIN-Compliant Systems CDC needs to contribute to more timely development of PHIN-compliant systems in all jurisdictions. A review of the literature evaluating the timeliness of reporting of infectious diseases found that reporting lag and the variability among states limit the usefulness of data. The inconsistency in reporting limits CDC's ability to identify and respond to multistate outbreaks in a timely manner. The review called for a more standardized approach in evaluating and describing surveillance-system timeliness (Jajosky and Groseclose, 2004). Although it did not look specifically at hepatitis B or hepatitis C, its conclusions are relevant to the present report.

Electronic Medical Records The reporting of relevant infectious-disease test results should be a component of electronic medical-record systems. CDC should support state and local jurisdictions in working with clinical and community health-center partners to develop algorithms for automatic viral-hepatitis disease reporting based on electronic medical records. It has already been shown to be effective in enhancing acute-HBV reporting without adding to the burden on medical providers (Klompas et al., 2008).

Case Investigation and Followup

Standards for case investigation and followup should be developed and implemented to ensure that newly diagnosed patients receive adequate information and referrals. An effective surveillance system should identify most of the diagnosed cases of both acute and chronic HBV and HCV infections. Identification of infected people by health departments should be the first step in getting them into appropriate care. Because of resource and system inadequacies, it is not. Most health departments indicated that they were unable to do more than follow up on potentially pregnant HBV-positive women (personal communication, Adult Viral Hepatitis Prevention Coordinators, May 2009). If state health departments had appropriate funding to follow up recently diagnosed cases of HBV and HCV infection directly, more people would be able to receive appropriate education and referral into the array of medical and social-service care that may be indicated.

Analyzing, Reporting, and Disseminating Findings

Once the capacity for state health departments to conduct HBV and HCV surveillance is improved, CDC should report accurate results that are based on the improved data. As discussed earlier in this chapter, there are important concerns about underreporting, particularly of the incidence of acute HCV infection. Until the quality of the data collected has improved, reports should clearly indicate the limitations of the data. For example,

- Trends in acute HBV and HCV infections should be interpreted with caution because of systematically missing cases that represent the burden of disease in particular risk groups.
- Discussions of data on acute HBV and HCV infections should reflect the issue of the large number of chronic infections to ensure appropriate understanding of the scope of the problem.
- Reported incidences should be presented as ranges rather than single numbers to reflect the uncertainty of the estimates.

Targeted Surveillance

Once core hepatitis B and hepatitis C surveillance activities are well established, supplemental or pilot projects should be tested. CDC should develop and support innovative supplemental surveillance programs.

Recommendation 2-3. The Centers for Disease Control and Prevention should support and conduct targeted active surveillance, including serologic testing, to monitor incidence and prevalence of hepatitis B virus and hepatitis C virus infections in populations not fully captured by core surveillance.

- Active surveillance should be conducted in specific (sentinel) geographic regions and populations.
- Appropriate serology, molecular biology, and followup will allow for distinction between acute and chronic hepatitis B and hepatitis C.

Enhanced Surveillance

Supplemental surveillance projects should be funded or conducted by CDC and should include serosurveillance among targeted populations. Serosurveillance projects will provide data for improved estimation of the scope of the problem in underrepresented populations such as certain racial and ethnic groups, and at-risk populations, including institutionalized, homeless, immigrant, and refugee populations. Enhanced surveillance projects should be structured to obtain information in both rural and urban regions of the United States. Serosurveillance programs should be flexible and allow researchers to focus on emerging behavioral risks, for example, in adolescents and young adults and in HIV-positive men who have sex with men (Klevens et al., 2009). Conducting serosurveillance or screening among at-risk populations in correctional facilities may provide opportunities to collect more detailed data and to refer people directly into appropriate medical care, including treatment for acute HCV infection (McGovern et al., 2006). Other enhanced surveillance projects should include

- Determining the level of care that patients receive after diagnosis, including medical and social-service referrals and treatment (Fleming et al., 2006).
- Following subsets of cases to improve understanding of natural history (Global Burden of Hepatitis C Working Group, 2004).
- Matching data on chronic hepatitis B and hepatitis C with cancer registries (Global Burden of Hepatitis C Working Group, 2004).
- Matching data on chronic HBV and HCV infections with HIV/AIDS data to determine the burden of coinfection in communities.
- Measuring the vaccination status of acute HBV infection cases and identifying missed opportunities for vaccination.
- Ensuring that viral hepatitis is addressed and integrated with appropriate projects for the National HIV Behavioral Surveillance System.
- Measuring HBV and HCV seroconversion rates in selected populations.

Partner Services

Partner services have been found to be effective in identifying undiagnosed cases of HIV (Hogben et al., 2007). Similar programs could potentially be useful identifying cases of hepatitis B and hepatitis C (CDC, 2008e; Hogben and Niccolai, 2009; Marcus et al., 2009). State and local health departments should be funded to pilot and evaluate partner-services programs for suspected acute and chronic cases of HBV infection and acute cases of HCV infection, especially in young people. Integration with existing partner service programs should be explored. Evaluation should focus on the efficacy of referral into care services and on screening of exposed partners—sexual partners for hepatitis B and drug-sharing partners for hepatitis B and hepatitis C (CDC, 2007).

REFERENCES

Allen, C. J., and M. J. Ferson. 2000. Notification of infectious diseases by general practitioners: A quantitative and qualitative study. *Medical Journal of Australia* 172(7):325-328.

Alter, M. J., W. L. Kuhnert, and L. Finelli. 2003. Guidelines for laboratory testing and result reporting of antibody to hepatitis C virus. Centers for Disease Control and Prevention. *Morbidity and Morality Weekly: Recommendations and Reports* 52(RR-3):1-13, 15; quiz CE11-CE14.

CDC (Centers for Disease Control and Prevention). 1996. Prevention of perinatal hepatitis B through enhanced case management—Connecticut, 1994-95, and the United States, 1994. *Morbidity and Mortality Weekly Report* 45(27):584-587.

———. 1999. Guidelines for national human immunodeficiency virus case surveillance, including monitoring for human immunodeficiency virus infection and acquired immunodeficiency syndrome. Centers for Disease Control and Prevention. *Morbidity and Morality Weekly: Recommendations and Reports* 48(RR-13):1-27, 29-31.

———. 2001a. *National hepatitis C prevention strategy: A comprehensive strategy for the prevention and control of hepatitis C virus infection and its consequences.* Atlanta, GA: CDC. http://www.cdc.gov/hepatitis/HCV/Strategy/PDFs/NatHepCPrevStrategy.pdf (accessed August 21, 2009).

———. 2001b. Updated guidelines for evaluating public health surveillance systems: Recommendations from the guidelines working group. *Morbidity and Mortality Weekly Report* 50(RR-13):1-36.

———. 2003a. *2003-2008 HIV prevention community planning guidance.* http://www.cdc.gov/hiv/topics/cba/resources/guidelines/hiv-cp/pdf/hiv-cp.pdf (accessed May 18, 2009).

———. 2003b. Hepatitis C virus transmission from an antibody-negative organ and tissue donor—United States, 2000-2002. *Morbidity and Mortality Weekly Report* 52(13):273-274, 276.

———. 2003c. Prevention and control of infections with hepatitis viruses in correctional settings. *Morbidity and Mortality Weekly Report* 52(RR01):1-33.

———. 2003d. Transmission of hepatitis B and C viruses in outpatient settings—New York, Oklahoma, and Nebraska, 2000-2002. *Morbidity and Mortality Weekly Report* 52(38):901-906.

———. 2005a. *Guidelines for viral hepatitis surveillance and case management.* Centers for Disease Control and Prevention.

———. 2005b. Transmission of hepatitis B virus among persons undergoing blood glucose monitoring in long-term-care facilities—Mississippi, North Carolina, and Los Angeles county, California, 2003-2004. *Morbidity and Mortality Weekly Report* 54(9):220-223.

———. 2006 (unpublished). 2006 assessment tool: Hepatitis C coordination and integration activities.

———. 2007. *Program announcement ps08-802: HIV/AIDS surveillance.* http://www.cdc.gov/od/pgo/funding/PS08-802.htm (accessed August 19, 2009).

———. 2008a. Acute hepatitis C virus infections attributed to unsafe injection practices at an endoscopy clinic—Nevada, 2007. *Morbidity and Mortality Weekly Report* 57(19):513-517.

———. 2008b. Automated detection and reporting of notifiable diseases using electronic medical records versus passive surveillance—Massachusetts, June 2006-July 2007. *Morbidity and Mortality Weekly Report* 57(14):373-376.

———. 2008c. Disease burden from hepatitis A, B, and C in the United States.

———. 2008d. *HIV infection reporting.* http://www.cdc.gov/hiv/topics/surveillance/reporting.htm (accessed July 28, 2009).

———. 2008e. Recommendations for partner services programs for HIV infection, syphilis, gonorrhea, and chlamydial infection. *Morbidity and Morality Weekly: Recommendations and Reports* 57(RR-9):1-83; quiz CE81-84.

———. 2008f. Use of enhanced surveillance for hepatitis C virus infection to detect a cluster among young injection-drug users—New York, November 2004-April 2007. *Morbidity and Mortality Weekly Report* 57(19):517-521.

———. 2009a. *Case definitions.* http://www.cdc.gov/ncphi/disss/nndss/casedef/case_definitions.htm (accessed August 21, 2009).

———. 2009b. *FAQs for health professionals: Hepatitis C.* http://www.cdc.gov/hepatitis/HCV/HCVfaq.htm (accessed August 21, 2009).

———. 2009c. Hepatitis C virus transmission at an outpatient hemodialysis unit—New York, 2001-2008. *Morbidity and Mortality Weekly Report* 58(8):189-194.

———. 2009d. HIV-associated behaviors among injecting-drug users—23 cities, United States, May 2005-February 2006. *Morbidity and Mortality Weekly Report* 58(13):329-332.

———. 2009e. *National electronic disease surveillance system.* http://www.cdc.gov/nedss/ (accessed July 28, 2009).

———. 2009f. *National electronic telecommunications system for surveillance.* http://www.cdc.gov/ncphi/disss/nndss/netss.htm (accessed July 28, 2009).

———. 2009g. *Perinatal hepatitis B prevention coordinators.* http://www.cdc.gov/hepatitis/Partners/PeriHepBCoord.htm (accessed August 21, 2009).

———. 2009h. (unpublished) *Report on the status of state viral hepatitis plans for the Institute of Medicine.*

———. 2009i. Status of state electronic disease surveillance systems—United States, 2007. *Morbidity and Mortality Weekly Report* 58(29):804-807.

CDC/CSTE. 2006. *Technical guidance for HIV/AIDS surveillance programs, volumes I-III* Centers for Disease Control and Prevention.

Chen, S. L., and T. R. Morgan. 2006. The natural history of hepatitis C virus (HCV) infection. *International Journal of Medical Sciences* 3(2):47-52.

Coleman, P. J., G. M. McQuillan, L. A. Moyer, S. B. Lambert, and H. S. Margolis. 1998. Incidence of hepatitis B virus infection in the United States, 1976-1994: Estimates from the national health and nutrition examination surveys. *Journal of Infectious Diseases* 178(4):954-959.

Cox, A. L., D. M. Netski, T. Mosbruger, S. G. Sherman, S. Strathdee, D. Ompad, D. Vlahov, D. Chien, V. Shyamala, S. C. Ray, and D. L. Thomas. 2005. Prospective evaluation of community-acquired acute-phase hepatitis C virus infection. *Clinical Infectious Diseases* 40(7):951-958.

CSTE (Council of State and Territorial Epidemiologists). 2009. *State reportable conditions assessment (SRCA).* http://www.cste.org/dnn/ProgramsandActivities/PublicHealthInformaticsOLD/StateReportableConditionsQueryResults/tabid/261/Default.aspx (accessed December 15, 2009).

Daniels, D., S. Grytdal, and A. Wasley. 2009a. Surveillance for acute viral hepatitis—United States, 2007. *Morbidity and Mortality Weekly Report: Surveillance Summaries* 58(3):1-27.

———. 2009b. Surveillance for acute viral hepatitis—United States, 2007. *Morbidity and Mortality Weekly Report: Surveillance Summaries* 58(3):1-27.

Department of Justice. 2009. *Office of Justice Programs, Bureau of Justice Statistics.* http://www.ojp.usdoj.gov/bjs/ (accessed August 30, 2009).

Deuffic-Burban S., T. Poynard, M. S. Sulkowski, and J. B. Wong. 2007. Estimating the future health burden of chronic hepatitis C and human immunodeficiency virus infections in the United States. *Journal of Viral Hepatitis* 14(2):107-115.

Effler, P., M. Ching-Lee, A. Bogard, M.-C. Ieong, T. Nekomoto, and D. Jernigan. 1999. Statewide system of electronic notifiable disease reporting from clinical laboratories: Comparing automated reporting with conventional methods. *Journal of the American Medical Association* 282(19):1845-1850.

Effler, P. V., M. C. Ieong, T. Tom, and M. Nakata. 2002. Enhancing public health surveillance for influenza virus by incorporating newly available rapid diagnostic tests. *Emerging Infectious Diseases* 8(1):23-28.

Fabrizi, F., A. Marzano, P. Messa, P. Martin, and P. Lampertico. 2008. Hepatitis B virus infection in the dialysis population: Current perspectives. *International Journal of Artificial Organs* 31(5):386-394.

Fairchild, A. L., R. Bayer, and J. Colgrove. 2008. Privacy, democracy and the politics of disease surveillance. *Public Health Ethics* 1(1):30-38.

Fleming, D. T., A. Zambrowski, F. Fong, A. Lombard, L. Mercedes, C. Miller, J. Poujade, A. Roome, A. Sullivan, and L. Finelli. 2006. Surveillance programs for chronic viral hepatitis in three health departments. *Public Health Reports* 121(1):23-35.

George, P. 2004 (unpublished). *New directions for hepatitis surveillance*. Division of Viral Hepatitis, CDC.

Ghany, M. G., D. B. Strader, D. L. Thomas, and L. Seeff. 2009. Diagnosis, management, and treatment of hepatitis c: An update. *Hepatology* 49(4):1335-1374.

Global Burden of Hepatitis C Working Group, GBHCWG. 2004. Global burden of disease (GBD) for hepatitis C. *Journal of Clinical Pharmacology* 44(1):20-29.

Glynn, M. K., L. M. Lee, and M. T. McKenna. 2007. The status of national HIV case surveillance, United States 2006. *Public Health Reports* 122(Suppl 1):63-71.

Guerrant, R. L., D. H. Walker, and P. F. Weller, eds. 2001. *Essentials of tropical infectious diseases*. Philadelphia, PA: Churchill Livingstone.

Hagan, H., N. Snyder, E. Hough, T. Yu, S. McKeirnan, J. Boase, and J. Duchin. 2002. Case-reporting of acute hepatitis B and C among injection drug users. *Journal of Urban Health* 79(4):579-585.

Hall, H. I., and E. D. Mokotoff. 2007. Setting standards and an evaluation framework for human immunodeficiency virus/acquired immunodeficiency syndrome surveillance. *Journal of Public Health Management and Practice* 13(5):519-523.

Hall, H. I., R. Song, J. E. Gerstle, 3rd, and L. M. Lee. 2006. Assessing the completeness of reporting of human immunodeficiency virus diagnoses in 2002-2003: Capture-recapture methods. *American Journal of Epidemiology* 164(4):391-397.

Hogben, M., and L. M. Niccolai. 2009. Innovations in sexually transmitted disease partner services. *Current Infectious Disease Reports* 11(2):148-154.

Hogben, M., T. McNally, M. McPheeters, and A. B. Hutchinson. 2007. The effectiveness of HIV partner counseling and referral services in increasing identification of HIV-positive individuals a systematic review. *American Journal of Preventive Medicine* 33(2 Suppl):S89-S100.

Hopkins, R. S. 2005. Design and operation of state and local infectious disease surveillance systems. *Journal of Public Health Management and Practice* 11(3):184-190.

Hutton, D. W., D. Tan, S. K. So, and M. L. Brandeau. 2007. Cost-effectiveness of screening and vaccinating Asian and Pacific Islander adults for hepatitis B. *Annals of Internal Medicine* 147(7):460-469.

Hyams, K. C. 1995. Risks of chronicity following acute hepatitis B virus infection: A review. *Clinical Infectious Diseases* 20(4):992-1000.

Jajosky, R. A., and S. L. Groseclose. 2004. Evaluation of reporting timeliness of public health surveillance systems for infectious diseases. *BMC Public Health* 4:29.

Kim, W. R. 2007. Epidemiology of hepatitis B in the United States. *Current Hepatitis Reports* 6(1):3-8.

Klein, S. J., C. A. Flanigan, J. G. Cooper, D. R. Holtgrave, A. F. Carrascal, and G. S. Birkhead. 2008. Wanted: An effective public health response to hepatitis C virus in the United States. *Journal of Public Health Management and Practice* 14(5):471-475.

Klevens, R. M., C. Vonderwahl, S. Speers, K. Alelis, K. Sweet, E. Rocchio, T. Poissant, T. Vogt, and K. Gallagher. 2009 (unpublished). *Hepatitis C virus infection from population-based surveillance in six U.S. sites, 2006-2007*.

Klompas, M., G. Haney, D. Church, R. Lazarus, X. Hou, and R. Platt. 2008. Automated identification of acute hepatitis b using electronic medical record data to facilitate public health surveillance. *PLoS ONE* 3(7):e2626.

Koff, R. S. 2004. Hepatitis B and hepatitis D. In *Infectious diseases*, edited by S. L. Gorbach, J. G. Bartlett, and N. R. Blacklow. Philadelphia, PA: Lippincott, Williams & Wilkins. Pp. 765-784.

Lanini, S., V. Puro, F. Lauria, F. Fusco, C. Nisii, and G. Ippolito. 2009. Patient to patient transmission of hepatitis B virus: A systematic review of reports on outbreaks between 1992 and 2007. *BMC Medicine* 7(1):15.

LaPorte, T., M. Conant, M. McGarty, S. Troppy, S. Barrus, S. Lett, M. O'Donnell, G. Haney, and A. DeMaria. 2008 (March). *Improved case finding of hepatitis B positive women of child-bearing age through implementation of a web-based surveillance system.* Paper presented at National Immunization Conference, Atlanta, Georgia.

Lazarus, R., K. P. Kleinman, I. Dashevsky, A. DeMaria, and R. Platt. 2001. Using automated medical records for rapid identification of illness syndromes (syndromic surveillance): The example of lower respiratory infection. *BMC Public Health* 1:9.

Maher, L., B. Jalaludin, K. G. Chant, R. Jayasuriya, T. Sladden, J. M. Kaldor, and P. L. Sargent. 2006. Incidence and risk factors for hepatitis C seroconversion in injecting drug users in Australia. *Addiction* 101(10):1499-1508.

Marcus, J. L., K. T. Bernstein, and J. D. Klausner. 2009. Updated outcomes of partner notification for human immunodeficiency virus, San Francisco, 2004-2008. *AIDS* 23(8): 1024-1026.

Margolis, H. S., P. J. Coleman, R. E. Brown, E. E. Mast, S. H. Sheingold, and J. A. Arevalo. 1995. Prevention of hepatitis B virus transmission by immunization. An economic analysis of current recommendations. *Journal of the American Medical Association* 274(15):1201-1208.

Mast, E. E., H. S. Margolis, A. E. Fiore, E. W. Brink, S. T. Goldstein, S. A. Wang, L. A. Moyer, B. P. Bell, and M. J. Alter. 2005. A comprehensive immunization strategy to eliminate transmission of hepatitis B virus infection in the United States: Recommendations of the advisory committee on immunization practices (ACIP) part 1: Immunization of infants, children, and adolescents. *Morbidity and Morality Weekly: Recommendations and Reports* 54(RR-16):1-31.

Mathei, C., G. Robaeys, P. van Damme, F. Buntinx, and R. Verrando. 2005. Prevalence of hepatitis C in drug users in Flanders: Determinants and geographic differences. *Epidemiology and Infection* 133(1):127-136.

Matthews, G. V., M. Hellard, J. Kaldor, A. Lloyd, and G. J. Dore. 2007. Further evidence of HCV sexual transmission among HIV-positive men who have sex with men: Response to Danta et al. *AIDS* 21(15):2112-2113.

McGovern, B. H., C. E. Birch, M. J. Bowen, L. L. Reyor, E. H. Nagami, R. T. Chung, and A. Y. Kim. 2009. Improving the diagnosis of acute hepatitis C infection using expanded viral load criteria. *Clinical Infectious Diseases* 49.

McGovern, B. H., A. Wurcel, A. Y. Kim, J. Schulze zur Wiesch, I. Bica, M. T. Zaman, J. Timm, B. D. Walker, and G. M. Lauer. 2006. Acute hepatitis C virus infection in incarcerated injection drug users. *Clinical Infectious Diseases* 42(12):1663-1670.

McMahon, B. J., W. L. M. Alward, D. B. Hall, W. L. Heyward, T. R. Bender, D. P. Francis, and J. E. Maynard. 1985. Acute hepatitis B virus infection: Relation of age to the clinical expression of disease and subsequent development of the carrier state. *Journal of Infectious Diseases* 151(4):599-603.

Mehta, S. H., A. Cox, D. R. Hoover, X. H. Wang, Q. Mao, S. Ray, S. A. Strathdee, D. Vlahov, and D. L. Thomas. 2002. Protection against persistence of hepatitis C. *Lancet* 359(9316):1478-1483.

Mosley, J. W., E. A. Operskalski, L. H. Tobler, W. W. Andrews, B. Phelps, J. Dockter, C. Giachetti, M. P. Busch, f. t. T.-t. V. Study, and R. E. D. S. Groups. 2005. Viral and host factors in early hepatitis C virus infection. *Hepatology* 42(1):86-92.

Nakashima, A. K., and P. L. Fleming. 2003. HIV/AIDS surveillance in the United States, 1981-2001. *Journal of Acquired Immune Deficiency Syndromes* 32(Suppl 1):S68-S85.

NASTAD (National Alliance of State and Territorial AIDS Directors). 2009 (unpublished). *Viral hepatitis surveillance survey.*

NIH (National Institutes of Health). 2002. NIH consensus statement on management of hepatitis C: 2002. *NIH Consensus and State-of-the-Science Statements* 19(3):1-46.

Onofrey, S., D. Church, D. Heisey-Grove, P. Briggs, T. Bertrand, and A. J. DeMaria. March 10-13, 2008. *Utilizing disease intervention specialist for follow-up on hepatitis C in individuals between the ages of 15 and 25 years: A 3-month pilot program.* Paper presented at 2008 National STD Prevention Conference, Chicago, IL.

Overhage, J. M., S. Grannis, and C. J. McDonald. 2008. A comparison of the completeness and timeliness of automated electronic laboratory reporting and spontaneous reporting of notifiable conditions. *American Journal of Public Health* 98(2):344-350.

Panackal, A. A., M. M'Ikanatha N, F. C. Tsui, J. McMahon, M. M. Wagner, B. W. Dixon, J. Zubieta, M. Phelan, S. Mirza, J. Morgan, D. Jernigan, A. W. Pasculle, J. T. Rankin, Jr., R. A. Hajjeh, and L. H. Harrison. 2002. Automatic electronic laboratory-based reporting of notifiable infectious diseases at a large health system. *Emerging Infectious Diseases* 8(7):685-691.

Pungpapong, S., W. R. Kim, and J. J. Poterucha. 2007. Natural history of hepatitis B virus infection: An update for clinicians. *Mayo Clinic Proceedings* 82(8):967-975.

Ruan, Y., G. Qin, L. Yin, K. Chen, H. Z. Qian, C. Hao, S. Liang, J. Zhu, H. Xing, K. Hong, and Y. Shao. 2007. Incidence of HIV, hepatitis C and hepatitis B viruses among injection drug users in southwestern China: A 3-year follow-up study. *AIDS* 21(Suppl 8):S39-S46.

Thacker, S. B. 2000. Historical development. In *Principles and Practice of Public Health Surveillance*, edited by S. Teutsch and R. E. Churchill. Oxford, United Kingdom: Oxford University Press.

Thompson, N. D., J. F. Perz, A. C. Moorman, and S. D. Holmberg. 2009. Nonhospital health care-associated hepatitis B and C virus transmission: United States, 1998-2008. *Annals of Internal Medicine* 150(1):33-39.

van de Laar, T., O. Pybus, S. Bruisten, D. Brown, M. Nelson, S. Bhagani, M. Vogel, A. Baumgarten, M. L. Chaix, M. Fisher, H. Gotz, G. V. Matthews, S. Neifer, P. White, W. Rawlinson, S. Pol, J. Rockstroh, R. Coutinho, G. J. Dore, G. M. Dusheiko, and M. Danta. 2009. Evidence of a large, international network of HCV transmission in HIV-positive men who have sex with men. *Gastroenterology* 136(5):1609-1617.

van den Berg, C. H., C. Smit, M. Bakker, R. B. Geskus, B. Berkhout, S. Jurriaans, R. A. Coutinho, K. C. Wolthers, and M. Prins. 2007. Major decline of hepatitis C virus incidence rate over two decades in a cohort of drug users. *European Journal of Epidemiology* 22(3):183-193.

Villano, S. A., D. Vlahov, K. E. Nelson, S. Cohn, and D. L. Thomas. 1999. Persistence of viremia and the importance of long-term follow-up after acute hepatitis C infection. *Hepatology* 29(3):908-914.

Vogt, M., T. Lang, G. Frosner, C. Klingler, A. F. Sendl, A. Zeller, B. Wiebecke, B. Langer, H. Meisner, and J. Hess. 1999. Prevalence and clinical outcome of hepatitis C infection in children who underwent cardiac surgery before the implementation of blood-donor screening. *New England Journal of Medicine* 341(12):866-870.

Vogt, R. L., R. Spittle, A. Cronquist, and J. L. Patnaik. 2006. Evaluation of the timeliness and completeness of a web-based notifiable disease reporting system by a local health department. *Journal of Public Health Management and Practice* 12(6):540-544.

Ward, J. 2008. FY 2008 domestic enacted funds. Presentation to the committee: December 4, 2008.

Ward, M., P. Brandsema, E. van Straten, and A. Bosman. 2005. Electronic reporting improves timeliness and completeness of infectious disease notification, the Netherlands, 2003. *Euro Surveillance* 10(1):27-30.

Wasley, A., J. T. Miller, and L. Finelli. 2007. Surveillance for acute viral hepatitis—United States, 2005. *Morbidity and Mortality Weekly Report: Surveillance Summaries* 56(3):1-24.

Wurtz, R., and B. J. Cameron. 2005. Electronic laboratory reporting for the infectious diseases physician and clinical microbiologist. *Clinical Infectious Diseases* 40(11):1638-1643.

3

Knowledge and Awareness About Chronic Hepatitis B and Hepatitis C

An estimated 0.8–1.4 million people in the United States are chronically infected with hepatitis B virus (HBV) and 2.7–3.9 million people are chronically infected with hepatitis C virus (HCV). However, there is relatively poor awareness about these infections among health-care providers, social-service providers, and the general public. Lack of awareness about the prevalence of chronic viral hepatitis in the United States and about the proper methods and target populations for screening and medical management of chronic hepatitis B and hepatitis C probably contributes to continuing transmission; missing of opportunities for prevention, including vaccination; missing of opportunities for early diagnosis and medical care; and poor health outcomes in infected people.

As discussed in Chapters 1 and 2, surveillance data on the numbers of people acutely and chronically infected with HBV and HCV are imprecise and can be difficult to interpret. The prevalence of chronic infections remains high for several reasons, and the aging of the chronically infected population has contributed to the tripling of liver-cancer incidence during the last three decades (Altekruse et al., 2009; McGlynn et al., 2006). The persistently high prevalence of chronic HBV infection can be attributed in part to immigration of chronically infected people from HBV-endemic regions—including East Asia, Southeast Asia, and sub-Saharan Africa—to the United States. The high prevalence of chronic HCV infection is due in part to the lack of access to preventive measures, such as harm-reduction programs, and lack of access to antiviral treatments in high-risk populations.

This chapter is divided into two sections. The first addresses knowledge and awareness about hepatitis B and hepatitis C in health-care providers and social-service providers; the second addresses the topic with reference to the general population and at-risk populations. Each section begins by describing what is known about the levels of knowledge and awareness about hepatitis B and hepatitis C and how gaps in education about these diseases are affecting prevention, screening and testing, and treatment opportunities. Those summaries are followed by the committee's recommendations for addressing the gaps and the rationale and supportive evidence for the recommendations.

KNOWLEDGE AND AWARENESS AMONG HEALTH-CARE AND SOCIAL-SERVICE PROVIDERS

The committee found that knowledge about chronic hepatitis B and hepatitis C among health-care providers, particularly primary-care providers (for example, physicians, physician assistants, and nurse practitioners), and social-service providers (for example, staff of drug-treatment programs, needle-exchange programs, and immigrant services centers) is generally poor. Although there have been no large-scale, controlled studies of health-care providers' knowledge about chronic hepatitis B and hepatitis C, it is clear that knowledge has been imperfect among providers in all the surveys whose results have been published. Subjects of deficient knowledge include

- The prevalence of chronic hepatitis B and hepatitis C in the general and high-risk populations in the United States.
- The clinical sequelae of chronic viral hepatitis.
- The characteristics of at-risk persons who should be tested for chronic HBV and HCV infection and vaccinated to protect them from hepatitis B.
- The approaches to primary and secondary prevention in addition to hepatitis B vaccination.
- The proper methods of testing and interpretation of test results.
- The proper followup management for chronic infection.

Provider guidelines for hepatitis screening, prevention, treatment, and followup have been in place for decades and are updated regularly (CDC, 1991, 1998, 2005, 2008b, 2008c; Ghany et al., 2009; Lok and McMahon, 2009; Mast et al., 2005, 2006). However, current studies of provider knowledge about chronic viral hepatitis have not identified why health-care providers fail to follow national recommended guidelines.

Hepatitis B

Studies have shown that many primary care providers cannot differentiate between adult populations that should be screened for chronic hepatitis B because of their high prevalence of chronic infection (for example, people born in geographic regions with high HBV endemicity; see Box 3-1) and populations that should be vaccinated against HBV because of their high risk of becoming newly infected (for example, health-care workers, men who have sex with men, prison inmates, and household and sexual contacts of chronically infected individuals) (Euler et al., 2003b; Ferrante et al., 2008; Lai et al., 2007).

In a survey of primary care providers in San Francisco, all 91 respondents correctly answered that Chinese immigrants have a higher prevalence of chronic hepatitis B than non-Hispanic white or US-born Chinese people. However, a portion of the same group incorrectly identified HIV-infected

---

BOX 3-1
Geographic Regions That Have Intermediate and High Hepatitis B Virus Endemicity

Africa: all countries

Asia and Middle East: all countries

South and Western Pacific: all countries and territories but only indigenous persons in Australia and New Zealand

Eastern Europe: all countries except Hungary

Western Europe: Greece, Malta, Portugal, and Spain and indigenous populations of Greenland

North America: Alaska natives and indigenous populations of northern Canada

Central America: all countries

South America: Argentina, Bolivia, Brazil, Ecuador, Guyana, Suriname, Venezuela, and Amazonian areas of Colombia and Peru

Caribbean: Antigua and Barbuda, Dominica, Dominican Republic, Grenada, Haiti, Jamaica, Puerto Rico, St. Kitts and Nevis, St. Lucia, St. Vincent and Grenadines, Trinidad and Tobago, and Turks and Caicos

---

SOURCE: Modified from Mast et al., 2006.

persons (16%), men who have sex with men (18%), and injection-drug users (IDUs; 23%) as having a higher prevalence of chronic hepatitis B than Chinese immigrants (Lai et al., 2007). In the same study, 30% of the respondents were not able to identify the correct test to use for diagnosing chronic HBV infection.

A cross-sectional survey conducted among 217 members of the New Jersey Academy of Family Physicians found that a higher proportion of family physicians recommended screening for hepatitis B among men who have sex with men (93%), IDUs (95%), and HIV-infected patients (96%) than for immigrants from Southeast Asia (68%) or sub-Saharan Africa (57%)—areas that are highly endemic for HBV with over 8% seroprevalence of hepatitis B surface antigen (HBsAg) (Ferrante et al., 2008). Only 50% of survey participants recommended screening household contacts of persons who had chronic HBV infection—an established high-risk population. Finally, 21% of the New Jersey family physicians did not know what step to take next if a patient tested positive for HBsAg or would refer such a patient to a specialist for followup (Ferrante et al., 2008). However, 83% of the respondents were interested in receiving education about chronic viral hepatitis.

Chu (2009) presented data at the 2009 International Symposium on Viral Hepatitis and Liver Disease that showed that only 18–30% of Asian American primary care providers who treat Asian American adult patients reported routinely testing them for HBV infection in their practice. That finding illustrates the incomplete knowledge even among primary care providers who themselves constitute a group at high risk for chronic HBV infection.

At the 2007 Society of General Internal Medicine annual meeting, Dulay et al. (2007) reported on the results of a multiple-choice hepatitis B knowledge survey completed by 196 attendees at a university-based continuing-medical-education conference for primary care providers, including nurse practitioners and physician assistants. Of the respondents, 55% were not able to identify HBsAg as the determinant for chronic HBV infection. Knowledge about the appropriate use of the HBsAg test was substantially higher among primary care providers who were Asian (68%) than those of other ethnicities (43%), among physicians (56%) than nonphysicians (23%), and among providers who had more years of experience or more time spent in the clinic. Some 44% of the respondents did not know that chronic HBV infection could be controlled with medication, and 25% incorrectly responded that chronic HBV infection is curable.

Given that the probability of developing chronic hepatitis B is highest when infants are exposed to HBV through their mothers at birth, both the US Preventive Services Task Force and the US Centers for Disease Control and Prevention (CDC) recommend testing all pregnant women for HBsAg during an early prenatal visit even if they have been previously vaccinated or tested (CDC, 1991; U.S. Preventive Services Task Force, 2009). Currently, only 27 states have maternal HBsAg screening laws (CDC, 2008c). State screening laws do not necessarily translate into higher testing rates, because they often do not include an enforcement mechanism or sanctions for noncompliance (Euler et al., 2003b). In a study of family physicians in New Jersey, a state with a maternal screening law, Ferrante et al. (2008) found that 22% of respondents indicated that they did not recommend testing pregnant women for HBV infection.

At the 2009 International Symposium on Viral Hepatitis and Liver Disease, Chao et al. (2009b) presented results of a study of perinatal health-care providers' knowledge about hepatitis B and the management of HBsAg-positive pregnant patients recommended by the Advisory Committee on Immunization Practices (ACIP). Questionnaires were mailed or administered to 100 practicing obstetrician/gynecologists (OB/GYNs) and 31 peripartum nurses in Santa Clara County, CA, an area with one of the largest annual numbers of HBsAg-positive pregnant women in the United States. Although most of the OB/GYNs reported that they tested pregnant women for HBsAg and properly advised HBsAg-positive women that their newborns should receive the hepatitis B vaccine and hepatitis B immunoglobulin within 12 hours of birth, overall knowledge about hepatitis B was low. Only 26% of OB/GYNs and 10% of peripartum nurses knew that the prevalence of chronic hepatitis B is higher in Asians than in other ethnic populations; only 33% of OB/GYNs and 17% of peripartum nurses knew that there is a high risk of HBV infection becoming chronic in exposed newborns; and only 22% of OB/GYNs and 37% of peripartum nurses knew about the risk of death conferred by chronic hepatitis B. Only 62% of the OB/GYNs referred their HBsAg-positive pregnant patients for chronic-hepatitis management.

Hepatitis C

Health-care providers' knowledge about hepatitis C appears to be similarly insufficient, although there is far less published research on this topic (Ascione et al., 2007; Ferrante et al., 2008; Shehab et al., 1999, 2001; Strauss et al., 2006).

In the study of New Jersey family physicians described above, Ferrante et al. (2008) found that although 95% would recommend testing of IDUs for HCV infection, only 81% would recommend HCV testing for people who received blood transfusions before 1992, and only 65% would recommend testing of incarcerated persons—all populations that are at high risk for HCV infection and that fall within national testing guidelines. Although HCV testing of pregnant women is not supported by any evidence-based recommendations or guidelines, 34% of family physicians surveyed by Ferrante et al. would nevertheless recommend it. Of the respondents, 31% did not know what to do next or would refer a patient to a specialist after a positive test for HCV antibody, and 2% incorrectly assured patients that those who tested positive were immune to HCV. Physicians in practice for more than 20 years were found to have the lowest level of knowledge about HCV risk factors, whereas those in practice for 5 years or less had the highest knowledge level.

A survey of 593 fellows of the American College of Obstetricians and Gynecologists (ACOG), half of whom considered themselves to be primary care providers, assessed screening and counseling practices for HCV infection. About half (49%) reported that they tested for HCV infection in all obstetric and gynecologic patients who self-reported ever having injected illicit drugs, and 35% tested all patients who reported having received blood transfusions before 1992 (Boaz et al., 2003). Nearly half counseled HCV-infected patients to avoid breastfeeding, and 70% counseled HCV-infected patients to use condoms with their steady sexual partners; both kinds of advice are inconsistent with recommendations of CDC (CDC, 1998) and ACOG (2000, as cited in Boaz et al., 2003). Only 64% recommended that patients who had HCV infection avoid alcohol, which has been found to increase the risk of disease progression (Ascione et al., 2007).

An earlier mailed survey of 1,412 primary care providers in the United States also assessed knowledge about risk factors for HCV infection and management of hepatitis C (Shehab et al., 2001). Nearly three-fourths (73%) of the respondents had seen fewer than five hepatitis C patients within the preceding year, and almost half (44%) had no experience with treatment for HCV infection. Almost all knew the most common risk factors for HCV infection—injection-drug use, blood transfusion during the 1980s, and multiple sex partners. One-fourth incorrectly indicated that blood transfusion continues to be a risk factor, and 19% erroneously believed that casual household contact is a major risk factor. Some 50% of the providers reported that they routinely ask their patients about risk factors for HCV infection; 78% test for HCV infection among patients who have increased liver enzymes with or without HCV risk factors, and 70% test all patients who have risk factors regardless of liver enzyme levels. When presented with a scenario on how to treat a hypothetical patient for chronic HCV infection, 27% of the respondents did not know which therapy to use. A previous study by the same researchers had also found substantial gaps in primary care providers' knowledge about hepatitis C (Shehab et al., 1999). The gaps persisted even though 95% of the respondents in the 2001 study reported having used at least one educational tool about hepatitis C in the preceding 2 years; this suggests that primary care providers misreport their exposure to educational materials about hepatitis C or that such materials do not communicate accurate information effectively.

HCV-positive patients perceive that health-care providers are judgmental toward those with HCV infection because of its association with illicit drug use (Janke et al., 2008). Numerous studies have shown that healthcare workers have extremely negative views of IDUs and characterize them as manipulative, unpleasant, and uncooperative (McLaughlin et al., 2000; Paterson et al., 2007). Such attitudes among health-care providers can have a number of deleterious effects, including discouraging of at-risk persons from accessing testing and other services and reducing the effectiveness of HCV education and counseling messages (Zickmund et al., 2003).

Additional research has examined HCV knowledge among drugtreatment providers. Research conducted with 104 members of the staffs of two drug-free and two methadone-maintenance treatment programs (MMTPs) in the New York metropolitan area demonstrated that knowledge about hepatitis C is inadequate (Strauss et al., 2006). Five of 20 items on an HCV knowledge assessment were not answered correctly by the majority of the participating staff, suggesting that staff may be systematically misinformed rather than merely uninformed about some important HCV issues that affect their clients. Total scores on the assessment averaged 70%, 71%, and 45% among the medically credentialed staff, noncredentialed staff in the MMTPs, and noncredentialed staff in the drug-free programs, respectively. The majority of those in the latter group had never participated in training specifically devoted to HCV; these staff may be sharing incorrect information with patients or, aware of their limitations in HCV knowledge, failing to provide patients much needed HCV information. It is critical that both medically credentialed and noncredentialed staff in the programs receive effective HCV training so that they can support their patients' HCV education and information needs appropriately.

Recommendation

Many providers are not aware of the high prevalence of chronic hepatitis B and hepatitis C in some populations. Improved understanding of risk factors for acute and chronic HBV and HCV infections and collection of data on them, including country of birth and ethnicity, and the use of risk-factor screening will lead to increased identification of cases, increased provision of preventive resources, increased vaccination to protect those at risk for hepatitis B infection, and reduction in disparities in the burden of chronic viral hepatitis.

On the basis of the evidence described above, the committee concludes that insufficient provider knowledge leads to critical missed opportunities for providers to educate patients about prevention of hepatitis B and hepatitis C, to identify patients who may be at risk for these infections, and to test for chronic HBV and HCV infection in patients and their sexual, family, and household contacts in the case of hepatitis B and in drug-use networks in the case of hepatitis C. To address that issue, the committee offers the following recommendation:

> **Recommendation 3-1. The Centers for Disease Control and Prevention should work with key stakeholders (other federal agencies, state and local governments, professional organizations, health-care organizations, and educational institutions) to develop hepatitis B and hepatitis C educational programs for health-care and social-service providers.**

Educational programs and materials for health-care and social-service providers should focus on improving provider awareness and adherence to practice guidelines for hepatitis B and hepatitis C. The educational programs should be targeted to primary care providers, appropriate social-service providers (such as staff of drug-treatment facilities and immigrant-services centers), and licensed and unlicensed alternative-medicine professionals (such as acupuncturists and traditional Chinese medicine practitioners) that serve at-risk populations. At-risk populations include foreign-born people from HBV- or HCV-endemic countries, clients of sexually-transmitted-disease (STD) clinics and HIV clinics, IDUs, others at risk because of a history of percutaneous exposures, and close contacts of people who have chronic hepatitis B and chronic hepatitis C.

The educational programs should include at least the following components:

- Information about the prevalence and incidence of acute and chronic hepatitis B and hepatitis C both in the general US population and in at-risk populations, particularly foreign-born populations in the case of hepatitis B, and IDUs and incarcerated populations in the case of hepatitis C.
- Guidance on screening for risk factors associated with hepatitis B and hepatitis C.
- Information about hepatitis B and hepatitis C prevention, hepatitis B immunization, and medical monitoring of chronically infected patients, specifically,
    - Information about methods of testing and interpretation of results.
    - Information about medical management and long-term care:
        - How to select candidates for antiviral therapy.
        - Importance of liver-cancer screening.
        - When to refer patients to a specialist.

- Information about prevention of HBV and HCV transmission in hospital and nonhospital health-care settings.
- Information about discrimination and stigma associated with hepatitis B and hepatitis C and guidance on reducing them.
- Information about health disparities related to hepatitis B and hepatitis C.

CDC should examine interventions that target several venues and types of providers, such as educational institutions, health-care facilities, substance-abuse service providers, and alternative-care providers.

Educational Institutions

Schools of medicine, nursing, physician assistants, complementary and alternative medicine, and public health should develop improved curricula to ensure that their graduates are knowledgeable about chronic hepatitis B and hepatitis C. The curricula should include information on disease prevalence, risk factors, preventive actions, appropriate diagnostics, selection of persons for testing, and appropriate followup for chronically infected patients and those susceptible to infection.

Continuing-medical-education courses and activities about viral hepatitis conducted online or at provider meetings should be regularly offered to family-practice physicians, internists, OB/GYNs, pediatricians, nurses, and physician assistants. Drug-treatment counselors' education and certification examinations should also include hepatitis B and hepatitis C. Questions about chronic hepatitis B should be included on board-certification or recertification examinations for internists, family-practice physicians, pediatricians, and OB/GYNs; and questions about chronic hepatitis C should be included in board examinations for internists and family-practice physicians. Although there has been no systematic effort to determine whether continuing-medical-education courses and certification examinations include questions about hepatitis B and hepatitis C, the shortcomings in knowledge among health-care providers suggest that current efforts are insufficient, and that new approaches are needed to improve knowledge.

Educational programs should include targeted outreach to and enrollment of providers who work in high-risk venues (for example, STD and HIV clinics) and in areas where there are many at-risk foreign-born clients, such as hospitals, clinics, and community health centers that serve large populations of Asian and Pacific Islander (API) and foreign-born patients from other highly endemic regions.

Hospital and Other Health-Care Facilities

Health-care workers and their patients are at risk for exposure to infected blood and body fluids and therefore vulnerable to infection with HBV and HCV. As discussed in Chapter 2, there have been several outbreaks of hepatitis B and hepatitis C in health-care settings in recent years (CDC, 2003b, 2003c, 2005, 2008a, 2009a; Fabrizi et al., 2008; Thompson et al., 2009). Hospitals and nonhospital health-care facilities (such as dialysis units, endoscopy clinics, and long-term-care facilities) should develop educational programs to reinforce the importance of adhering to recommended standard precautions and procedures to prevent the transmission of bloodborne infections in both inpatient and outpatient health-care settings (Thompson et al., 2009). Health-care workers should be routinely vaccinated to protect them from hepatitis B. Although the ACIP recommends that health-care workers receive the hepatitis B vaccine, and the Occupational Safety and Health Administration requires employers to offer the hepatitis B vaccine to all health-care workers who may be exposed to blood (29 CFR 1910.1030), about 25% of health-care workers remain unvaccinated (Simard et al., 2007). Successful interventions to prevent exposures known to transmit bloodborne infections have included general safety training; training specific to prevention of needle-stick injuries; modification of practice, staffing, and workload adjustments; and use of protective devices, such as needles that automatically retract (Clarke et al., 2002; Holodnick and Barkauskas, 2000; Hooper and Charney, 2005; Stringer et al., 2002; Trim, 2004).

Substance-Abuse–Related Service Providers

Staff of drug-treatment programs, needle-exchange programs, and correctional facilities should be participants in viral-hepatitis educational programs. Studies have shown that IDUs who used needle-exchange programs or who had been in drug treatment were more likely than others to report their HCV-antibody status accurately (Hagan et al., 2006). Very high proportions of IDUs have been in jail or prison (Milloy et al., 2008); therefore, periods of incarceration may present a prime opportunity for providing hepatitis C education to this high-risk population. In many communities that have needle-exchange programs, the majority of IDUs have participated in them (Hagan et al., 1999; Lorvick et al., 2006). Over the period during which a person may inject illicit drugs, the likelihood that he or she has been in a drug-treatment program rises (Galai et al., 2003; Hagan et al., 1999). Thus, the committee believes that providing standardized education to staff of drug-treatment and needle-exchange programs and correctional facilities will increase the likelihood that at-risk and HCV-infected persons in these settings receive consistent and accurate information.

Alternative-Care Providers

Alternative-care providers would also benefit from participating in educational programs about viral hepatitis. In California, four annual educational symposia, in 2004–2007, were arranged by a collaboration of academic, professional, and community-based organizations to improve HBV-related knowledge among traditional Chinese medicine practitioners and acupuncturists—providers who serve a largely API population, a patient population that has a high prevalence of chronic hepatitis B and the associated risk of hepatocellular carcinoma (Chang et al., 2007). A precourse survey was administered; about half the participants did not know ways to prevent HBV transmission, the age group most likely to develop chronic infection, which blood test to use to diagnose chronic infection, or the risk of death from liver disease or cancer in people who had chronic hepatitis B. The postcourse survey showed a statistically significant improvement in HBV-related knowledge: about 80% of participants were able to answer questions about prevention and diagnosis of and treatment for HBV infection correctly.

COMMUNITY KNOWLEDGE AND AWARENESS

The committee has found that knowledge and awareness about hepatitis B and hepatitis C are lacking in members of the public and, most important, in members of specific at-risk populations. Lack of knowledge and awareness about hepatitis B and hepatitis C in the community often leads to misinformation, missing of opportunities for prevention and treatment, and stigmatization of infected populations. The consequences for members of at-risk communities are important in that missing opportunities for prevention can lead to infection of additional people with HBV and HCV. Once infected, they frequently are unaware of their infection and so run the risk of unknowingly infecting others and of not receiving appropriate medical management. Although there have been no large-scale, population-based, controlled studies of community knowledge about hepatitis B and hepatitis C, all published surveys have shown that knowledge about these diseases is sparse.

Hepatitis B

As mentioned earlier, APIs are at high risk for chronic hepatitis B. A number of studies have assessed awareness and knowledge about hepatitis B in API populations, including Vietnamese, Cambodian, Korean, and Chinese Americans, who are known to have a higher prevalence of chronic HBV infection than the general US population (Hwang et al., 2008; Ma et al., 2007b, 2008; Taylor, 2006; Taylor et al., 2000, 2002, 2004, 2005a, 2005b; Thompson et al., 2002; Wu et al., 2007). For example, among Vietnamese Americans, about 64% had never heard of the hepatitis B vaccine (Ma et al., 2007b), about 70% were unaware that Asian Americans are at high risk for chronic hepatitis B (Hwang et al., 2008), most were uninformed about routes of HBV transmission (Taylor et al., 2000, 2005a, 2005b), and only one-third had a doctor's recommendation to undergo HBV testing (Taylor et al., 2004). In populations of low socioeconomic status, fewer than 10% had been tested for or vaccinated against HBV (Ma et al., 2007a, 2007b). In a group of Cambodian Americans, fewer than 50% had ever heard of or been tested for HBV, and fewer than 25% knew that chronic infection is lifelong and incurable (Taylor et al., 2002).

Misinformation about HBV transmission creates obstacles for prevention and treatment. In qualitative interviews, most Korean Americans expressed the belief that sharing of contaminated food and eating utensils was the most common route of HBV transmission, whereas few mentioned that HBV can be sexually or parenterally transmitted, and none mentioned vertical mother-to-child transmission (Choe et al., 2005). Among Chinese Americans, fewer than half had been tested or vaccinated (Taylor et al., 2006; Thompson et al., 2002), up to 53% believed HBV could be transmitted by contaminated food (Wu et al., 2007), up to 61% were unaware that chronic hepatitis B is typically asymptomatic, and 46% believed that there is a curative treatment for chronic hepatitis B (Wu et al., 2007); about 65% of those who were chronically infected were unaware of their infection status (Lin et al., 2007).

The committee was unable to find studies that looked at hepatitis B awareness among other foreign-born immigrants from highly endemic regions such as sub-Saharan Africa, the Middle East, and Eastern European nations (see Box 3-1). Some educational resources have been translated into a few languages. For example, New York City has translated its hepatitis B educational materials into Chinese, Korean, Spanish, and French (New York Department of Health and Mental Hygiene, 2008).

The incarcerated population has a high risk of being infected with HBV. About 30% of patients who had acute hepatitis B reported a history of incarceration before HBV infection (Charuvastra et al., 2001; Goldstein et al., 2002). Knowledge about HBV transmission in this population is poor and results in missing of opportunities for vaccination and prevention. A voluntary, anonymous survey of 153 male and female inmates of the Rhode Island Department of Corrections revealed that over half the 30% who reported having risk factors for HBV infection did not consider themselves to be at risk for hepatitis B (Vallabhaneni et al., 2004), and 44% of the inmates were not aware that HBV can be transmitted through unprotected sexual activity.

Several studies have found that knowledge about hepatitis B is low among men who have sex with men, another population at high risk for HBV infection (McCusker et al., 1990; Neighbors et al., 1999; Rhodes et al., 2000). A 1990 study found that 68% of men who have sex with men and are patients at a community health center reported that they were aware of the vaccine, and 25% of those who knew about it had been vaccinated (McCusker et al., 1990). Most of the participants who knew about the hepatitis B vaccine had learned about it from newspapers targeting the gay population (64%); a minority had learned about it from health-care providers (44%), friends (37%), and brochures from health-care facilities or gay organizations (36%). A 1999 study had similar findings: 33% of the participants were unaware of the hepatitis B vaccine, and 63% had not been tested for hepatitis B; of those who were aware of the vaccine, only 22% had received the full vaccine series (Neighbors et al., 1999). A similarly low level of hepatitis B knowledge was found among patrons of gay bars in Birmingham, Alabama, where 32% reported having no information about hepatitis, 96% reported engaging in high-risk sexual behavior, and those who had not been vaccinated against HBV (58% of respondents) had much poorer knowledge about hepatitis B prevention than those who had been vaccinated (Rhodes et al., 2000).

Stigma

For many people born outside the United States, a cultural stigma is attached to a diagnosis of chronic hepatitis B. For example, in China, there is pervasive discrimination against people who are chronically infected with hepatitis B, who are frequently expelled from schools, fired from jobs, and shunned by other community members despite the recent passage of national antidiscrimination laws (China Digital Times, 2009). In a 2007 survey covering 10 major cities in China, hepatitis B was cited as one of the top three reasons for job discrimination (China Daily, 2007). Given the deeply ingrained stigma of hepatitis B in some endemic countries, it is not surprising that many immigrants remain reluctant to undergo testing and seek medical attention for a positive test result even after moving to the United States. Because that cultural aversion to hepatitis B testing and management is due largely to a lack of knowledge about routes of HBV transmission and means of prevention, any effort to deliver viral-hepatitis services to the foreign-born population must include an educational component to dispel myths (for example, that HBV can be transmitted through food, water, and casual contact) and to establish facts, particularly ones that encourage testing, vaccination, and followup.

Education Programs

Several educational programs targeting API communities have been successful in disseminating hepatitis B awareness and promoting prevention. Successful programs often build on community partnerships and combine educational resources with increased access to testing, prevention, and care for participants (CDC, 2006; Chao et al., 2009a; Juon et al., 2008; Lin et al., 2007). The Hepatitis B Initiative is a community-based hepatitis B outreach program that partnered with nine Korean American and Chinese American churches in the Baltimore and Washington, DC, metropolitan area to provide culturally and linguistically tailored, faith-based HBV education, testing, and vaccination (Juon et al., 2008). The initiative has generated community support and awareness through word of mouth, articles in local Asian ethnic media, educational sessions and luncheons for API community leaders, and a national conference for API pastors. In 2003–2006, the program tested 1,775 participants for HBV and found that 2% were chronically infected and 61% were not vaccinated. Among 924 unvaccinated participants, nearly all received the first dose of hepatitis B vaccine, 89% received the second, and 79% completed the three-dose series. The Asian American Hepatitis B Program, a collaboration of community groups and academic and community health centers in New York City, provides hepatitis B screening, vaccination, and treatment. The program found that about 15% of newly tested persons had chronic HBV infection, all of whom were born outside the United States and half of whom had been in the country for more than 10 years (CDC, 2006).

The Jade Ribbon Campaign is a program focused on reducing the nationwide health disparity in hepatitis B. This program sponsors community HBV screening and education clinics and partners with over 400 community-based organizations and federal and state agencies to provide culturally and linguistically tailored information and multimedia public-service announcements about hepatitis B burden, risk factors, transmission, prevention, detection, treatment, and followup to the API community and health professionals (Asian Liver Center, 2009; CDC, 2009b). The program's clinics have found that about 45% of participants were not vaccinated against HBV, 9–13% of participants were chronically infected, and up to two-thirds of those who were chronically infected were unaware of their infection status. Of those who said that they had been vaccinated against HBV, 20% were unprotected and 5% chronically infected (Chao et al., 2009a; Lin et al., 2007). This model has been adapted by a number of cities around the country (Chang et al., 2009; Fernandez, 2008; Hsu et al.,

2007; Larkin, 2007; McBride, 2008; *San Francisco HepB Free*, 2009; Tsai et al., 2008; Zola et al., 2009).

As discussed in Chapter 4, the ACIP recommends that all newborns, previously unvaccinated children and adolescents, and previously unvaccinated adults at high risk for infection be vaccinated against hepatitis B (Mast et al., 2005, 2006). The latter group includes adults at risk for infection by sexual exposure, IDUs, household contacts of chronically infected persons, developmentally disabled persons in long-term-care facilities, persons at risk for occupational exposure to HBV, hemodialysis patients, persons with chronic liver disease, and travelers to HBV-endemic regions, including Asia, Africa, much of Eastern Europe, the Amazon Basin, the Caribbean, and the Pacific Islands (see Box 4-1). There is a shortage of hepatitis B education, vaccine promotion, and awareness programs for nearly all those at-risk populations, and programs need to be developed to target HIV-positive people, IDUs, and people from highly HBV-endemic regions (Rein et al., 2009). Although a handful of studies have evaluated cross-sectional hepatitis B knowledge levels in some of the populations, the committee knows of no programs that have demonstrated a quantitative improvement in knowledge about hepatitis B after the implementation of a targeted, evidence-based educational program.

A potential model to target at-risk populations is to develop pilot sites similar to CDC's Racial and Ethnic Approaches to Community Health, REACH 2010. The REACH 2010 program provided grants to communities to address services for specified illnesses in particular racial and ethnic populations. The program targeted blacks, American Indians, Alaska Natives, Asian Americans, Hispanics, and Pacific Islanders—all populations that have a high prevalence or incidence of hepatitis B and some hepatitis C also. Viral hepatitis was not part of the program (Collins, 2006; Giles et al., 2004).

Hepatitis C

Although fewer studies have been conducted to assess awareness of hepatitis C in specific populations, the literature suggests that knowledge about this disease is poor. In a cohort of 3,768 women who had or were at risk for HIV infection, about one-fourth of those with chronic HCV infection were not aware of their infection status (Cohen et al., 2007). Younger and black women were less likely to be aware of their HCV infection status, whereas women who had past alcohol treatment, a history of injection-drug use, or increased alanine aminotransferase (a liver enzyme) were more likely to be aware that they were positive for HCV infection. Of those aware of their chronic HCV infection, the health-care providers of 47% had recommended that they have a liver biopsy, and 56% of these had undergone a biopsy; 39% of those who were aware of their HCV infection status had been offered treatment, and 57% of these had received treatment.

Similarly, in the Collaborative Injection Drug User Study Drug User Intervention Trial (DUIT), which enrolled 3,004 young IDUs in five US cities, 72% of anti-HCV-positive and 46% of anti-HCV-negative IDUs were not aware of their HCV serologic status (Hagan et al., 2006). History of drug treatment or needle exchange was associated with increased awareness of HCV serologic status, so these programs may be key locations for provision of HCV screening in this population. In a questionnaire survey given to 150 patients who were seeking substance-abuse treatment at a Department of Veterans Affairs medical center, 90% of patients who were HCV-infected were not aware of their status, and 41% of the IDUs did not know or were unsure of how HCV is transmitted or about the complications of hepatitis C (Dhopesh et al., 2000).

Stein et al. (2001) surveyed 306 former IDUs about their knowledge of HCV transmission, infection status, and risk of liver disease. They found that nearly all the participants knew that HCV is transmitted by sharing contaminated needles. Among people who had not been tested or did not know their test results, some 82% were HCV seropositive. One-third of the people reporting that they were seronegative were actually seropositive—a demonstration that, as in other surveys, self-reported infection status is unreliable. Of respondents, 81% estimated their risk of developing liver disease, specifically cirrhosis, in the next 10 years at 50% or greater.

The risk associated with the shared use of injection paraphernalia other than syringes is poorly understood (Rhodes et al., 2004). Among IDUs who have chronic HCV infection and are aware of their infection, the pattern is similar: the majority understand that they can transmit their infection by passing on their used syringes to others, but there is less certainty regarding the shared use of cookers, cottons, and rinse water (Rhodes and Treloar, 2008; Wright et al., 2005).

There is substantial confusion among IDUs regarding the interpretation of HCV screening tests. In an Australian study, 42% of IDUs believed that being antibody-positive meant that they were immune to HCV infection (O'Brien et al., 2008). Misunderstanding of the meaning of antibody-test results was also observed in a qualitative study of IDUs in London, England (Rhodes et al., 2004).

Stigma

A number of studies have examined the psychologic consequences of HCV infection and concluded that hepatitis C is a highly stigmatized disease, owing in large part to its association with injection-drug use (Conrad et al., 2006; Crofts et al., 1997; Dunne and Quayle, 2001; Grundy and

Beeching, 2004). There is also a public perception that HCV is highly contagious and that it is life-threatening in most cases (Conrad et al., 2006); this has led to discrimination on the part of people who inappropriately perceive themselves to be at risk from casual contact with an HCV-positive person. In a study of patients in a liver clinic in Iowa, 57% of HCV-positive people reported having experienced stigma associated with their infection (Zickmund et al., 2003). Many patients who have HCV infection wish to disclose their HCV status to family, intimate partners, and others in an effort to protect them from infection and to obtain psychosocial support. Even in work settings, people have been eager to disclose their HCV status so that in the event of injury co-workers would take extra care in avoiding exposure to contaminated blood. However, many people report that informing others of their HCV status has led to inappropriate reactions, such as "[I'm] not allowed to use the cups because they don't really know . . . how to pass it on" (Conrad et al., 2006). In another study, a patient reported that "they didn't want me drinking out of the water fountain" (Zickmund et al., 2003).

Education Programs

Although only a handful of studies have examined the influence of education on HCV-related risk behavior in IDUs, the results are consistent in showing that enhanced education and counseling are associated with safer injection practices (Garfein et al., 2007; Latka et al., 2008; Tucker et al., 2004). In the DUIT study by Garfein et al. (2007), young HIV-seronegative and HCV-seronegative IDUs were enrolled in a randomized trial of an intervention that sought to train them to be peer educators. The goals of the peer-education intervention (PEI) were to develop mastery over knowledge and skills necessary for prevention of HIV and HCV infection so that they could pass the knowledge on to their peers. Behavior change was measured in the PEI subjects and in subjects randomized to an equal-attention control group. Reductions in injection risk behavior were observed in both study arms, but the PEI group reported significantly greater reductions.

A parallel study, the Study to Reduce Intravenous Exposures (STRIVE), enrolled young HCV-seropositive IDUs (most of whom were chronically infected) and randomized them into a PEI or control condition. Significantly greater reductions in injection practices that could transmit HCV to other IDUs were observed in the PEI group (Latka et al., 2008). Thus, enhanced education and skill-building can lead to safer injection practices and may contribute to avoidance of infection in susceptible IDUs and reduction in transmission of infection to other IDUs. That strategy parallels the Prevention for Positives initiatives for HIV (CDC, 2003a).

Patients in drug-treatment programs have considerable needs for education about hepatitis C. In spite of the disproportionate prevalence of HCV infection in drug users, research conducted with 280 patients who never injected drugs (non-injection-drug users, NIDUs) and past or current IDUs in 14 US drug-treatment programs showed that many remain uninformed or misinformed about the disease (Strauss et al., 2007). The 280 participating patients scored, on the average, 56% on a 20-item true–false HCV knowledge assessment, demonstrating inadequate knowledge about hepatitis C. IDUs scored significantly higher, on the average, than did NIDUs (60% vs 51%), but their scores also suggest many gaps in their knowledge about hepatitis C. Fewer than half of all the patients correctly endorsed facts concerning HCV transmission, the duration of hepatitis C treatment, the potential effectiveness of hepatitis C medication in active drug users, the course of HCV infection, and the possibility of spontaneous clearance of the infection.

To address the knowledge gaps, all the programs offered at least one form of hepatitis C education: all offered one-on-one sessions with staff, 12 of the programs offered hepatitis C education in a group format, and 11 offered education through pamphlets and books. However, only 60% of all the participating patients used any of their programs' hepatitis C education services. Those who did avail themselves of the hepatitis C education opportunities generally assessed them favorably. Of all the patients, many were unaware that hepatitis C education was offered in their programs through individual sessions with staff, group meetings, and books and pamphlets (42%, 49%, and 46% of the patients, respectively), and 22% were unaware that any hepatitis C education opportunities existed (Strauss et al., 2007). Thus, efforts need to focus especially on ensuring that all drug-treatment program patients are made aware of and encouraged to use hepatitis C education services in their programs. Such awareness and encouragement, however, will be useful only if staff of drug-treatment programs have up-to-date knowledge about the virus and treatment options so that they can share hepatitis C information with their patients accurately.

Recommendation

On the basis of the above findings, the committee offers the following recommendation to increase educational and awareness opportunities about hepatitis B and hepatitis C.

Recommendation 3-2. The Centers for Disease Control and Prevention should work with key stakeholders to develop, coordinate, and evaluate innovative and effective outreach and education programs to target at-risk populations and to increase awareness in the general population about hepatitis B and hepatitis C.

CDC should work with other federal agencies and state and local governments to form partnerships with health-care providers, private organizations (including employers and nonprofit organizations), schools, and appropriate community organizations to develop awareness programs and campaigns to educate the general public and at-risk populations about hepatitis B and hepatitis C. The programs should include shared resources that are linguistically and culturally appropriate and support integration of education about viral hepatitis and liver health into other health programs that serve at-risk populations. Successful programs like those discussed above should serve as models for interventions and existing materials, such as the American Congress of Obstetricians and Gynecologists patient education materials on viral hepatitis (American College of Obstetricians and Gynecologists, 2007, 2008, 2009), should be used as a basis for producing linguistically and culturally relevant materials.

Innovative approaches should be developed to address populations that have access to few educational programs including foreign-born people from the highly HBV endemic regions, men who have sex with men, IDUs, and household and sexual contacts of people who are chronically infected with HBV and HCV.

Programs should be evaluated to ensure that they are effectively targeting the general public and at-risk people and populations. The general public should be targeted because HBV and HCV infections occur in people not easily identifiable as belonging to an at-risk population or people who fail to report potential risk factors (Daniels et al., 2009). The results of evaluation of the programs will inform future initiatives. The programs should incorporate interventions that meet the following goals:

- Promote better understanding of HBV and HCV infections, transmission, prevention, and treatment in at-risk and general populations.
- Promote increased hepatitis B vaccination rates among children and at-risk adults.
- Educate pregnant women and women of childbearing age about hepatitis B prevention.
- Reduce perinatal HBV infections and improvement of at-birth immunization rates.
- Increase testing rates in at-risk populations.
- Reduce stigmatization of chronically infected people.
- Promote safe injections among IDUs and safe drug use among NIDUs.
- Provide culturally and linguistically appropriate educational information for all persons who have tested positive for chronic HBV or HCV infections and those who are receiving treatment.

- Encourage notification of household and sexual contacts of infected people to be tested for HBV and HCV and encourage hepatitis B vaccination of close contacts.

General Public Awareness and Education

Lack of knowledge about HBV and HCV transmission contributes to the stigma of infection and is a barrier to testing, prevention, and care. Public HIV-awareness campaigns led to reduced stigma and discrimination toward patients with HIV infection (Brown et al., 2003). As in the case of HIV/AIDS, increasing general public knowledge about hepatitis B and hepatitis C can be expected to reduce discrimination toward infected people, reduce transmission, and increase early diagnosis and treatment that ultimately save lives.

Broader community education should include print and multimedia educational materials about viral hepatitis for the public, large employers, and health insurers. It should work to mobilize and facilitate a grassroots movement among community stakeholders, including health-care providers, employers, mainstream and ethnic media, community-based organizations, and students. Large employers, such as multinational corporations, are potentially important partners in hepatitis prevention and control in that they provide health benefits to about two-thirds of Americans who have health insurance and are commonly employers of foreign-born people from HBV-endemic countries both in the United States and overseas.

The lack of knowledge and awareness about hepatitis B and hepatitis C in the general population suggests that integration of viral-hepatitis and liver-health education into existing health-education curricula in schools will help to eliminate the stigma of those chronically infected and improve prevention of viral hepatitis. There is evidence that adolescents are unaware of hepatitis B and hepatitis C risks and how to prevent becoming infected (Moore-Caldwell et al., 1997; Slonim et al., 2005). Many schools already require health education on HIV, which has transmission routes similar to those of hepatitis B and hepatitis C (CDC, 2008b). Several school-based programs have been demonstrated to reduce HIV risk in students and could serve as models for viral hepatitis education initiatives (Gaydos et al., 2008; Kennedy et al., 2000).

Community-Based Outreach to Foreign-Born

Immigrants from HBV-endemic countries make up the largest population of people who have chronic hepatitis B in the United States, and it is essential that they receive culturally and linguistically tailored information about transmission and risks of HBV infection and that it promote testing, vaccination, and medical management.

Rein et al. (2009) estimated that there are 55 active community-based hepatitis B outreach programs in the country that were targeting mostly APIs, of which they contacted 31. Although those programs have done much to inform APIs about hepatitis B, there is a need for additional programs that target APIs, given the burden of hepatitis B within that population.

There is also a need for education programs that target foreign-born people from other HBV-endemic regions. The models used by programs designed for APIs could be modified to address the needs of other populations. Community-based education and screening programs—including outreach at cultural festivals, health fairs, and places of worship—have been shown to be effective in improving APIs' knowledge about hepatitis B (Chao et al., 2009a; Hsu et al., 2007; Juon et al., 2008; Lin et al., 2007) and could potentially be effective with other ethnic populations. Each year, around 20,000 people are tested through those programs, and HBsAg is detected in about 8% of the tested population (Rein et al., 2009). Some 30% of the programs were supported by local government funding, 27% by state funding, and 10% by federal funding. Other sources include pharmaceutical and insurance companies, research and service grants, community hospitals, and other private funding sources (Rein et al., 2009).

Rein et al. (2009) also found that there were few or no hepatitis B outreach programs in most regions of the United States (the Southeast, the Midwest, and the Southwest outside of California and the Houston area). Education and prevention programs should be expanded to provide services in underserved regions of the United States given that the highest rates of acute hepatitis B incidence are in the south (Daniels et al., 2009).

Correctional Facilities

About 2 million people are incarcerated in the US correctional system. The major risk factors for viral hepatitis in people in correctional facilities are injection-drug use, tattooing, and sexual activity (see Chapters 4 and 5 for additional information about incarcerated populations). Because people in the correctional system are more likely to be infected or to become infected with HBV and HCV than the US general population, it is important to provide educational opportunities about hepatitis B and hepatitis C in correctional facilities. Increased knowledge and awareness about the diseases will lead to a greater understanding among inmates about how to prevent them, the advantages of hepatitis B vaccination, why they should be tested for chronic hepatitis B and hepatitis C, and what to do about a positive test result for either infection. Niveau (2006) reviewed risk factors for acquiring infectious diseases in correctional settings and found that effective preventive measures included information dissemination and education. Inmate peer-based health education has been effective in primary prevention of HIV (Hammett, 2006). The addition of hepatitis education to existing peer-based inmate educational programs is feasible and will probably incur minimal additional cost. Boutwell et al. (2005) called education of prisoners about hepatitis C as part of a larger program of prevention, testing, and treatment a "cornerstone of the public health response to the hepatitis C epidemic in the United States" and recommended research into program implementation.

Drug-Treatment Facilities and Needle-Exchange Programs

Drug-treatment and needle-exchange programs reach a substantial proportion of active injectors who have HCV infection or are at risk of acquiring it. Because the programs have regular, long-term contact with many IDUs, there are multiple opportunities to disseminate information about hepatitis B and hepatitis C, including the benefits of hepatitis B vaccination, how to avoid reinfection with HCV, and the importance of followup care for those chronically infected.

Although education programs developed for needle exchange, drug treatment, and corrections facilities will reach substantial proportions of those at risk, important segments of IDU populations will not be reached by them. Women and young people who inject drugs are less likely than others to attend needle-exchange and drug-treatment programs (Bluthenthal et al., 2000; Miller et al., 2001). Novel programs are needed that will access the hidden injectors, and outreach and peer-education programs are potentially effective ways to achieve this goal.

Perinatal Facilities That Care for Pregnant Women

The risk of chronic infection after exposure to HBV is highest in early life, and most people who have chronic hepatitis B were infected at birth or during early childhood. Each year in the United States, about 24,000 HBsAg-positive women give birth and about 1,000 newborns develop chronic HBV infection (Ward, 2008). The latter occurs largely because of failure to adhere to ACIP recommendations and timely administration of the birth dose of the hepatitis B vaccine and hepatitis B immunoglobulin.

Although it is recommended that household contacts be tested because of high risk of infection, fewer than 50% are tested, and fewer than 50% of those tested and found to be HBV-negative or of unknown status are vaccinated (Euler et al., 2003a). Therefore, perinatal-care facilities and their staffs (including OB/GYNs and their clinic staffs) provide an excellent opportunity to educate pregnant women about the importance of HBsAg testing, interpretation of the results, and the importance of newborn hepatitis B vaccination. The women should be given culturally and linguistically appropriate educational information about the importance of administration of the birth dose of the hepatitis B vaccine and hepatitis B immunoglobulin within 12 hours of birth if needed, completion of the hepatitis B vaccine series by the age of 6 months, and postvaccination testing. There is a need to develop a novel program to educate pregnant women in perinatal-care facilities about hepatitis B to prevent perinatal transmission, to refer women who are chronically infected for medical care, and to refer family and household contacts for testing, vaccination, and care if needed.

REFERENCES

Altekruse, S. F., K. A. McGlynn, and M. E. Reichman. 2009. Hepatocellular carcinoma incidence, mortality, and survival trends in the United States from 1975 to 2005. *Journal of Clinical Oncology* 27(9):1485-1491.

American College of Obstetricians and Gynecologists. 2007. ACOG practice bulletin no. 86: Viral hepatitis in pregnancy. *Obstetrics and Gynecology* 110(4):941-956.

———. 2008. *Hepatitis B virus in pregnancy.* http://www.acog.org/publications/patient_education/bp093.cfm (accessed August 21, 2009).

———. 2009. *Protecting yourself against hepatitis B.* http://www.acog.org/publications/patient_education/bp125.cfm (accessed October 24, 2009).

Ascione, A., T. Tartaglione, and G. G. Di Costanzo. 2007. Natural history of chronic hepatitis C virus infection. *Digestive and Liver Disease* 39(Suppl 1):S4-S7.

Asian Liver Center. 2009. *Information resources.* http://liver.stanford.edu/Public/index.html (accessed August 21, 2009).

Boaz, K., A. E. Fiore, S. J. Schrag, B. Gonik, and J. Schulkin. 2003. Screening and counseling practices reported by obstetrician-gynecologists for patients with hepatitis C virus infection. *Infectious Diseases in Obstetrics and Gynecology* 11(1):39-44.

Bluthenthal, R. N., A. H. Kral, L. Gee, E. A. Erringer, and B. R. Edlin. 2000. The effect of syringe exchange use on high-risk injection drug users: A cohort study. *AIDS* 14(5):605-611.

Boutwell, A. E., S. A. Allen, and J. D. Rich. 2005. Opportunities to address the hepatitis C epidemic in the correctional setting. *Clinical Infectious Diseases* 40(s5):S367-S372.

Brown, L., K. Macintyre, and L. Trujillo. 2003. Interventions to reduce HIV/AIDS stigma: What have we learned? *AIDS Education and Prevention* 15(1):49-69.

CDC (Centers for Disease Control and Prevention). 1991. Hepatitis B virus: A comprehensive strategy for eliminating transmission in the United States through universal childhood vaccination: recommendations of the Immunization Practices Advisory Committee. *Mobility and Mortality Weekly Report* 40(No. RR-13):1-25.

———. 1998. Recommendations for prevention and control of hepatitis C virus (HCV) infection and HCV-related chronic disease. Centers for Disease Control and Prevention. *Morbidity and Morality Weekly: Recommendations and Reports* 47(RR-19):1-39.

———. 2003a. Advancing HIV prevention: New strategies for a changing epidemic—United States, 2003. *Morbidity and Mortality Weekly Report* 52(15):329-332.

———. 2003b. Hepatitis C virus transmission from an antibody-negative organ and tissue donor—United States, 2000-2002. *Morbidity and Mortality Weekly Report* 52(13):273-274, 276.

———. 2003c. Transmission of hepatitis B and C viruses in outpatient settings—New York, Oklahoma, and Nebraska, 2000-2002. *Morbidity and Mortality Weekly Report* 52(38): 901-906.

———. 2005. Transmission of hepatitis B virus among persons undergoing blood glucose monitoring in long-term-care facilities—Mississippi, North Carolina, and Los Angeles county, California, 2003-2004. *Morbidity and Mortality Weekly Report* 54(9):220-223.

———. 2006. Screening for chronic hepatitis B among Asian/Pacific Islander populations—New York City, 2005. *Morbidity and Mortality Weekly Report* 55(18):505-509.

———. 2008a. Acute hepatitis C virus infections attributed to unsafe injection practices at an endoscopy clinic—Nevada, 2007. *Morbidity and Mortality Weekly Report* 57(19): 513-517.

———. 2008b. HIV prevention education and HIV-related policies in secondary schools—selected sites, United States, 2006. *Morbidity and Mortality Weekly Report* 57(30): 822-825.

———. 2008c. *Maternal hepatitis B screening and reporting requirements.* http://www2a.cdc.gov/nip/stateVaccApp/StateVaccsApp/HepatitisScreenandReport.asp (accessed November 7, 2008).

———. 2009a. Hepatitis C virus transmission at an outpatient hemodialysis unit—New York, 2001-2008. *Morbidity and Mortality Weekly Report* 58(8):189-194.

———. 2009b. *Patient education resources.* http://www.cdc.gov/hepatitis/B/PatientEduB.htm (accessed September 9, 2009).

Chang, E. T., S. Y. Lin, E. Sue, M. Bergin, J. Su, and S. K. So. 2007. Building partnerships with traditional Chinese medicine practitioners to increase hepatitis B awareness and prevention. *Journal of Alternative and Complementary Medicine* 13(10):1125-1127.

Chang, E. T., E. Sue, J. Zola, and S. K. So. 2009. 3 for life: A model pilot program to prevent hepatitis B virus infection and liver cancer in Asian and Pacific Islander Americans. *American Journal of Health Promotion* 23(3):176-181.

Chao, S. D., E. T. Chang, P. V. Le, W. Prapong, M. Kiernan, and S. K. So. 2009a. The Jade Ribbon Campaign: A model program for community outreach and education to prevent liver cancer in Asian Americans. *Journal of Immigrant and Minority Health* 11(4):281-290.

Chao, S. D., C. Cheung, A. Yue, and S. K. So. 2009b. *Low hepatitis B knowledge among perinatal healthcare providers serving county with nation's highest rate of births to mothers chronically infected with hepatitis B.* Paper presented at Poster presentation at the 13th Internationational Symposium on Viral Hepatitis and Liver Disease, Washington, DC. March 20-24, 2009.

Charuvastra, A., J. Stein, B. Schwartzapfel, A. Spaulding, E. Horowitz, G. Macalino, and J. D. Rich. 2001. Hepatitis B vaccination practices in state and federal prisons. *Public Health Reports* 116(3):203-209.

China Daily. 2007 (June 14). *Discrimination in job market common.* http://www.china.org.cn/english/features/cw/213887.htm (accessed March 30, 2009).

China Digital Times. 2009. *China news tagged with: hepatitis B.* http://chinadigitaltimes.net/china/hepatitis-b/ (accessed August 21, 2009).

Choe, J. H., N. Chan, H. H. Do, E. Woodall, E. Lim, and V. M. Taylor. 2005. Hepatitis B and liver cancer beliefs among Korean immigrants in western Washington. *Cancer* 104(12 Suppl):2955-2958.

Chu, D. 2009. *Hepatitis B virus screening practices of Asian-American primary care physicians who treat Asian adults living in the United States.* Paper presented at oral presentation at the 13th International Symposium on Viral Hepatitis and Liver Disease, Washington, DC. March 20-24, 2009.

Clarke, S. P., J. L. Rockett, D. M. Sloane, and L. H. Aiken. 2002. Organizational climate, staffing, and safety equipment as predictors of needlestick injuries and near-misses in hospital nurses. *American Journal of Infection Control* 30(4):207-216.

Cohen, M. H., D. Grey, J. A. Cook, K. Anastos, E. Seaberg, M. Augenbraun, P. Burian, M. Peters, M. Young, and A. French. 2007. Awareness of hepatitis C infection among women with and at risk for HIV. *Journal of General Internal Medicine* 22(12):1689-1694.

Collins, J. 2006. Addressing racial and ethnic disparities: Lessons from the REACH 2010 communities. *Journal of Health Care for the Poor and Underserved* 17(2 Suppl):1-5.

Conrad, S., L. E. Garrett, W. G. Cooksley, M. P. Dunne, and G. A. MacDonald. 2006. Living with chronic hepatitis C means "you just haven't got a normal life any more." *Chronic Illness* 2(2):121-131.

Crofts, N., R. Louie, and B. Loff. 1997. The next plague: Stigmatization and discrimination related to Hepatitis C virus infection in Australia. *Health and Human Rights* 2(2):86-97.

Daniels, D., S. Grytdal, and A. Wasley. 2009. Surveillance for acute viral hepatitis—United States, 2007. *Morbidity and Mortality Weekly Report: Surveillance Summaries* 58(3):1-27.

Dhopesh, V. P., K. R. Taylor, and W. M. Burke. 2000. Survey of hepatitis B and C in addiction treatment unit. *American Journal of Drug and Alcohol Abuse* 26:703.

Dulay, M., J. Zola, J. Hwang, A. Baron, and C. Lai. 2007. Are primary care clinicians knowledgeable about screening for chronic hepatitis B infection? Presented at the 30th annual meeting of the Society of General Internal Medicine (SGIM), Toronto, Canada. *Journal of General Internal Medicine* 22(Suppl 1):100.

Dunne, E. A., and E. Quayle. 2001. The impact of iatrogenically acquired Hepatitis C infection on the well-being and relationships of a group of Irish women. *Journal of Health Psychology* 6(6):679-692.

Euler, G. L., J. Copeland, and W. W. Williams. 2003a. Impact of four urban perinatal hepatitis B prevention programs on screening and vaccination of infants and household members. *American Journal of Epidemiology* 157(8):747-753.

Euler, G. L., K. G. Wooten, A. L. Baughman, and W. W. Williams. 2003b. Hepatitis B surface antigen prevalence among pregnant women in urban areas: Implications for testing, reporting, and preventing perinatal transmission. *Pediatrics* 111(5):1192-1197.

Fabrizi, F., A. Marzano, P. Messa, P. Martin, and P. Lampertico. 2008. Hepatitis B virus infection in the dialysis population: Current perspectives. *International Journal of Artificial Organs* 31(5):386-394.

Fernandez, E. 2008. Hepatitis B plan seeks to aid high-risk groups. *San Francisco Chronicle*, September 19, 2008.

Ferrante, J. M., D. G. Winston, P. H. Chen, and A. N. de la Torre. 2008. Family physicians' knowledge and screening of chronic hepatitis and liver cancer. *Family Medicine* 40(5):345-351.

Galai, N., M. Safaeian, D. Vlahov, A. Bolotin, and D. D. Celentano. 2003. Longitudinal patterns of drug injection behavior in the ALIVE study cohort, 1988-2000: Description and determinants. *American Journal of Epidemiology* 158(7):695-704.

Garfein, R. S., E. T. Golub, A. E. Greenberg, H. Hagan, D. L. Hanson, S. M. Hudson, F. Kapadia, M. H. Latka, L. J. Ouellet, D. W. Purcell, S. A. Strathdee, and H. Thiede. 2007. A peer-education intervention to reduce injection risk behaviors for HIV and hepatitis C virus infection in young injection drug users. *AIDS* 21(14):1923-1932.

Gaydos, C. A., Y.-H. Hsieh, J. S. Galbraith, M. Barnes, G. Waterfield, and B. Stanton. 2008. Focus-on-teens, sexual risk-reduction intervention for high-school adolescents: Impact on knowledge, change of risk-behaviours, and prevalence of sexually transmitted diseases. *International Journal of STD and AIDS* 19(10):704-710.

Ghany, M. G., D. B. Strader, D. L. Thomas, and L. Seeff. 2009. Diagnosis, management, and treatment of Hepatitis C: An update. *Hepatology* 49(4):1335-1374.

Giles, W. H., P. Tucker, L. Brown, C. Crocker, N. Jack, A. Latimer, Y. Liao, T. Lockhart, S. McNary, M. Sells, and V. B. Harris. 2004. Racial and ethnic approaches to community health (REACH 2010): An overview. *Ethnicity and Disease* 14(3 Suppl 1):S5-S8.

Goldstein, S. T., M. J. Alter, I. T. Williams, L. A. Moyer, F. N. Judson, K. Mottram, M. Fleenor, P. L. Ryder, and H. S. Margolis. 2002. Incidence and risk factors for acute hepatitis B in the United States, 1982-1998: Implications for vaccination programs. *Journal of Infectious Diseases* 185(6):713-719.

Grundy, G., and N. Beeching. 2004. Understanding social stigma in women with hepatitis C. *Nursing Standard* 19(4):35-39.

Hagan, H., J. Campbell, H. Thiede, S. Strathdee, L. Ouellet, F. Kapadia, S. Hudson, and R. S. Garfein. 2006. Self-reported hepatitis C virus antibody status and risk behavior in young injectors. *Public Health Reports* 121(6):710-719.

Hagan, H., J. P. McGough, H. Thiede, N. S. Weiss, S. Hopkins, and E. R. Alexander. 1999. Syringe exchange and risk of infection with hepatitis B and C viruses. *American Journal of Epidemiology* 149(3):203-213.

Hammett, T. M. 2006. HIV/AIDS and other infectious diseases among correctional inmates: Transmission, burden, and an appropriate response. *American Journal of Public Health* 96(6):974-978.

Holodnick, C. L., and V. Barkauskas. 2000. Reducing percutaneous injuries in the or by educational methods. *AORN Journal* 72(3):461-464, 468-472, 475-466.

Hooper, J., and W. Charney. 2005. Creation of a safety culture: Reducing workplace injuries in a rural hospital setting. *AAOHN Journal* 53(9):394-398.

Hsu, C. E., L. C. Liu, H. S. Juon, Y. W. Chiu, J. Bawa, U. Tillman, M. Li, J. Miller, and M. Wang. 2007. Reducing liver cancer disparities: A community-based hepatitis-B prevention program for Asian-American communities. *Journal of the National Medical Association* 99(8):900-907.

Hwang, J. P., C. H. Huang, and J. K. Yi. 2008. Knowledge about hepatitis B and predictors of hepatitis B vaccination among Vietnamese American college students. *Journal of American College Health* 56(4):377-382.

Janke, E. A., S. McGraw, G. Garcia-Tsao, and L. Fraenkel. 2008. Psychosocial issues in hepatitis C: A qualitative analysis. *Psychosomatics* 49(6):494-501.

Juon, H. S., C. Strong, T. H. Oh, T. Castillo, G. Tsai, and L. D. Oh. 2008. Public health model for prevention of liver cancer among Asian Americans. *Journal of Community Health* 33(4):199-205.

Kennedy, M. G., Y. Mizuno, R. Hoffman, C. Baume, and J. Strand. 2000. The effect of tailoring a model HIV prevention program for local adolescent target audiences. *AIDS Education and Prevention* 12(3):225-238.

Lai, C. L., and M. F. Yuen. 2007. The natural history of chronic hepatitis B. *Journal of Viral Hepatitis* 14(Suppl 1):6-10.

Larkin, M. 2007. Hepatitis B awareness spread on the web. *The Lancet Infectious Diseases* 7(6):383.

Latka, M. H., H. Hagan, F. Kapadia, E. T. Golub, S. Bonner, J. V. Campbell, M. H. Coady, R. S. Garfein, M. Pu, D. L. Thomas, T. K. Thiel, and S. A. Strathdee. 2008. A randomized intervention trial to reduce the lending of used injection equipment among injection drug users infected with hepatitis C. *American Journal of Public Health* 98(5):853-861.

Lin, S. Y., E. T. Chang, and S. K. So. 2007. Why we should routinely screen Asian American adults for hepatitis B: A cross-sectional study of Asians in California. *Hepatology* 46(4):1034-1040.

Lok, A. S., and B. J. McMahon. 2009. Chronic hepatitis B: Update 2009. *Hepatology* 50(3):661-662.

Lorvick, J., R. N. Bluthenthal, A. Scott, M. L. Gilbert, K. S. Riehman, R. L. Anderson, N. M. Flynn, and A. H. Kral. 2006. Secondary syringe exchange among users of 23 California syringe exchange programs. *Substance Use and Misuse* 41(6-7):865-882.

Ma, G. X., C. Y. Fang, S. E. Shive, J. Toubbeh, Y. Tan, and P. Siu. 2007a. Risk perceptions and barriers to hepatitis B screening and vaccination among Vietnamese immigrants. *Journal of Immigrant and Minority Health* 9(3):213-220.

Ma, G. X., S. E. Shive, C. Y. Fang, Z. Feng, L. Parameswaran, A. Pham, and C. Khanh. 2007b. Knowledge, attitudes, and behaviors of hepatitis B screening and vaccination and liver cancer risks among Vietnamese Americans. *Journal of Health Care for the Poor and Underserved* 18(1):62-73.

Ma, G. X., S. E. Shive, J. I. Toubbeh, Y. Tan, and D. Wu. 2008. Knowledge, attitudes, and behaviors of Chinese hepatitis B screening and vaccination. *American Journal of Health Behavior* 32(2):178-187.

Mast, E. E., H. S. Margolis, A. E. Fiore, E. W. Brink, S. T. Goldstein, S. A. Wang, L. A. Moyer, B. P. Bell, and M. J. Alter. 2005. A comprehensive immunization strategy to eliminate transmission of hepatitis B virus infection in the United States: Recommendations of the Advisory Committee on Immunization Practices (ACIP) part 1: Immunization of infants, children, and adolescents. *Morbidity and Mortality Weekly Report Recommandations and Reports* 54(RR-16):1-31.

Mast, E. E., C. M. Weinbaum, A. E. Fiore, M. J. Alter, B. P. Bell, L. Finelli, L. E. Rodewald, J. M. Douglas, Jr., R. S. Janssen, and J. W. Ward. 2006. A comprehensive immunization strategy to eliminate transmission of hepatitis B virus infection in the United States: Recommendations of the advisory committee on immunization practices (ACIP) part II: Immunization of adults. *Morbidity and Morality Weekly: Recommendations and Reports* 55(RR-16):1-33; quiz CE31-34.

McBride, G. 2008. Hepatitis B virus-induced liver cancer in Asian Americans: A preventable disease. *Journal of the National Cancer Institute* 100(8):528-529.

McCusker, J., E. M. Hill, and K. H. Mayer. 1990. Awareness and use of hepatitis B vaccine among homosexual male clients of a Boston community health center. *Public Health Reports* 105(1):59-64.

McGlynn, K. A., R. E. Tarone, and H. B. El-Serag. 2006. A comparison of trends in the incidence of hepatocellular carcinoma and intrahepatic cholangiocarcinoma in the United States. *Cancer Epidemiology, Biomarkers and Prevention* 15(6):1198-1203.

McLaughlin, D. F., H. McKenna, and J. C. Leslie. 2000. The perceptions and aspirations illicit drug users hold toward health care staff and the care they receive. *Journal of Psychiatric and Mental Health Nursing* 7(5):435-441.

Miller, M., A. Eskild, I. Mella, H. Moi, and P. Magnus. 2001. Gender differences in syringe exchange program use in Oslo, Norway. *Addiction* 96(11):1639-1651.

Milloy, M. J., E. Wood, W. Small, M. Tyndall, C. Lai, J. Montaner, and T. Kerr. 2008. Incarceration experiences in a cohort of active injection drug users. *Drug and Alcohol Review* 27(6):693-699.

Moore-Caldwell, S. Y., M. J. Werner, L. Powell, and J. W. Greene. 1997. Hepatitis B vaccination in adolescents: Knowledge, perceived risk, and compliance. *Journal of Adolescent Health* 20(4):294-299.

Neighbors, K., C. Oraka, L. Shih, and P. Lurie. 1999. Awareness and utilization of the hepatitis B vaccine among young men in the Ann Arbor area who have sex with men. *Journal of American College Health* 47(4):173-178.

New York Department of Health and Mental Hygiene. 2008. *Hepatitis B: The facts booklet.* http://www.nyc.gov/html/doh/html/cd/cdhepb.shtml (accessed October 28, 2009).

Niveau, G. 2006. Prevention of infectious disease transmission in correctional settings: A review. *Public Health* 120(1):33-41.

O'Brien, S., C. Day, E. Black, and K. Dolan. 2008. Injecting drug users' understanding of hepatitis C. *Addictive Behaviors* 33(12):1602-1605.

Paterson, B. L., M. Backmund, G. Hirsch, and C. Yim. 2007. The depiction of stigmatization in research about hepatitis C. *International Journal on Drug Policy* 18(5):364-373.

Rein, D. B., S. B. Lesesne, P. J. Leese, and C. M. Weinbaum. 2010. Community-based hepatitis B screening programs in the United States in 2008. *Journal of Viral Hepatitis* 17(1):28-33.

Rhodes, S. D., R. J. Diclemente, L. J. Yee, and K. C. Hergenrather. 2000. Hepatitis B vaccination in a high risk MSM population: The need for vaccine education. *Sexually Transmitted Infections* 76(5):408-409.

Rhodes, T., and C. Treloar. 2008. The social production of hepatitis C risk among injecting drug users: A qualitative synthesis. *Addiction* 103(10):1593-1603.

Rhodes, T., M. Davis, and A. Judd. 2004. Hepatitis C and its risk management among drug injectors in London: Renewing harm reduction in the context of uncertainty. *Addiction* 99(5):621-633.

San Francisco HepB Free. 2009. http://sfhepbfree.org (accessed September 9, 2009).

Shehab, T. M., S. S. Sonnad, and A. S. F. Lok. 2001. Management of hepatitis C patients by primary care physicians in the USA: Results of a national survey. *Journal of Viral Hepatitis* 8(5):377-383.

Shehab, T. M., S. S. Sonnad, M. Jeffries, N. Gunaratnum, and A. S. Lok. 1999. Current practice patterns of primary care physicians in the management of patients with hepatitis C. *Hepatology* 30(3):794-800.

Simard, E. P., J. T. Miller, P. A. George, A. Wasley, M. J. Alter, B. P. Bell, and L. Finelli. 2007. Hepatitis B vaccination coverage levels among healthcare workers in the United States, 2002-2003. *Infection Control and Hospital Epidemiology* 28(7):783-790.

Slonim, A. B., A. J. Roberto, C. R. Downing, I. F. Adams, N. J. Fasano, L. Davis-Satterla, and M. A. Miller. 2005. Adolescents' knowledge, beliefs, and behaviors regarding hepatitis B: Insights and implications for programs targeting vaccine-preventable diseases. *Journal of Adolescent Health* 36(3):178-186.

Stein, M. D., J. Maksad, and J. Clarke. 2001. Hepatitis C disease among injection drug users: Knowledge, perceived risk and willingness to receive treatment. *Drug and Alcohol Dependence* 61(3):211-215.

Strauss, S. M., J. M. Astone-Twerell, C. Munoz-Plaza, D. C. Des Jarlais, M. Gwadz, H. Hagan, A. Osborne, and A. Rosenblum. 2006. Hepatitis C knowledge among staff in U.S. drug treatment programs. *Journal of Drug Education* 36(2):141-158.

———. 2007. Drug treatment programs patients' hepatitis C virus (HCV) education needs and their use of available HCV education services. *BMC Health Services Research* 7(39).

Stringer, B., C. Infante-Rivard, and J. A. Hanley. 2002. Effectiveness of the hands-free technique in reducing operating theatre injuries. *Occupational and Environmental Medicine* 59(10):703-707.

Taylor, V. M., J. H. Choe, Y. Yasui, L. Li, N. Burke, and J. C. Jackson. 2005a. Hepatitis B awareness, testing, and knowledge among Vietnamese American men and women. *Journal of Community Health* 30(6):477-490.

Taylor, V. M., J. C. Jackson, N. Chan, A. Kuniyuki, and Y. Yasui. 2002. Hepatitis B knowledge and practices among Cambodian American women in Seattle, Washington. *Journal of Community Health* 27(3):151-163.

Taylor, V. M., J. C. Jackson, M. Pineda, P. Pham, M. Fischer, and Y. Yasui. 2000. Hepatitis B knowledge among Vietnamese immigrants: Implications for prevention of hepatocellular carcinoma. *Journal of Cancer Education* 15(1):51-55.

Taylor, V. M., S. P. Tu, E. Woodall, E. Acorda, H. Chen, J. Choe, L. Li, Y. Yasui, and T. G. Hislop. 2006. Hepatitis B knowledge and practices among Chinese immigrants to the United States. *Asian Pacific Journal of Cancer Prevention* 7(2):313-317.

Taylor, V. M., Y. Yasui, N. Burke, J. H. Choe, E. Acorda, and J. C. Jackson. 2005b. Hepatitis B knowledge and testing among Vietnamese-American women. *Ethnicity and Disease* 15(4):761-767.

Taylor, V. M., Y. Yasui, N. Burke, T. Nguyen, A. Chen, E. Acorda, J. H. Choe, and J. C. Jackson. 2004. Hepatitis B testing among Vietnamese American men. *Cancer Detection and Prevention* 28(3):170-177.

Thompson, M. J., V. M. Taylor, J. C. Jackson, Y. Yasui, A. Kuniyuki, S. P. Tu, and T. G. Hislop. 2002. Hepatitis B knowledge and practices among Chinese American women in Seattle, Washington. *Journal of Cancer Education* 17(4):222-226.

Thompson, N. D., J. F. Perz, A. C. Moorman, and S. D. Holmberg. 2009. Nonhospital health care-associated hepatitis B and C virus transmission: United States, 1998-2008. *Annals of Internal Medicine* 150(1):33-39.

Trim, J. C. 2004. Raising awareness and reducing the risk of needlestick injuries. *Professional Nurse* 19(5):259-264.

Tsai, N. C., P. S. Holck, L. L. Wong, and A. A. Ricalde. 2008. Seroepidemiology of hepatitis B virus infection: Analysis of mass screening in Hawaii. *Hepatology International* 2(4):478-485.

Tucker, T., C. L. Fry, N. Lintzeris, S. Baldwin, A. Ritter, S. Donath, and G. Whelan. 2004. Randomized controlled trial of a brief behavioural intervention for reducing hepatitis C virus risk practices among injecting drug users. *Addiction* 99(9):1157-1166.

U.S. Preventive Services Task Force. 2009. Screening for hepatitis B virus infection in pregnancy: U.S. Preventive Services Task Force reaffirmation recommendation statement. *Annals of Internal Medicine* 150(12):869-873, W154.

Vallabhaneni, S., G. E. Macalino, S. E. Reinert, B. Schwartzapfel, F. A. Wolf, and J. D. Rich. 2004. Prisoners' attitudes toward hepatitis B vaccination. *Preventive Medicine* 38(6):828-833.

Ward, J. W. 2008. Time for renewed commitment to viral hepatitis prevention. *American Journal of Public Health* 98(5):779-781.

Wright, N. M., C. N. Tompkins, and L. Jones. 2005. Exploring risk perception and behaviour of homeless injecting drug users diagnosed with hepatitis C. *Health & Social Care in the Community* 13(1):75-83.

Wu, C. A., S. Y. Lin, S. K. So, and E. T. Chang. 2007. Hepatitis B and liver cancer knowledge and preventive practices among Asian Americans in the San Francisco bay area, California. *Asian Pacific Journal of Cancer Prevention* 8(1):127-134.

Zickmund, S., E. Y. Ho, M. Masuda, L. Ippolito, and D. R. LaBrecque. 2003. "They treated me like a leper." Stigmatization and the quality of life of patients with hepatitis C. *Journal of General Internal Medicine* 18(10):835-844.

Zola, J., E. M. Bachus, M. Bergin, T. Fang, and S. So. March 30-April 2, 2009. *San Francisco Hep B Free: A proactive approach to promoting hepatitis B immunization in conjunction with screening and care.* Poster presentation at the 43rd National Immunization Conference Dallas, Texas.

4

Immunization

Hepatitis B is a vaccine-preventable disease for which a safe and effective vaccine has been available for nearly three decades. The first part of this chapter reviews current federal vaccination recommendations and state vaccination requirements for hepatitis B. It also summarizes what is known about hepatitis B vaccination rates in specific populations (for example, infants, children, and adults, including subgroups of at-risk adults, such as incarcerated people and occupationally exposed people). The committee identified missed opportunities for hepatitis B vaccination and makes recommendations to increase the vaccination rate among various populations.

A vaccine for hepatitis C does not exist. The second part of this chapter summarizes current efforts to develop a hepatitis C vaccine and challenges that have been encountered. The committee makes a recommendation about hepatitis C vaccine development.

HEPATITIS B VACCINE

The first hepatitis B vaccine, a plasma-derived vaccine, was licensed by the US Food and Drug Administration (FDA) in 1981 (IOM, 1994). By the late 1980s, the plasma-derived vaccine was replaced with a recombinant version, which expresses the hepatitis B surface antigen (HBsAg) and is produced in *Saccharomyces cerevisiae* (common baker's yeast). The recombinant vaccine was licensed by FDA in 1986 and is the type of hepatitis B vaccine currently used in the United States. It is an anticancer vaccine: by preventing hepatitis B, it prevents hepatocellular carcinoma.

Hepatitis B vaccine is available both as single-antigen formulations and as multiantigen formulations in fixed combination with other vaccines (Mast et al., 2005). The two single-antigen vaccines are Recombivax HB® (Merck & Co., Inc., Whitehouse Station, NJ) and Engerix-B® (GlaxoSmithKline Biologicals, Rixensart, Belgium). Of the three licensed combination vaccines, Twinrix® (GlaxoSmithKline Biologicals, Rixensart, Belgium) is used for vaccination of adults, and Comvax® (Merck & Co., Inc., Whitehouse Station, NJ) and Pediarix® (GlaxoSmithKline Biologicals, Rixensart, Belgium) are used for vaccination of infants and young children. Twinrix contains recombinant HBsAg and inactivated hepatitis A virus. Comvax contains recombinant HBsAg and *Haemophilus influenzae* type b (Hib) polyribosylribitol phosphate conjugated to *Neisseria meningitidis* outer-membrane protein complex. Pediarix contains recombinant HBsAg, diphtheria and tetanus toxoids and acellular pertussis adsorbed (DTaP), and inactivated poliovirus.

The hepatitis B vaccine is administered in a three-dose series: two priming doses administered 1 month apart and a third dose administered 6 months after the second (Mast and Ward, 2008). Alternative schedules have been used successfully. Administration of the three-dose series results in protective concentrations of anti-HBs in more than 95% of healthy infants, children, and adolescents and in more than 90% of healthy adults aged 40 years old and younger. Immunogenicity drops below 90% in adults over the age of 40 years. The hepatitis B vaccine has a pre-exposure efficacy of 80–100% and a postexposure efficacy of 70–95%, depending on whether hepatitis B immune globulin (HBIG) is given with the vaccine. The duration of immunity appears to be long-lasting, and booster doses of the vaccine are not routinely recommended (Mast and Ward, 2008).

HBIG is derived from plasma and is used prophylactically to prevent infection with the hepatitis B virus (HBV). It provides passively acquired antibody to hepatitis B surface antigen (anti-HBsAg) and temporary protection (3–6 months). HBIG is typically used as an adjunct to hepatitis B vaccine for postexposure immunoprophylaxis to prevent HBV infection (Mast et al., 2005). HBIG administered alone is the primary means of protection after an HBV exposure for people who do not respond to hepatitis B vaccination. It is also used after liver transplantation for end-stage hepatitis B to prevent recurrence of the disease in the transplanted liver.

Current Vaccination Recommendations, Requirements, and Rates

The Advisory Committee on Immunization Practices (ACIP) provides advice and guidance to the US Department of Health and Human Services and the US Centers for Disease Control and Prevention (CDC) on the control of vaccine-preventable diseases. It develops written recommendations for the routine administration of vaccines to children and adults in the civilian population. The ACIP recommendations for who should receive the hepatitis B vaccine are summarized in Box 4-1. The American Academy of Pediatrics in its Report of the Committee on Infectious Diseases follows the ACIP recommendations for the hepatitis B vaccine (American Academy of Pediatrics, 2009).

Perinatal Vaccination

ACIP first recommended universal hepatitis B vaccination of infants in 1991 (ACIP, 1991). Despite the recommendation, each year about 1,000 newborns in the United States acquire chronic HBV infection (Ward, 2008), a number that has not declined in the last decade. That constitutes an important gap that needs to be addressed in future prevention efforts.

ACIP currently recommends that the first dose—that is, the birth dose—be administered before hospital discharge in infants born to HbsAg-negative women and within 12 hours of birth in infants born to women who are HbsAg-positive or of unknown status (Mast et al., 2005). It also recommends that infants born to HBsAg-positive mothers should be given HBIG within 12 hours of birth. There is no evidence of appreciable benefit if HBIG is administered more than 72 hours after birth. The timely identification of HBsAg-positive mothers to prevent perinatal transmission underscores the need for rapid hepatitis B tests (discussed further in Chapter 5). The hepatitis B vaccine series should be completed by the age of 18 months (see Table 4-1). Depending on which type of vaccine (single-antigen or combination) is administered, the series can consist of three or four vaccinations.

Current ACIP hepatitis B vaccine recommendations for preterm infants who weigh less than 2,000 g are summarized in Table 4-2. For preterm infants, the first dose of the vaccine is given within 12 hours of birth if the mother is HBsAg-positive or is of unknown status. If the mother is known to be HbsAg-negative, the first dose is administered at the age of 1 month or at hospital discharge (Mast et al., 2005). The preterm-infant schedule is based on the recognition that preterm infants have a decreased response to hepatitis B vaccine administered before the age of 1 month.

Data from National Immunization Surveys demonstrate that national newborn hepatitis B vaccination coverage did not change appreciably after implementation of the 2005 ACIP hepatitis B vaccination recommendation (CDC, 2009b). Using National Immunization Survey data that were collected before implementation of the 2005 ACIP hepatitis B vaccination recommendation, CDC estimated that the national newborn hepatitis B vaccination coverage was 46%, 47.9%, and 42.8% at the age of 1 day in the 2004, 2005, and 2006 surveys (CDC, 2008c, 2009b). Using data

> **BOX 4-1**
> **Summary of ACIP Hepatitis B Vaccination Recommendations**
>
> **Vaccination of infants**
>
> *At birth*
> - Infants born to mothers who are HbsAg-positive should receive hepatitis B vaccine and HBIG within 12 hours of birth.
> - Infants born to mothers whose HBsAg status is unknown should receive hepatitis B vaccine within 12 hours of birth. The mother should have blood drawn as soon as possible to determine her HBsAg status; if she is HbsAg-positive, the infant should receive HBIG as soon as possible (no later than the age of 1 week).
> - Full-term infants who are medically stable, weigh over 2,000 g, and are born to HBsAg-negative mothers should receive single-antigen hepatitis B vaccine before hospital discharge.
> - Preterm infants weighing less than 2,000 g and born to HbsAg-negative mothers should receive the first dose of vaccine 1 month after birth or at hospital discharge.
>
> *After the birth dose*
> - All infants should complete the hepatitis B vaccine series with either single-antigen vaccine or combination vaccine according to a recommended vaccination schedule.
> - Infants born to HBsAg-positive mothers should be tested for HBsAg and antibody to HBsAg after completion of the hepatitis B vaccine series at the age of 9–18 months.
>
> **Vaccination of children and adolescents**
> - All unvaccinated children and adolescents less than 19 years old should receive the hepatitis B vaccine series.

from the 2007 National Immunization Survey, which were collected after implementation of the 2005 ACIP recommendation, CDC estimates that the national newborn hepatitis B vaccine coverage was 46% at the age of 1 day (CDC, 2009b).

As noted above, despite the ACIP recommendation to vaccinate all newborns, about 1,000 newborns each year become chronically infected with HBV. Even with the ACIP recommendation, birth doses of the hepati-

Vaccination of adults

Persons at risk for infection by sexual exposure
- Sex partners of HbsAg-positive persons.
- Sexually active persons who are not in a long-term, mutually monogamous relationship (for example, persons with more than one sex partner during the previous 6 months).
- Persons seeking evaluation or treatment for a sexually transmitted disease.
- Men who have sex with men.

Persons at risk for infection by percutaneous or mucosal exposure to blood
- Current or recent injection-drug users.
- Household contacts of HBsAg-positive persons.
- Residents and staff of facilities for developmentally disabled persons.
- Health-care and public-safety workers who have a reasonably anticipated risk of exposure to blood or blood-contaminated body fluids.
- Persons with end-stage renal disease, including predialysis, hemodialysis, peritoneal-dialysis, and home-dialysis patients.
- Incarcerated persons.

Others
- International travelers to regions that have high or intermediate levels (HBsAg prevalence of at least 2%) of endemic HBV infection.
- Persons who have chronic liver disease.
- Persons who have HIV infection.
- All other persons who are seeking protection from HBV infection.

Abbreviations: ACIP, Advisory Committee on Immunization Practices; HBsAg, hepatitis B surface antigen; HBIG, hepatitis B immune globulin.
SOURCE: Adapted from Mast et al., 2005, 2006.

tis B vaccine are being missed or delayed, which the committee believes is due to the lack of a delivery-room policy for hepatitis B vaccination. Missing or delaying the birth dose for infants born to HBsAg-positive women substantially increases the risk that they will develop chronic hepatitis B. To reduce the incidence of perinatal HBV infections, the committee offers the following recommendation:

TABLE 4-1 Hepatitis B Vaccine Schedules for Newborns, by Maternal HBsAg Status—ACIP Recommendations

Maternal HbsAg Status	Single-Antigen (Stand-alone) Vaccine		Single Antigen (Stand-alone) + Combination Vaccine	
	Dose	Age	Dose	Age
Positive	1[a]	Birth (up to 12 hours)	1[a]	Birth (up to 12 hours)
	HBIG[b]	Birth (up to 12 hours)	HBIG	Birth (up to 12 hours)
	2	1–2 months	2	2 months
	3[c]	6 months	3	4 months
			4[c]	6 months (Pediarix) or 12–15 months (Comvax)
Unknown[d]	1[a]	Birth (up to 12 hours)	1[a]	Birth (up to 12 hours)
	2	1–2 months	2	2 months
	3[c]	6 months	3	4 months
			4[c]	6 months (Pediarix) or 12–15 months (Comvax)
Negative	1[a,e]	Birth (before discharge)	1[a,e]	Birth (before discharge)
	2	1–2 months	2	2 months
	3[c]	6–18 months	3	4 months
			4[c]	6 months (Pediarix) or 12–15 months (Comvax)

[a] Recombivax HB or Engerix-B should be used for the birth dose. Comvax and Pediarix cannot be administered at birth or before the age of 6 weeks.

[b] HBIG (0.5 mL) administered intramuscularly in a separate site from vaccine.

[c] Final dose in vaccine series should not be administered before the age of 24 weeks.

[d] Mothers should have blood drawn and tested for HBsAg as soon as possible after admission for delivery; if mother is found to be HbsAg-positive, infant should receive HBIG as soon as possible but no later than the age of 7 days.

[e] On a case-by-case basis and only in rare circumstances, first dose may be delayed until after hospital discharge for an infant who weighs ≤2,000 g and whose mother is HbsAg-negative, but only if physician's order to withhold birth dose and copy of mother's original HBsAg-negative laboratory report are documented in infant's medical record.

Abbreviations: HBsAg, hepatitis B surface antigen; ACIP, Advisory Committee on Immunization Practices; HBIG, hepatitis B immune globulin.
SOURCE: Mast et al., 2005.

IMMUNIZATION

TABLE 4-2 Hepatitis B Immunization Management of Preterm Infants Who Weigh Less Than 2,000 g, by Maternal HBsAg Status—ACIP Recommendations

Maternal HBsAg Status	Recommendation
Positive	HBIG + hepatitis B vaccine (within 12 hours of birth) Continue vaccine series beginning at age of 1–2 months according to recommended schedule for infants born to HBsAg-positive mothers (see Table 4-1) Do not count birth dose as part of vaccine series Test for HBsAg and antibody to HBsAg after completion of vaccine series at age of 9–18 months (that is, next well-child visit)
Unknown	HBIG + hepatitis B vaccine (within 12 hours of birth) Test mother for HBsAg Continue vaccine series beginning at age of 1–2 months according to recommended schedule based on mother's HBsAg result (see Table 4-1) Do not count birth dose as part of vaccine series
Negative	Delay first dose of hepatitis B vaccine until age of 1 month or hospital discharge Complete vaccine series (see Table 4-1)

Abbreviations: ACIP, Advisory Committee on Immunization Practices; HBIG, hepatitis B immune globulin; HBsAg, hepatitis B surface antigen.
SOURCE: Mast et al., 2005.

Recommendation 4-1. All infants weighing at least 2,000 grams and born to hepatitis B surface antigen-positive women should receive single-antigen hepatitis B vaccine and hepatitis B immune globulin in the delivery room as soon as they are stable and washed. The recommendations of the Advisory Committee on Immunization Practices should remain in effect for all other infants.

Administration of prophylaxis in the delivery room is not novel. In the United States, vitamin K prophylaxis for vitamin K–deficiency bleeding and tetracycline or erythromycin for prophylaxis of neonatal gonococcal infections are routinely given to infants in the delivery room (American Academy of Pediatrics, 1961, 1980; Workowski and Berman, 2006). The World Health Organization recommends that the birth dose of the hepatitis B vaccine be administered as soon after birth as possible (WHO, 2006). A pilot project in The Lao People's Democratic Republic demonstrated almost 100% coverage when the hepatitis B vaccine was administered in the delivery room (WHO, 2006). When mothers were asked to take their newborns to a vaccination room for their hepatitis B vaccine birth dose, vaccine coverage was low.

Childhood Vaccination

ACIP recommends that unvaccinated children and adults under 19 years old be given the hepatitis B vaccine series (Mast et al., 2005). Studies have found racial and ethnic disparities in childhood vaccination rates: Asian and Pacific Islander (API), Hispanic, and black children had lower vaccination rates than non-Hispanic white children (CDC, 2000; Darling et al., 2005; Jenkins et al., 2000; Morita et al., 2008; Szilagyi et al., 2002). However, when poverty was controlled for, the estimates did not remain significantly lower for any racial or ethnic population than for non-Hispanic white children (CDC, 2009c).

Studies have also found geographic variability in vaccination coverage (Darling et al., 2005; Morita et al., 2008; Szilagyi et al., 2002). The disparities are seen state by state and within regions. For instance, in 2008, Maryland had the highest percentage of children who were up to date[1] on their vaccinations with a rate of 82.3%, compared with Montana with a rate of 59.2% (CDC, 2009c). Szilagyi et al. (2002) looked at the use of reminder and recall interventions by primary-care providers to increase immunization rates for children under 2 years old. Before the intervention, the baseline geographic disparity was an 18% difference between inner-city children (55%) and suburban children (73%). Within 3 years of the establishment of the intervention, the vaccination rates had increased in all areas, including 84% in the inner city and 88% in the suburbs.

All but three states—Alabama, Montana, and South Dakota—have a childhood hepatitis B vaccination mandate for daycare or school entry (Immunization Action Coalition, 2009). A retrospective cohort study of Chicago public-school children found that the hepatitis B vaccination school-entry mandate led to an increase in the vaccination rate among all children and substantially decreased the disparity in the vaccination rate between white children and black and Hispanic children (Morita et al., 2008). Before the school-entry mandate, the study found immunizations rates in non-Hispanic white, black, and Hispanic children of 89%, 76%, and 74%, respectively. After the mandate was enacted, the rates changed to

---

[1] The immunization series used in these data includes the following vaccinations—4 or more doses of DTaP, 3 or more doses of poliovirus vaccine, 1 or more dose of any measles-containing vaccine, 3 or more doses of Hib vaccine, 3 or more doses of hepatitis B vaccine, as well as 1 or more dose of varicella vaccine (CDC, 2009c).

88%, 81%, and 87%, respectively. Although a disparity in the vaccinations rates persisted, the gap was narrowed (Szilagyi et al., 2002).

Other studies also have found that school-entry mandates are effective in increasing hepatitis B vaccination rates (CDC, 2001b; Koff, 2000; Olshen et al., 2007; Zimet et al., 2008) although such mandates may not be as effective in children in daycare (Stanwyck et al., 2004). CDC (2007) found that about 75% of states reported at least 95% hepatitis B vaccination coverage of children in kindergarten in 2006-2007. Another study reported that hepatitis B vaccine series coverage for children 19-35 months old in 2000-2002 ranged from 49% to 82%, depending on the state (Luman et al., 2005).

Special attention needs to be given to vaccination coverage of foreign-born children from countries that have a high prevalence of hepatitis B; because of their high risk of prior infection, laboratory testing is indicated to determine HBV-infection status.

Recommendation 4-2. All states should mandate that the hepatitis B vaccine series be completed or in progress as a requirement for school attendance.

Parents of foreign-born children from HBV-endemic countries should be given information about testing for HBV and should have their children tested before vaccination.

Adult Vaccination

Hepatitis B vaccination for adults is recommended to high-risk populations—people at risk for HBV infection from infected household contacts and sex partners, from occupational exposure to infected blood or body fluids, and from travel to regions with high or intermediate levels of endemic HBV infection (Mast et al., 2006). The estimated chance that an acute HBV infection will become chronic decreases with increasing age (see Table 4-3). The probability that an acute HBV infection in a 1-year-old will become chronic is 88.5%, but only 9.0% in a 19-year-old (Edmunds et al., 1993). Universal hepatitis B vaccination for adults is not recommended (that is, people born before 1991 do not need to receive the hepatitis B vaccine unless they are at risk for HBV infection). It is not cost-effective; that is, the health benefits achieved do not justify the cost compared with other potential health-care interventions (Gold et al., 1996). Interventions in the United States that cost less than $100,000 per quality adjusted life year (QALY) gained are generally considered to be cost-effective (Owens, 1998; WHO, 2009). Universal hepatitis B vaccination is not cost-effective even in adult Asians and Pacific Islanders, who have a higher prevalence of HBV

TABLE 4-3 Estimated Chance That an Acute Hepatitis B Infection Becomes Chronic with Age

Age (years)	Estimated Chance That Acute HBV Infection Becomes Chronic (%)
1	88.5
2	52.5
3	41.3
4	34.6
5	29.8
6	26.1
7	23.3
8	20.9
9	19.0
10	17.3
11	15.9
12	14.7
13	13.6
14	13.0
15	11.7
16	11.0
17	10.3
18	9.6
19	9.0

NOTE: Calculated using a formula from Edmunds et al., 1993.

infection than the general US population (Hutton et al., 2007). However, ring vaccination—vaccination of the close contacts of people found to be chronically infected with HBV—is cost-effective (Hutton et al., 2007).

Figure 4-1 shows estimated cost effectiveness of hepatitis B vaccination for different age groups and different incidences of acute hepatitis B. The leftmost line of the graph represents a recent estimate of acute HBV incidence in the general US population (Hutton et al., 2007). This estimate is expressed as the annual percentage of people in the population who acquire acute HBV infection. At that incidence, hepatitis B vaccination of adults in the general US population costs more than $100,000 per QALY gained, and is not considered to be cost-effective.

In 2004, just over half (54.6%) the adults at high risk for HBV infection had received the hepatitis B vaccine, including about 75% of health-care workers and 64% of public-safety workers for whom vaccination is recommended (CDC, 2006; Simard et al., 2007). Of adults with acute hepatitis B, 61% reported having missed an opportunity for vaccination (Williams et al., 2005). Low coverage of high-risk adults is attributed to the lack of dedicated vaccine programs, limited vaccine supply, inadequate funding, and noncompliance by the involved populations (Mast et al., 2006).

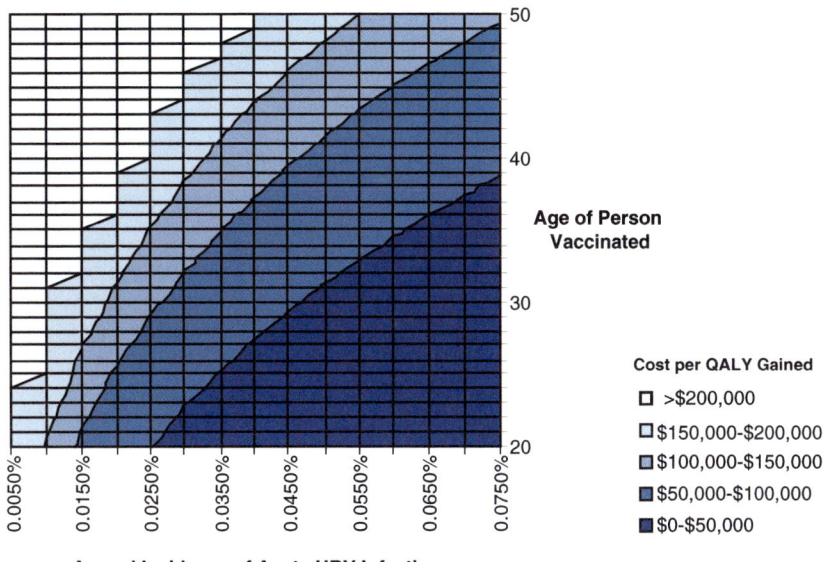

FIGURE 4-1 Estimated cost of adult hepatitis B vaccination per quality adjusted life year (QALY) gained for different age groups and different rates of acute hepatitis B virus (HBV) infection incidence. Incidence is expressed as the annual percentage of the population becoming acutely infected with HBV (for example, incidence of 0.005% means that 5 persons per 100,000 are acutely infected with HBV each year, and incidence of 0.075% means that 75 persons per 100,000 are acutely infected with HBV each year). Shadings show different levels of cost per QALY gained. Interventions are more cost-effective as one moves down (lower age) and to the right (higher incidence). Interventions that cost less than approximately $100,000 per QALY gained are generally considered cost-effective in the United States (Owens, 1998; WHO, 2009). The leftmost line, incidence of 0.0050%, is based on a recent estimate of acute hepatitis B incidence in the general US population (Hutton et al., 2007). Analysis performed by D. Hutton using the model developed in Hutton et al., 2007.

Adults at Risk from Sexual Exposure In a national sample of 500 sexually-transmitted-disease (STD) clinics, the percentage that offered the hepatitis B vaccine increased from 25% to 45% (p = 0.02) from 1997 to 2001, and the percentage of the clinics that considered all patients eligible for the vaccine rose from 9% to 26% (p = 0.023) during the same period (Gilbert et al., 2005). However, declining hepatitis B vaccination rates were reported in a study of six STD clinics in the United States (Harris et al., 2007). The researchers collected data on patient visits and hepatitis B vaccinations for the period 1997–2005 and found that vaccination rates declined during the later years. Possible reasons for the decline include fiscal constraints and increasing rates of prior vaccination.

Several studies have reported that when STD clinics offered the hepatitis B vaccine, many patients at high risk for HBV infection opted to be vaccinated. A study of 194 STD clinic patients found that 62% had not previously been vaccinated for hepatitis B, and 50% of the 62% elected to receive the vaccination (Samoff et al., 2004). A national program to vaccinate adults at STD clinics for hepatitis B is likely to be cost saving to society (Miriti et al., 2008). In an anonymous HIV-testing program in Madison, WI, 86% of patients were considered to be at high risk for HBV infection; 51% of the 86% initiated hepatitis B vaccination, and 80% who initiated vaccination completed the vaccine series (Savage et al., 2000).

Foreign-born people from HBV-endemic countries who reside in the United States are at risk for HBV infection from sexual exposures. Continuing sexual transmission of HBV in these communities is likely. Thus, foreign-born adults may be at high risk for acquiring hepatitis B, and women may transmit the virus to their newborns. Foreign-born adults would benefit from laboratory testing to determine their infection status and subsequent hepatitis B vaccination of susceptible people.

Adults at Risk from Injection-Drug Use CDC estimates that injection-drug users (IDUs) account for 15% of acute HBV infections in the United States (Daniels et al., 2009). The incidence of HBV infection in susceptible IDUs ranges from 10 to 30 per 100 person-years (Des Jarlais et al., 2003; Hagan et al., 1999). Hepatitis B vaccine coverage rates in IDUs are low and estimated to be 3–20% (Altice et al., 2005; Kuo et al., 2004; Lum et al., 2008) (see Table 4-4). The highest reported vaccination rate in US IDUs was 22%, in new injectors studied in 2000–2002 (Lum et al., 2003). In a study conducted in San Francisco, only 13% of IDUs over 30 years old had ever been offered hepatitis B vaccination compared with 25% of younger injectors (Seal et al., 2000).

On-site hepatitis B vaccination achieves higher success rates in IDUs than referral to other locations (summarized in Table 4-4). In a multisite study of IDUs in five US cities, IDUs participating in a randomized clinical trial to reduce HIV and HCV transmission were offered hepatitis B vaccination under a variety of conditions. Vaccine uptake was highest when it was provided on site and during the initial study visit (Campbell et al., 2007). A New Haven mobile health van at a needle-exchange program found that 66% of those initially offered the hepatitis B vaccine completed all three doses (Altice et al., 2005). Des Jarlais et al. (2001) reported a 31% completion rate in Alaskan IDUs given an off-site referral compared with 83% in

IDUs offered on-site vaccination and a $5–10 incentive at a New York City needle-exchange program.

The committee believes that the hepatitis B vaccination rate in the high-risk IDU population is unacceptably low. Studies of vaccine protocols show that completion rates are substantially higher when vaccination is offered at such a location as a needle-exchange program. Using a modeling approach, Hu et al. (2008) found that hepatitis B vaccination of IDUs who participate in needle-exchange programs in the United States is likely to be cost-saving to society.

Incarcerated Populations Hennessey et al. (2009) reported that only 12% of inmates at three jails in Chicago, Detroit, and San Francisco had serologic evidence of hepatitis B vaccination compared with a 25% self-reported vaccination rate in the US population. The study also found an unexpectedly high rate of chronic hepatitis B infections (3.6%) and the lowest rate of hepatitis B vaccination (10%) among Hispanic inmates.

Twenty states require that inmates receive at least some immunizations, including the hepatitis B vaccine (CDC, 2008a). Four of those states require vaccination of all inmates, and 16 require only that juvenile inmates be vaccinated. Several studies reported that if offered the hepatitis B vaccine, most inmates (60–93%) would agree to be vaccinated (Rotily et al., 1997; Vallabhaneni et al., 2004). Alternative vaccination schedules may be effective for inmates. In a study of inmates in Denmark, 63% completed the hepatitis B vaccination series on an accelerated 3-week schedule compared with 20% of those on a 6-month schedule (Christensen et al., 2004).

According to CDC, 28.8% of patients who had acute hepatitis B reported a history of incarceration before HBV infection (Goldstein et al., 2002). Thus, immunization of incarcerated people could potentially prevent nearly one-third of all acute hepatitis B cases in the United States. Although most prison systems in the United States do not provide universal hepatitis B vaccination for inmates, Charuvastra et al. (2001) noted that 25 of 26 states that responded to a survey reported that they would routinely vaccinate their inmates against HBV infection if funding for vaccination were available.

Although the length of stay is shorter in jails than in prisons, offering hepatitis B vaccination to jail inmates is feasible and provides a benefit to the community after the inmates are released. Using an accelerated schedule increases the completion rate (Christensen et al., 2004). Substantial protection is provided after even one or two of the three doses of the series. It is important to have a health-record system that tracks immunizations so that the vaccine series can be continued if later incarcerations occur. Ideally, immunizations administered in jails will be captured in an adult immunization registry (see discussion on immunization-information systems below) so

TABLE 4-4 Studies of Hepatitis B Vaccination Rates in Injection-Drug Users

Reference	Location	Sample; Design
Cross-sectional studies of vaccination rates		
Seal et al., 2000	San Francisco, CA	135 under 30 years old, 96 at least 30 years old
		Cross-sectional
Lum et al., 2008	San Francisco, CA	831 young IDUs
		Cross-sectional
Kuo et al., 2004	Baltimore, MD	324 IDUs, NIDUs
		Cross-sectional
Additional vaccination studies		
Campbell et al., 2007	5 US cities	3,181
		Cohort; vaccination protocol varied by city
Altice et al., 2005	New Haven, CT; mobile health van at SEP	134 HBV-negative IDUs
		Observational
Des Jarlais et al., 2001	Anchorage, AK; New York City	AK cohort referred to clinic (350); New York City cohort offered on-site vaccination at SEP (36) + small cash incentives
		Cohort
Hutchinson et al., 2004	Glasgow, Scotland, prison vaccination, community assessment	In 1999, offered HBV vaccination to all inmates; surveyed new injectors (within 5 years)

Abbreviations: HBV, hepatitis B virus; IDU, injection-drug user; NIDU, non-injection-drug user; SEP, syringe-exchange program.

Percentage Previously Vaccinated	Percentage Ever Offered Vaccination	Percentage Completed Vaccination Series
	25% under 30 years old, 13% at least 30 years old	
22%; 18% among HCV positive		
10% IDUs; 14% NIDUs		
		Vaccination highest where available on site (83% had at least one dose); incentives did not affect vaccination rates
3%		94% had one dose; 77% had two doses; 66% had three doses 30/36 (83%) offered on site had all three doses vs 31% of those referred to clinic
1993, 16% 1994, 19% 1999, 15% 2002, 52% (56% received hepatitis B vaccine while in prison)		

that the vaccine series can be completed at other sites, such as drug-treatment centers and STD clinics.

Hepatitis B vaccination of inmates costs the correctional system $415 per HBV infection averted, but it provides additional postincarceration savings to society as a whole (Pisu et al., 2002).

Other At-Risk Adults

HIV-infected people. At a clinic that serves primarily HIV-infected patients in Jacksonville, FL, 45% of 1,576 HIV-infected patients were considered to be at risk for HBV infection (Bailey et al., 2008), and 30% of those at risk were not offered hepatitis B vaccine by their health-care providers. Routine hepatitis B vaccination at HIV clinics is highly cost-effective, with a cost of $4,400 per QALY gained (Kim et al., 2006). Similarly, hepatitis B vaccination at STD testing, counseling, and treatment sites has been demonstrated to be highly cost-effective (Miriti et al., 2008).

Institutionalized populations. Vellinga et al. (1999) reviewed the literature and reported that among institutionalized developmentally disabled people in the United States, the prevalence of anti-HBs antibody ranged from 36% to 63% in residents who had Down syndrome and from 48% to 69% in people who had other intellectual disabilities. HBsAg prevalence was very high—27–51% in people who had Down syndrome and 6–9% in people who had other intellectual disabilities—and this suggests that many residents of institutions are immunized by natural infection rather than by vaccination. The committee did not find data on rates of hepatitis B vaccination of institutionalized developmentally disabled people. Because they are at risk for hepatitis B, they would benefit from vaccination.

Occupational exposure to hepatitis B virus. Only 75% of health-care workers (HCWs) in the United States—a population at high risk for HBV infection—have received the three-dose vaccine series in 2002-2003 (Simard et al., 2007). The vaccination rate was highest in physicians and nurses (81%) and lowest among black HCWs (67.6%).

Identifying At-Risk Adults

As discussed above, recommendations regarding childhood hepatitis B vaccination are aimed at achieving universal coverage, and recommendations regarding adult vaccination focus on the identification of risk populations for targeted immunization efforts. The identification of at-risk adults has proved problematic (CDC, 2006), and current CDC recommendations have emphasized both site-based and individual-based risk assessment to improve hepatitis B vaccine coverage (Mast et al., 2006). A key to the success of such an approach is the routine availability of hepatitis B vaccine in settings where a high proportion of persons who have risk factors are seen (such as STD clinics), in primary-care and specialty-care medical settings, and in occupational-health programs.

Identification of at-risk people is particularly challenging in medical settings in that risks must be assessed in individual patients. In many health-care settings, physicians and other providers might not be comfortable in asking direct questions to elicit risk history with respect to sexual or percutaneous exposures (Ashton et al., 2002; Bull et al., 1999; Maheux et al., 1995). Time constraints during medical appointments and inadequate provider education in the assessment of risk histories also might lead to insufficient assessment of risk history. In addition, there may be discrepancies between a patient's self-assessment of risk and a health-care provider's documented assessment (Fishbein et al., 2006). Therefore, the ACIP recommends that hepatitis B vaccination be offered to any adult who requests it, regardless of a provider's assessment of risk (Mast et al., 2006).

Recommendation

In 2007, there were more than 40,000 new acute HBV infections in adults (Daniels et al., 2009). To reduce the incidence of HBV infection in adults, the committee offers the following recommendation:

Recommendation 4-3. Additional federal and state resources should be devoted to increasing hepatitis B vaccination of at-risk adults.

- Correctional institutions should offer hepatitis B vaccination to all incarcerated persons. Accelerated schedules for vaccine administration should be considered for jail inmates.
- Organizations that serve high-risk people should offer the hepatitis B vaccination series.
- Efforts should be made to improve identification of at-risk adults. Health-care providers should routinely seek risk histories from adult patients through direct questioning and self-assessment.
- Efforts should be made to increase rates of completion of the vaccine series in adults.
- Federal and state agencies should determine gaps in hepatitis B vaccine coverage among at-risk adults annually and estimate the resources needed to fill the gaps.

Immunization-Information Systems

Immunization registries are databases that allow the collection and consolidation of vaccination data from multiple health-care providers. They also make it possible to generate reminder and recall notifications and assess vaccination coverage in defined geographic areas. Immunization-information systems (IISs) are registries that have additional capabilities, such as vaccine management, adverse-event reporting, lifespan vaccination histories, and linkages with electronic data (CDC, 2005). According to a report of the National Vaccine Advisory Committee (NVAC), IISs have been demonstrated to improve immunization coverage, support vaccine safety, increase timeliness of immunization, and help in the study of immunization effectiveness in children (Hinman et al., 2007). IISs can also prevent unnecessary immunizations by giving providers a single source for patients' immunization histories (Yawn et al., 1998), reduce "no-show" rates, reduce vaccine waste, save staff costs by avoiding manual review of multiple records, aid in the establishment of Healthcare Effectiveness Data and Information Set (HEDIS) performance measures, and avoid costs associated with the National Immunization Survey (NIS) (Bartlett et al., 2007).

The development of IISs began in 1993 when CDC started to award planning grants to develop registries in every state (CDC, 2001a). President Clinton established the national Childhood Immunization Initiative by directing the secretary of health and human services to work with states to build "an integrated immunization registry system." That initiative led to the Initiative on Immunization Registries, which was spearheaded by the NVAC with support from CDC's National Immunization Program and the Department of Health and Human Services National Vaccine Program Office (Bartlett et al., 2007). Since 1994, CDC's National Center for Immunization and Respiratory Diseases (formerly the National Immunization Program) has provided funding to 64 grantees (all 50 states, 6 cities, and the US territories) through Section 317 of the Public Health Service Act for the development of IISs. From 1994 through 2001, $181.3 million was allocated by CDC, and an additional $20 million was provided by the Robert Wood Johnson Foundation (CDC, 2001a). Only one state had reported no efforts to develop and implement an IIS as of December 31, 2005 (Hinman et al., 2007). However, three other states did not report to CDC in 2005 the percentage of children younger than 6 years old who participated in an IIS, and this might indicate inadequacy of IISs in those states.

CDC has indicated a commitment to support the continued development and expansion of state and community IISs (CDC, 2008b) and has a goal of including more than 95% of children under 6 years old in grantee IISs by 2010. To address wide variation in the performance of IISs nationally, CDC required detailed business plans from grantees in 2006 to describe operational and financial objectives of the systems. In addition, a technical work group was established to develop approaches to measuring performance of the systems against 12 functional standards (Hinman et al., 2007). There are also plans to develop an IIS certification process.

As the state and community IISs develop, they are increasingly used for broader purposes, such as emergency preparedness and response (Boom et al., 2007), monitoring the impact of vaccine shortages (Allred et al., 2006), and monitoring the use of new vaccines. There have also been calls to integrate IISs with other child-information systems—such as vital registration, newborn dried-blood spot screening, and early hearing detection and intervention (Saarlas et al., 2004)—and to expand the systems to include adolescents and adults. The NVAC reported that as of 2005, 87% of CDC grantees included adolescents in their IISs, and 75% included information on persons 50 years old and older (Hinman et al., 2007).

In 2009, the NVAC issued new recommendations for federal adult immunization programs (HHS, 2009).One recommendation was that CDC and the Health Resources and Services Administration (HRSA) devote resources to the inclusion of adult immunization records in all grantee IISs, and another was that all grantees be required to implement adult immunization activities and adopt ACIP recommendations for routine adult immunization.

> **Recommendation 4-4. States should be encouraged to expand immunization-information systems to include adolescents and adults.**
>
> - Systems should allow the sharing of information between states so that immunization status can be tracked when people move from state to state.
> - Vaccine registries should include adult populations, such as incarcerated persons, IDUs, and people who have STDs.
> - Data sharing on vaccination status should be established between correctional facilities and public-health departments.

Barriers to Hepatitis B Vaccination

Mistrust of Vaccination

Like other childhood vaccinations, hepatitis B vaccination is sometimes refused because patients or parents of children have concerns about the safety of a vaccine (Allred et al., 2005; Gust et al., 2008; Smith et al., 2006a). The committee is unaware of credible evidence of serious harms caused by the hepatitis B vaccine in its many forms. In a 2002 scientific review by the Institute of Medicine, the hepatitis B vaccine was not found to be associated with adverse health outcomes (IOM, 2002). The committee believes that it is one of the safest vaccines available. The efforts of groups opposed to vaccination present a serious obstacle to comprehensive vaccination coverage, which is essential for the prevention and control of hepatitis B in the United States.

Payment for Vaccines

Insurance Coverage

Health-insurance coverage for the nonelderly population (less than 65 years old) is provided by employers (63%) and public programs (11% by the Medicaid/Children's Health Insurance Program and 2% by other public programs) or is acquired by individuals in the private market (5%) (Holahan and Cook, 2008). Some 17% of Americans under 65 years old were reported as chronically uninsured in 2007, but as many as one-third of Americans were uninsured for at least some of the time in 2007-2008 (Families USA, 2009b). Robust coverage for vaccinations, including hepatitis B vaccination, is provided by public insurance plans (Table 4-5). Private insurance plans have variable coverage for vaccinations and various degrees of cost-sharing. Insurance coverage for vaccinations also varies substantially with age: children under 5 years old and people 65 years old and over have high rates of private or public coverage (89% and nearly 100%, respectively). People 18-64 years old have much lower rates (50%) because of lack of insurance, inadequate insurance, and the absence of a public safety net for recommended adult vaccinations (IOM, 2003).

Insurance coverage has been demonstrated to have an important impact on access to preventive and other health services and on health outcomes (IOM, 2009). Studies in children involving various vaccine series, including hepatitis B vaccine, and in adults transitioning to Medicare have shown notable increases in vaccination rates in those with insurance coverage (IOM, 2009). In an NIS sample of children 19-24 months old, recommended vaccination completion rates were found in 76% of the children covered by private insurance, 70% of the children covered by Medicaid or the Children's Health Insurance Program (CHIP), and 53% of uninsured children (Smith et al., 2006b).

Public Vaccine Programs and Insurance

Vaccines for Children program. Children with no private insurance may be covered up to the age of 18 years by the Vaccines for Children (VFC) program administered by CDC (CDC, 2003). The VFC program was created by the Omnibus Budget Reconciliation Act of 1993 as a new entitlement program to be a required part of each state's Medicaid plan. The program began in October 1994. The Office of Management and Budget approves funding for the VFC program. Funding is through the Centers for Medicare and Medicaid Services to CDC, and awards are made to eligible grantees. The VFC program provides a vaccination entitlement for Medicaid-eligible, uninsured, American Indian and Alaska Native, and underinsured children who receive vaccines at federally qualified health centers (FQHCs). The VFC program negotiates vaccine prices at the federal level and allocates credits to states to distribute vaccines free of charge. The program does not cover any of the practice-based costs associated with the administration of the vaccines. Payment for vaccine administration is generally sought from specific insurance programs, such as Medicaid, or from parents of VFC-eligible, non-Medicaid children (CDC, 2003).

Section 317 Immunization Grant program. The Section 317 Immunization Grant Program is a federal discretionary grants program for states and other US jurisdictions (CDC, 2009d). It was established by the 1962 Vaccination Assistance Act and was the primary source of federal funds for vaccine purchase until it was supplanted by the VFC program in 1993. Unlike the VFC program, Section 317 provides federal funds for both vaccine purchase and vaccine-related infrastructure, such as population needs assessments, surveillance, compliance monitoring, training, and school-based delivery systems. The program targets immunization coverage for underinsured children and youths not eligible for the VFC program and to a small degree uninsured and underinsured adults. In 2007, CDC created the Adult Hepatitis B Vaccine Initiative by using savings from Section 317 funds to provide free vaccine for high-risk adults in various community settings. Funding for vaccine costs totaled $36 million in the first 2 years; this resulted in the delivery of over 581,000 doses, 343,000 of which reportedly were administered. The initiative involves 56 grantees that enroll 2,437 sites, of which 38% are local health departments, 20% STD clinics, 13% primary-care loci, 11% jails or prisons, and 18% other sites, including substance-abuse and HIV centers (personal communication, J. Ward, CDC, July 30, 2009). However, Section 317 funding for adult vaccination initiatives does not support the infrastructure and medical-supply costs to deliver vaccines to people at highest risk.

Children's Health Insurance Program. The federal CHIP was established in 1997 under Title IX of the Social Security Act and was expanded in the Children's Health Insurance Program Reauthorization Act of 2009 (CMS, 2009). It is a federal block-grant program that requires state matching funds to expand health-care coverage to children under 18 years old and pregnant women who do not meet income eligibility requirements for

TABLE 4-5 Public Health-Insurance Plans

	Coverage	Medical Management
US Department of Veterans Affairs 7.9 million beneficiaries	Hepatitis B, hepatitis C	Dedicated hepatitis program
FEHBP 8 million beneficiaries	Hepatitis B, hepatitis C	Coverage similar to private plans
MEDICARE Parts A, B, C, D 49 million beneficiaries	Hepatitis B, hepatitis C	Yes
MEDICAID, EPSDT 43 million beneficiaries	Hepatitis B, hepatitis C	Yes
VFC	Hepatitis B	No
SECTION 317 Immunization Program	Hepatitis B	No
CHIP 7.4 million child, 334,000 adult beneficiaries	Hepatitis B	Yes

[a]Household income limitations apply.

[b]Covers children under 6 years old and pregnant women whose family income is no more than 133% of federal poverty level and children 6–18 years old below 100% of federal poverty level.

Abbreviations: EPSDT, Early Periodic Screening, Diagnosis, and Treatment program; FEHBP, Federal Employees Health Benefits Program; VFC, Vaccines for Children; CHIP, Children's Health Insurance Program.

Vaccination	Target Audience	Cost Structure
100%	Veterans[a]	No cost-sharing except for non-service-connected veterans
Coverage similar to private plans	Federal employees	Coverage similar to private plans
High-risk group coverage	People at least 65 years old, disabled, people with end-stage renal disease	Coinsurance or copayment applies only after yearly deductible has been met
Yes	Low-income people, families with children, SSI recipients, pregnant women[b]	States have option to impose nominal copayment for beneficiaries on basis of income
Yes	Children up to 18 years old who are uninsured, Medicaid-eligible, underinsured, American Indians, Alaska Natives	Covers cost of vaccines but not administration; providers can charge administration fee for non–Medicaid-eligible children
Yes	Children, adolescents not served by VFC program; small percentage (about 5%) used for adults	Can be used for infrastructure; annual appropriations vary
Yes	Insurance benefits for children up to 18 years old (for families making no more than $44,100/year) whose income is too high for Medicaid, too low for private insurance	Block grant program: federal match more than Medicaid match

Medicaid but cannot afford private health insurance. CHIP is available to citizens and some legal immigrants, and states can charge a premium for coverage and impose cost-sharing based on income. States have the option of using the grant money to establish independent insurance programs or to expand eligibility criteria for Medicaid; in the latter case, the coverage must conform to Medicaid requirements. Currently, 39 states have programs that are not expansions of Medicaid. Non-Medicaid CHIP programs must provide coverage for ACIP-recommended immunizations, including hepatitis B, and must meet a federally established minimal overall coverage.

Public programs for adults. Nonelderly adults have more limited access to publicly funded vaccination programs and public insurance benefits than children. Adults enrolled in Medicaid make up 25% of enrollees and are provided coverage for vaccinations, but the coverage varies between states. Most states provide coverage based on ACIP standards, including hepatitis B immunization. However, cost-sharing is common, and payment of providers varies from fixed-fee schedules, which allow separate billing for vaccine administration (Rosenbaum et al., 2003). Elderly adults covered under Medicare and enrolled in Medicare Part B are covered for hepatitis B vaccination if they fall into ACIP-designated high-risk or intermediate-risk populations. The Medicare Part B deductible must be met, and the relevant copayment or coinsurance is applicable to the hepatitis B coverage (CMS, 2008).

Federal law generally restricts coverage for adults under CHIP to pregnant women but does permit coverage of adults without dependent children under special waivers from the federal government. Eleven states are providing coverage to low-income adults under such waivers. The 2009 CHIP reauthorization act will phase out funding for such waivers by 2011 and thereby eliminate this public source of adult-vaccination coverage (Families USA, 2009a). Public Health Service Section 317 grants amounted to $527 million in 2008 and allow vaccination coverage for uninsured and underinsured adults. Nearly all the money, however, was used for vaccinating children and youths. In 2005, it was reported that less than 5% of Section 317 funding was used for adult-vaccination efforts (Mootrey, 2007).

Private Insurance Plans

Employers provide over 66% of all health insurance for 177 million Americans under the age of 65 years (U.S. Census Bureau, 2007). Trends in private health-insurance coverage have reflected a shift from comprehensive coverage with low out-of-pocket costs (health maintenance organizations, HMOs) to broader access, network-driven, and higher-cost–sharing health plans (preferred provider organization, PPOs) (Figure 4-2). The latter offer free choice of providers and hospitals but require out-of-pocket spending (deductibles) by the consumer before coverage under the plan, cost-sharing when the plan does provide coverage (flat dollar copayments or coinsurance payments), and different levels of coverage for the same service when acquired in-network versus out-of-network. PPO insurance arrangements now cover more than 58% of all persons who have employment-based health insurance (Figure 4-2).

Coverage for hepatitis B and other ACIP-recommended vaccinations is routine in HMOs but variable in PPOs and other private insurance plans. There is little or no cost-sharing for vaccinations and other preventive services in HMOs, whereas it is greater in PPOs and other health plans because of applicable deductibles and coinsurance or copayments. Cost-sharing is greatest in health plans that have very high deductibles (high-deductible health plans, HDHPs). In 2008, 8% of all privately insured Americans were covered by HDHPs with annual deductibles of $1,000 or more (Kaiser Family Foundation and HRET, 2008). HDHPs can pose formidable barriers to preventive care and vaccination unless these services are specifically exempted from the deductible or enrollees are provided a separate source of funds to pay for them (for example, a reimbursement arrangement or a

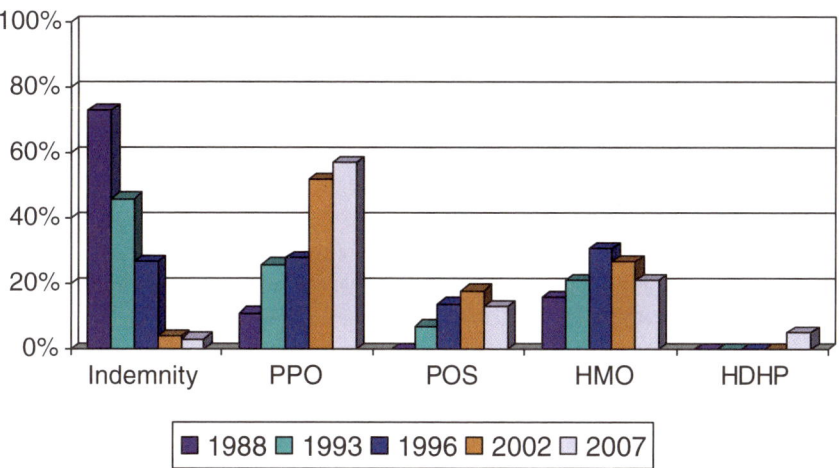

FIGURE 4-2 Trends in private health-insurance coverage.
Abbreviations: PPO, preferred provider organization; POS, point of service; HMO, health maintenance organization; HDHP, high-deductible health plan.
SOURCES: HIAA, 1988; Kaiser Family Foundation and HRET, 2008; KPMG, 1996.

funded health savings account). To ensure vaccination coverage for children under private insurance arrangements, most states have mandates for childhood immunizations. The regulations may also prohibit cost-sharing in the form of deductibles or coinsurance for those services (American Academy of Pediatrics, 2008). State mandates for recommended adult vaccinations are less common. Employers that use national health plans are exempted from the state mandates because their health-benefit plans operate under the federal Employee Retirement Security Act which pre-empts state laws that govern these plans.

Gaps and Barriers

Coverage for hepatitis B vaccination and other ACIP-recommended vaccinations is greater for children and youths than for adults. Federal and state funding for hepatitis B vaccination and other vaccinations provides a safety net for the poorest children and youths, but no such program, such as an adult version of the VFC program, exists for uninsured or underinsured adults. Public Health Section 317 provides a potential vehicle for filling that void, but funding has been increased only modestly since 2003 (Rodewald, 2008), and only recently has adult hepatitis B vaccination become a target for some of the Section 317 funds. CDC has reported to Congress that it would take about $1.6 billion—or 3 times the amount of current Section 317 funding—to fill gaps in coverage and support to states to provide a rigorous national vaccination program for children, adolescents, and adults, including $335 million for payments to providers for all vaccine administration (CDC, 2009d). In that report, CDC included only $49 million for hepatitis B vaccine purchase for 675,000 high-risk adults in a total high-risk population of 4.5 million people who visit STD-HIV and drug-treatment centers—a 15% uptake. If uptake at those venues reached 74% for the first dose, as was observed at a San Diego STD clinic that combined free vaccination with counseling (CDC, 2002), the cost for hepatitis B vaccine purchase alone would approach $80 million.

Except for Medicaid's Early Periodic Screening, Diagnosis, and Treatment entitlement, public-health insurance often contains cost-sharing, which may create a barrier to vaccination for some people. Adults covered by Medicaid and Medicare and those being phased out of CHIP coverage must share the costs of hepatitis B vaccination. Families of non-Medicaid VFC-covered children may be responsible for the administration portion of the vaccination cost.

Private health insurance has gaps for vaccination coverage because it does not universally cover all ACIP-recommended vaccinations for children and adults. Furthermore, most privately insured persons are required to pay to receive vaccinations. More than two-thirds of privately insured persons are enrolled in non-HMO health plans that require deductibles to be met before plan coverage and require out-of-pocket expenditures for services.

Recommendation 4-5. Private and public insurance coverage for hepatitis B vaccination should be expanded.

- Public Health Section 317 should be expanded with sufficient funding to become the public safety net for underinsured and uninsured adults to receive the hepatitis B vaccination.
- All private insurance plans should include coverage for all ACIP-recommended vaccinations. Hepatitis B vaccination should be free of any deductible so that first-dollar coverage exists for this preventive service.

Vaccine Accessibility

The hepatitis B vaccine is available at some physician offices, designated health clinics, and some community-based outreach programs. However, many health-care providers' offices do not offer vaccination, and many US cities do not have health clinics or community-based programs that provide the hepatitis B vaccine (Rein et al., 2010). Making the vaccine available through nontraditional settings, such as pharmacies, would probably increase hepatitis B immunization rates in the United States. Previous studies have shown that use of nontraditional settings, such as pharmacies and supermarkets, to deliver vaccines to US adults results in increased accessibility and convenience, reduced cost, and increased public awareness of the need for adult immunization (Postema and Breiman, 2000). That strategy is also likely to be cost-saving (Prosser et al., 2008). The involvement of community pharmacies in vaccine distribution and administration has been growing in recent years (Westrick et al., 2009), and enlisting their participation in public delivery of the hepatitis B vaccine is a natural progression.

Vaccine-Supply Concerns

Several studies of vaccine supply in the United States have expressed concerns regarding vaccine shortages (Jacobson et al., 2006; Klein and Myers, 2006; Santoli et al., 2004). Reasons for vaccine shortages include cessation of production by manufacturers due to lack of profitability, liability issues, problems with vaccine production, and unanticipated vaccine demands (Klein and Myers, 2006; Santoli et al., 2004). From 2000 to 2004, there were shortages of six pediatric vaccines: combined tetanus–diphtheria toxoids (November 2000–June 2002), diphtheria–tetanus–acellular pertussis (March 2001–July 2002), pneumococcal conjugate (September 2001–March 2003 and February 2004–September 2004), measles–mumps–rubella (October 2001–July 2002), and varicella (October 2001–August 2002) (Jacobson et al., 2006).

Although there has not been a national shortage of the hepatitis B vaccine, temporary supply problems occurred with this vaccine in 2008 (adult and dialysis formulations of Recombivax HB) and 2009 (pediatric formulations of Recombivax HB and Pediatric Engerix-B) (CDC, 2009a). A shortage was avoided because other manufacturers were able to provide an adequate supply of the vaccine in adult and dialysis formulations, and CDC released doses of pediatric vaccine from its stockpile.

Recommendation 4-6. The federal government should work to ensure an adequate, accessible, and sustainable hepatitis B vaccine supply.

HEPATITIS C VACCINE

Efforts are going on to develop a vaccine for hepatitis C, and several candidates are in phase I and phase II clinical trials (Inchauspe and Michel, 2007). Although some vaccines are being developed to treat people with chronic HCV infection (that is, therapeutic vaccines), this section focuses on vaccines to *prevent* chronic HCV infection. An incomplete understanding of how chronic HCV infection is spontaneously controlled in some people and antigenic variability of the virus remain barriers to development of a vaccine to prevent chronic hepatitis C.

Feasibility of Preventing Chronic Hepatitis C

The outcomes of HCV infections in humans and chimpanzees suggest that it may be possible to develop a vaccine to prevent HCV infection. Spontaneous clearance of the virus in 15–45% of persons after acute HCV infection demonstrates that immunity can prevent chronic infection and its long-term consequences, such as cirrhosis and hepatocellular carcinoma (HCC) (Alter et al., 1992; Barrera et al., 1995; Villano et al., 1999; Vogt et al., 1999). It also seems that immunity can be conditioned by prior exposure: humans and chimpanzees that recover from HCV infection appear to control a second infection better (the peak of viremia is lower than in the initial infection, and the chance of recovery is greater compared with that in persons not previously infected) (Lanford et al., 2004; Major et al., 2002; Mehta et al., 2002). In addition, IDUs who recovered from earlier HCV infections and have continuing HCV exposure have substantially less viremia than those who have similar exposure but had no earlier infection

(Mehta et al., 2002). Some hepatitis C vaccine candidates have shown similar potential (Forns et al., 2000; Weiner et al., 2001).

Although those clinical observations suggest that it is possible to develop a vaccine to prevent chronic HCV infection, there are important challenges. Immunity produced by natural infection does not prevent reinfection (that is, it is not sterilizing); such immunity reduces the frequency of chronic infection but does not prevent it (Farci et al., 1992). Moreover, the immunologic correlates of those critical clinical outcomes are not sufficiently understood for rational design or evaluation of vaccine products. Marked genetic variability in some HCV epitopes creates an especially formidable challenge if immunity to them is necessary for protection.

Need for a Vaccine to Prevent Chronic Hepatitis C

Although HCV infections occur in the general population of the United States and other economically developed countries, the incidence is probably too low to justify universal HCV vaccination. A hepatitis C vaccine is most likely to benefit populations that are at highest risk, include IDUs, health-care workers who perform high-risk procedures, and some men who report high-risk sexual practices with other men. A vaccine that prevents chronic HCV infection not only might reduce the likelihood of long-term disease, such as cirrhosis or HCC, but might reduce the likelihood of secondary transmission by reducing the infection reservoir. It may not be possible to produce a vaccine that prevents HCV infection, but a product that prevents acute HCV infections from becoming chronic would probably achieve many of the same benefits. In cases where acute HCV infection does not resolve within a few months, early treatment can prevent most cases from evolving into chronic HCV infection. However, because most acute HCV infections are not recognized, a vaccine is further likely to be of greatest benefit to populations in whom acute infection is rarely recognized and treated (for example, IDUs).

Cost Effectiveness of a Hepatitis C Vaccine

Estimates of the cost effectiveness of hepatitis C vaccination depend on a number of factors, including the cost of the vaccine, the target population's incidence, and projections of its effectiveness and duration. Several studies have evaluated the potential cost effectiveness of an HCV vaccine that prevents acute (and chronic) infection. Krahn et al. (2005) calculated that if a hepatitis C vaccine with 80% efficacy was available, had a duration of effectiveness equivalent to that of the hepatitis B vaccine, and was cost-equivalent to that of the current hepatitis A vaccine ($51 per dose plus administration fees), it would be cost saving to vaccinate IDUs. The authors also reported that vaccination of average-risk school-age children with such a vaccine would be cost-effective. The cost would be about $18,000 per QALY gained. Massad et al. (2009), on the basis of HCV incidence data for Sao Paolo, Brazil, calculated that a 100% effective hepatitis C vaccine that provides lifelong immunity and costs $300 per dose would cost $748,991 per death averted. If only high-risk people (for example, IDUs) were vaccinated, the cost would be $131,305 per death averted. If the hepatitis C vaccine had only 80% efficacy and lifelong duration, it would cost $242,667 per death averted if given only to high-risk people.

The committee recognizes the need for a safe, effective, and affordable hepatitis C vaccine. Such a vaccine could substantially enhance hepatitis C prevention efforts.

Recommendation 4-7. Studies to develop a vaccine to prevent chronic hepatitis C virus infection should continue.

REFERENCES

ACIP (Advisory Committee on Immunization Practices). 1991. Hepatitis B virus: A comprehensive strategy for eliminating transmission in the United States through universal childhood vaccination. Recommendations of the immunization practices advisory committee (ACIP). *Morbidity and Morality Weekly: Recommendations and Reports* 40(RR-13):1-25.

Allred, N. J., K. M. Shaw, T. A. Santibanez, D. L. Rickert, and J. M. Santoli. 2005. Parental vaccine safety concerns: Results from the national immunization survey, 2001-2002. *American Journal of Preventive Medicine* 28(2):221-224.

Allred, N. J., J. M. Stevenson, M. Kolasa, D. L. Bartlett, R. Schieber, K. S. Enger, and A. Shefer. 2006. Using registry data to evaluate the 2004 pneumococcal conjugate vaccine shortage. *American Journal of Preventive Medicine* 30(4):347-350.

Alter, M. J., H. S. Margolis, K. Krawczynski, F. N. Judson, A. Mares, W. J. Alexander, P. Y. Hu, J. K. Miller, M. A. Gerber, R. E. Sampliner, et al. 1992. The natural history of community-acquired hepatitis C in the United States. The sentinel counties chronic non-A, non-B hepatitis study team. *New England Journal of Medicine* 327(27):1899-1905.

Altice, F. L., R. D. Bruce, M. R. Walton, and M. I. Buitrago. 2005. Adherence to hepatitis B virus vaccination at syringe exchange sites. *Journal of Urban Health* 82(1):151-161.

American Academy of Pediatrics. 1961. Vitamin K compounds and the water-soluble analogues: Use in therapy and prophylaxis in pediatrics. *Pediatrics* 28:501-507.

———. 1980. Prophylaxis and treatment of neonatal gonococcal infections. *Pediatrics* 65(5): 1047-1048.

———. 2008. *State legislation report.* http://www.aap.org/advocacy/stategrpt.pdf (accessed August 21, 2009).

———. 2009. Section 3. Summaries of infectious diseases: hepatitis B. Edited by L. K. Pickering, C. J. Baker, D. W. Kimberlin, and S. S. Long, *Red book: 2009 report of the committee on infectious diseases.* Elk Grove Village, IL: American Academy of Pediatrics.

Ashton, M. R., R. L. Cook, H. C. Wiesenfeld, M. A. Krohn, T. Zamborsky, S. H. Scholle, and G. E. Switzer. 2002. Primary care physician attitudes regarding sexually transmitted diseases. *Sexually Transmitted Diseases* 29(4):246-251.

Bailey, C. L., V. Smith, and M. Sands. 2008. Hepatitis B vaccine: A seven-year study of adherence to the immunization guidelines and efficacy in HIV-1-positive adults. *International Journal of Infectious Diseases* 12(6):e77-e83.

Barrera, J. M., M. Bruguera, M. G. Ercilla, C. Gil, R. Celis, M. P. Gil, M. del Valle Onorato, J. Rodes, and A. Ordinas. 1995. Persistent hepatitis C viremia after acute self-limiting posttransfusion hepatitis C. *Hepatology* 21(3):639-644.

Bartlett, D. L., M. L. Washington, A. Bryant, N. Thurston, and C. A. Perfili. 2007. Cost savings associated with using immunization information systems for vaccines for children administrative tasks. *Journal of Public Health Management and Practice* 13(6):559-566.

Boom, J. A., A. C. Dragsbaek, and C. S. Nelson. 2007. The success of an immunization information system in the wake of Hurricane Katrina. *Pediatrics* 119(6):1213-1217.

Bull, S. S., C. Rietmeijer, J. D. Fortenberry, B. Stoner, K. Malotte, N. Vandevanter, S. E. Middlestadt, and E. W. Hook, 3rd. 1999. Practice patterns for the elicitation of sexual history, education, and counseling among providers of STD services: Results from the gonorrhea community action project (GCAP). *Sexually Transmitted Diseases* 26(10): 584-589.

Campbell, J. V., R. S. Garfein, H. Thiede, H. Hagan, L. J. Ouellet, E. T. Golub, S. M. Hudson, D. C. Ompad, and C. Weinbaum. 2007. Convenience is the key to hepatitis A and B vaccination uptake among young adult injection drug users. *Drug and Alcohol Dependence* 91(Suppl 1):S64-S72.

CDC (Centers for Disease Control and Prevention). 2000. Vaccination coverage among adolescents 1 year before the institution of a seventh grade school entry vaccination requirement—San Diego, California, 1998. *Morbidity and Mortality Weekly Report* 49(5):101-102, 111.

———. 2001a. Development of community- and state-based immunization registries. CDC response to a report from the National Vaccine Advisory Committee. *Morbidity and Morality Weekly: Recommendations and Reports* 50(RR-17):1-17.

———. 2001b. Effectiveness of a middle school vaccination law—California, 1999-2001. *Morbidity and Mortality Weekly Report* 50(31):660-663.

———. 2002. Hepatitis B vaccination among high-risk adolescents and adults—San Diego, California, 1998-2001. *Morbidity and Mortality Weekly Report* 51(28):618-621.

———. 2003. *Vaccines for children: Program management.* http://www.cdc.gov/vaccines/programs/vfc/projects/program-mgmt.htm#pm (accessed August 27, 2009).

———. 2005. Immunization information system progress—United States, 2004. *Morbidity and Mortality Weekly Report* 54(45):1156-1157.

———. 2006. Hepatitis b vaccination coverage among adults—United States, 2004. *Morbidity and Mortality Weekly Report* 55(18):509-511.

———. 2007. Vaccination coverage among children in kindergarten—United States, 2006–07 school year. *Morbidity and Mortality Weekly Report* 56(32):819-821.

———. 2008a. *Immunization administration requirements for correctional inmates and residents.* http://www2a.cdc.gov/nip/stateVaccApp/StateVaccsApp/AdministrationbyPatientType.asp?PatientTypetmp=Correctional%20Inmates%20and%20Residents (accessed July 11, 2008).

———. 2008b. Immunization information systems progress—United States, 2006. *Morbidity and Mortality Weekly Report* 57(11):289-291.

———. 2008c. Newborn hepatitis B vaccination coverage among children born January 2003-June 2005—United States. *Morbidity and Mortality Weekly Report* 57(30):825-828.

———. 2009a. *Current vaccine shortages and delays.* http://www.cdc.gov/vaccines/vac-gen/shortages/default.htm (accessed June 11, 2009).

———. 2009b. *Hepatitis B vaccine birth dose rates, national immunization survey.* http://www.cdc.gov/Hepatitis/Partners/PeriHepBCoord.htm (accessed December 14, 2009).

———. 2009c. National, state, and local area vaccination coverage among children aged 19-35 months—United States, 2008. *Morbidity and Mortality Weekly Report* 58(33): 921-926.

———. 2009d. *Report to congress on section 317 immunization program. Senate appropriations committee.* http://www.317coalition.org/legislativeupdate/senate317reportfinal.pdf (accessed August 21, 2009).

Charuvastra, A., J. Stein, B. Schwartzapfel, A. Spaulding, E. Horowitz, G. Macalino, and J. D. Rich. 2001. Hepatitis B vaccination practices in state and federal prisons. *Public Health Reports* 116(3):203-209.

Christensen, P. B., N. Fisker, H. B. Krarup, E. Liebert, N. Jaroslavtsev, K. Christensen, and J. Georgsen. 2004. Hepatitis B vaccination in prison with a 3-week schedule is more efficient than the standard 6-month schedule. *Vaccine* 22(29-30):3897-3901.

CMS (Centers for Medicare and Medicaid Services). 2008. *Adult immunizations.* http://www.cms.hhs.gov/MLNProducts/downloads/Adult_Immunization.pdf (accessed August 21, 2009).

———. 2009. *Overview of the Children's Health Insurance Program (CHIP).* http://www.cms.hhs.gov/LowCostHealthInsFamChild/ (accessed August 27, 2009).

Daniels, D., S. Grytdal, and A. Wasley. 2009. Surveillance for acute viral hepatitis—United States, 2007. *Morbidity and Mortality Weekly Report: Surveillance Summaries* 58(3): 1-27.

Darling, N. J., L. E. Barker, A. M. Shefer, and S. Y. Chu. 2005. Immunization coverage among Hispanic ancestry, 2003 national immunization survey. *American Journal of Preventive Medicine* 29(5):421-427.

Des Jarlais, D. C., T. Diaz, T. Perlis, D. Vlahov, C. Maslow, M. Latka, R. Rockwell, V. Edwards, S. R. Friedman, E. Monterroso, I. Williams, and R. S. Garfein. 2003. Variability in the incidence of human immunodeficiency virus, hepatitis B virus, and hepatitis C virus infection among young injecting drug users in New York city. *American Journal of Epidemiology* 157(5):467-471.

Des Jarlais, D. C., D. G. Fisher, J. C. Newman, B. N. Trubatch, M. Yancovitz, D. Paone, and D. Perlman. 2001. Providing hepatitis B vaccination to injection drug users: Referral to health clinics vs on-site vaccination at a syringe exchange program. *American Journal of Public Health* 91(11):1791-1792.

Edmunds, W. J., G. F. Medley, D. J. Nokes, A. J. Hall, and H. C. Whittle. 1993. The influence of age on the development of the hepatitis B carrier state. *Proceedings. Biological Sciences* 253(1337):197-201.

Families USA. 2009a. *CHIPRA 101: Overview of the CHIP reauthorization legislation.* Washington, DC: Families USA.

———. 2009b. *Hidden health tax: American pay a premium.* Washington, DC: Families USA.

Farci, P., H. J. Alter, S. Govindarajan, D. C. Wong, R. Engle, R. R. Lesniewski, I. K. Mushahwar, S. M. Desai, R. H. Miller, N. Ogata, et al. 1992. Lack of protective immunity against reinfection with hepatitis C virus. *Science* 258(5079):135-140.

Fishbein, D. B., B. C. Willis, W. M. Cassidy, D. Marioneaux, C. Bachino, T. Waddington, and P. Wortley. 2006. Determining indications for adult vaccination: Patient self-assessment, medical record, or both? *Vaccine* 24(6):803-818.

Forns, X., P. J. Payette, X. Ma, W. Satterfield, G. Eder, I. K. Mushahwar, S. Govindarajan, H. L. Davis, S. U. Emerson, R. H. Purcell, and J. Bukh. 2000. Vaccination of chimpanzees with plasmid DNA encoding the hepatitis C virus (HCV) envelope e2 protein modified the infection after challenge with homologous monoclonal HCV. *Hepatology* 32(3):618-625.

Gilbert, L. K., J. Bulger, K. Scanlon, K. Ford, D. Bergmire-Sweat, and C. Weinbaum. 2005. Integrating hepatitis B prevention into sexually transmitted disease services: U.S. sexually transmitted disease program and clinic trends—1997 and 2001. *Sexually Transmitted Diseases* 32(6):346-350.

Gold, M. R., J. E. Siegel, L. B. Russell, and M. C. Weinstein, eds. 1996. *Cost-effectiveness in health and medicine.* New York: Oxford University Press.

Goldstein, S. T., M. J. Alter, I. T. Williams, L. A. Moyer, F. N. Judson, K. Mottram, M. Fleenor, P. L. Ryder, and H. S. Margolis. 2002. Incidence and risk factors for acute hepatitis B in the United States, 1982-1998: Implications for vaccination programs. *Journal of Infectious Diseases* 185(6):713-719.

Gust, D. A., N. Darling, A. Kennedy, and B. Schwartz. 2008. Parents with doubts about vaccines: Which vaccines and reasons why. *Pediatrics* 122(4):718-725.

Hagan, H., J. P. McGough, H. Thiede, N. S. Weiss, S. Hopkins, and E. R. Alexander. 1999. Syringe exchange and risk of infection with hepatitis B and C viruses. *American Journal of Epidemiology* 149(3):203-213.

Harris, J. L., T. S. Jones, and J. Buffington. 2007. Hepatitis B vaccination in six STD clinics in the United States committed to integrating viral hepatitis prevention services. *Public Health Reports* 122(Suppl 2):42-47.

Hennessey, K. A., A. A. Kim, V. Griffin, N. T. Collins, C. M. Weinbaum, and K. Sabin. 2009. Prevalence of infection with hepatitis B and C viruses and co-infection with HIV in three jails: A case for viral hepatitis prevention in jails in the United States. *Journal of Urban Health* 86(1):93-105.

HHS (Department of Health and Human Services). 2009. *National Vaccine Advisory Committee recommendations for federal adult immunization programs regarding immunization delivery, assessment, research, and safety monitoring.* http://www.hhs.gov/nvpo/nvac/NVACAdultImmunizationsWorkingGroupJune2009.html (accessed September 10, 2009).

HIAA (Health Insurance Association of America). 1988. Survey from the Health Insurance Association of America.

Hinman, A. R., G. A. Urquhart, and R. A. Strikas. 2007. Immunization information systems: National Vaccine Advisory Committee progress report, 2007. *Journal of Public Health Management and Practice* 13(6):553-558.

Holahan, J., and A. Cook. 2008. *The decline in the uninsured in 2007: Why did it happen and can it last?* Commission on Medicaid and the Uninsured, Kaiser Family Foundation.

Hu, Y., L. E. Grau, G. Scott, K. H. Seal, P. A. Marshall, M. Singer, and R. Heimer. 2008. Economic evaluation of delivering hepatitis B vaccine to injection drug users. *American Journal of Preventive Medicine* 35(1):25-32.

Hutchinson, S. J., S. Wadd, A. Taylor, S. M. Bird, A. Mitchell, D. S. Morrison, S. Ahmed, and D. J. Goldberg. 2004. Sudden rise in uptake of hepatitis B vaccination among injecting drug users associated with a universal vaccine programme in prisons. *Vaccine* 23(2):210-214.

Hutton, D. W., D. Tan, S. K. So, and M. L. Brandeau. 2007. Cost-effectiveness of screening and vaccinating Asian and Pacific Islander adults for hepatitis B. *Annals of Internal Medicine* 147(7):460-469.

Immunization Action Coalition. 2009. *State information. Hepatitis B prevention mandates: Prenatal, daycare, and k-12.* http://www.immunize.org/laws/hepb.asp (accessed June 9, 2009).

Inchauspe, G., and M. L. Michel. 2007. Vaccines and immunotherapies against hepatitis B and hepatitis C viruses. *Journal of Viral Hepatitis* 14(Suppl 1):97-103.

IOM (Institute of Medicine). 1994. *Adverse events associated with childhood vaccines: Evidence bearing on causality.* Edited by K. R. Stratton, C. J. Howe, and R. B. J. Johnston. Washington, DC: National Academy Press.

———. 2002. *Immunization safety review: Hepatitis B vaccine and demyelinating neurological disorders.* Edited by K. Stratton, D. Almario, and M. C. McCormick. Washington, DC: The National Academies Press.

———. 2003. *Financing vaccines in the 21st century: Assuring access and availability. Public and private insurance coverage.* Washington, DC: The National Academies Press.

———. 2009. *America's uninsured crisis. Consequences for health and healthcare.* Washington, DC: The National Academies Press.

Jacobson, S. H., E. C. Sewell, and R. A. Proano. 2006. An analysis of the pediatric vaccine supply shortage problem. *Health Care Management Science* 9(4):371-389.

Jenkins, C. N., S. J. McPhee, C. Wong, T. Nguyen, and G. L. Euler. 2000. Hepatitis B immunization coverage among Vietnamese-American children 3 to 18 years old. *Pediatrics* 106(6):E78.

Kaiser Family Foundation and HRET. 2008. *Employer health benefits 2008 annual survey.* The Kaiser Family Foundation and Health Research & Educational Trust.

Kim, S.-Y., K. Billah, T. A. Lieu, and M. C. Weinstein. 2006. Cost effectiveness of hepatitis B vaccination at HIV counseling and testing sites. *American Journal of Preventive Medicine* 30(6):498-498.

Klein, J. O., and M. G. Myers. 2006. Vaccine shortages: Why they occur and what needs to be done to strengthen vaccine supply. *Pediatrics* 117(6):2269-2275.

Koff, R. S. 2000. Hepatitis B school-based vaccination programmes in the USA: A model for hepatitis A and B. *Vaccine* 18(Suppl 1):S77-S79.

KPMG. 1996. Survey of employer-sponsored health benefits, 1993.

Krahn, M. D., A. John-Baptiste, Q. Yi, A. Doria, R. S. Remis, P. Ritvo, and S. Friedman. 2005. Potential cost-effectiveness of a preventive hepatitis C vaccine in high risk and average risk populations in Canada. *Vaccine* 23(13):1549-1558.

Kuo, I., D. W. Mudrick, S. A. Strathdee, D. L. Thomas, and S. G. Sherman. 2004. Poor validity of self-reported hepatitis B virus infection and vaccination status among young drug users. *Clinical Infectious Diseases* 38(4):587-590.

Lanford, R. E., B. Guerra, D. Chavez, C. Bigger, K. M. Brasky, X. H. Wang, S. C. Ray, and D. L. Thomas. 2004. Cross-genotype immunity to hepatitis C virus. *Journal of Virology* 78(3):1575-1581.

Lum, P. J., J. A. Hahn, K. P. Shafer, J. L. Evans, P. J. Davidson, E. Stein, and A. R. Moss. 2008. Hepatitis B virus infection and immunization status in a new generation of injection drug users in San Francisco. *Journal of Viral Hepatitis* 15(3):229-236.

Lum, P. J., K. C. Ochoa, J. A. Hahn, K. Page Shafer, J. L. Evans, and A. R. Moss. 2003. Hepatitis B virus immunization among young injection drug users in San Francisco, Calif: The UFO study. *American Journal of Public Health* 93(6):919-923.

Luman, E. T., L. E. Barker, M. M. McCauley, and C. Drews-Botsch. 2005. Timeliness of childhood immunizations: A state-specific analysis. *American Journal of Public Health* 95(8):1367-1374.

Maheux, B., N. Haley, M. Rivard, and A. Gervais. 1995. STD risk assessment and risk-reduction counseling by recently trained family physicians. *Academic Medicine* 70(8):726-728.

Major, M. E., K. Mihalik, M. Puig, B. Rehermann, M. Nascimbeni, C. M. Rice, and S. M. Feinstone. 2002. Previously infected and recovered chimpanzees exhibit rapid responses that control hepatitis C virus replication upon rechallenge. *Journal of Virology* 76(13):6586-6595.

Massad, E., F. A. Coutinho, E. Chaib, and M. N. Burattini. 2009. Cost-effectiveness analysis of a hypothetical hepatitis C vaccine compared to antiviral therapy. *Epidemiology and Infection* 137(2):241-249.

Mast, E. E., and J. W. Ward. 2008. Chapter 13. Hepatitis B vaccines. In *Vaccines*. 5th ed, edited by S. A. Plotkin, W. A. Orenstein, and P. A. Offit: Elsevier Health Sciences.

Mast, E. E., H. S. Margolis, A. E. Fiore, E. W. Brink, S. T. Goldstein, S. A. Wang, L. A. Moyer, B. P. Bell, and M. J. Alter. 2005. A comprehensive immunization strategy to eliminate transmission of hepatitis B virus infection in the United States: Recommendations of the advisory committee on immunization practices (ACIP) part 1: Immunization of infants, children, and adolescents. *Morbidity and Morality Weekly: Recommendations and Reports* 54(RR-16):1-31.

Mast, E. E., C. M. Weinbaum, A. E. Fiore, M. J. Alter, B. P. Bell, L. Finelli, L. E. Rodewald, J. M. Douglas, Jr., R. S. Janssen, and J. W. Ward. 2006. A comprehensive immunization strategy to eliminate transmission of hepatitis B virus infection in the United States: Recommendations of the advisory committee on immunization practices (ACIP) part II: Immunization of adults. *Morbidity and Morality Weekly: Recommendations and Reports* 55(RR-16):1-33.

Mehta, S. H., A. Cox, D. R. Hoover, X. H. Wang, Q. Mao, S. Ray, S. A. Strathdee, D. Vlahov, and D. L. Thomas. 2002. Protection against persistence of hepatitis C. *Lancet* 359(9316):1478-1483.

Miriti, M. K., K. Billah, C. Weinbaum, J. Subiadur, R. Zimmerman, P. Murray, R. Gunn, and J. Buffington. 2008. Economic benefits of hepatitis B vaccination at sexually transmitted disease clinics in the U.S. *Public Health Reports* 123(4):504-513.

Mootrey, G. T. 2007. *Presentation. Adult immunization at CDC.* www.hhs.gov/nvpo/nvac/documents/2007oct/Mootrey.ppt (accessed August 21, 2009).

Morita, J. Y., E. Ramirez, and W. E. Trick. 2008. Effect of a school-entry vaccination requirement on racial and ethnic disparities in hepatitis B immunization coverage levels among public school students. *Pediatrics* 121(3):e547-e552.

Olshen, E., B. E. Mahon, S. Wang, and E. R. Woods. 2007. The impact of state policies on vaccine coverage by age 13 in an insured population. *Journal of Adolescent Health* 40(5):405-411.

Owens, D. K. 1998. Interpretation of cost-effectiveness analyses. *Journal of General Internal Medicine* 13(10):716-717.

Pisu, M., M. I. Meltzer, and R. Lyerla. 2002. Cost-effectiveness of hepatitis B vaccination of prison inmates. *Vaccine* 21(3-4):312-321.

Postema, A. S., and R. F. Breiman. 2000. Adult immunization programs in nontraditional settings: Quality standards and guidance for program evaluation. *Morbidity and Morality Weekly: Recommendations and Reports* 49(RR-1):1-13.

Prosser, L. A., M. A. O'Brien, N. A. Molinari, K. H. Hohman, K. L. Nichol, M. L. Messonnier, and T. A. Lieu. 2008. Non-traditional settings for influenza vaccination of adults: Costs and cost effectiveness. *Pharmacoeconomics* 26(2):163-178.

Rein, D. B., S. B. Lesesne, P. J. Leese, and C. M. Weinbaum. 2010. Community-based hepatitis B screening programs in the United States in 2008. *Journal of Viral Hepatitis* 17(1):28-33.

Rodewald, L. 2008. *Vaccination financing: Program funding and pressures, 317 operations funding: FY08-FY09.* Presentation at AIM program managers meeting. http://cdc.confex.com/recording/cdc/nic2009/ppt/free/4db77adf5df9fff0d3caf5cafe28f496/paper18425_5.ppt#930,5,Section (accessed November 19, 2008).

Rosenbaum, S., L. Stewart, M. Cox, and A. Lee. 2003. *Medicaid coverage of immunizations for noninstitutionalized adults.* Washington, DC: Center for Health Services Policy Research, George Washington University.

Rotily, M., C. Vernay-Vaisse, M. Bourliere, A. Galinier-Pujol, S. Rousseau, and Y. Obadia. 1997. HBV and HIV screening, and hepatitis B immunization programme in the prison of Marseille, France. *International Journal of STD and AIDS* 8(12):753-759.

Saarlas, K. N., A. R. Hinman, D. A. Ross, W. C. Watson, Jr., E. L. Wild, T. M. Hastings, and P. A. Richmond. 2004. All kids count 1991-2004: Developing information systems to improve child health and the delivery of immunizations and preventive services. *Journal of Public Health Management and Practice* (Suppl):S3-S15.

Samoff, E., A. Dunn, N. VanDevanter, S. Blank, and I. B. Weisfuse. 2004. Predictors of acceptance of hepatitis B vaccination in an urban sexually transmitted diseases clinic. *Sexually Transmitted Diseases* 31(7):415-420.

Santoli, J. M., J. O. Klein, G. Peter, and W. A. Orenstein. 2004. Disruptions in the supply of routinely recommended childhood vaccines in the United States. *Pediatric Infectious Disease Journal* 23(6):553-554.

Savage, R. B., M. J. Hussey, and M. B. Hurie. 2000. A successful approach to immunizing men who have sex with men against hepatitis B. *Public Health Nursing* 17(3):202-206.

Seal, K. H., K. C. Ochoa, J. A. Hahn, J. P. Tulsky, B. R. Edlin, and A. R. Moss. 2000. Risk of hepatitis B infection among young injection drug users in San Francisco: Opportunities for intervention. *Western Journal of Medicine* 172(1):16-20.

Simard, E. P., J. T. Miller, P. A. George, A. Wasley, M. J. Alter, B. P. Bell, and L. Finelli. 2007. Hepatitis B vaccination coverage levels among healthcare workers in the United States, 2002-2003. *Infection Control and Hospital Epidemiology* 28(7):783-790.

Smith, P. J., A. M. Kennedy, K. Wooten, D. A. Gust, and L. K. Pickering. 2006a. Association between health care providers' influence on parents who have concerns about vaccine safety and vaccination coverage. *Pediatrics* 118(5):e1287-1292.

Smith, P. J., J. Stevenson, and S. Y. Chu. 2006b. Associations between childhood vaccination coverage, insurance type, and breaks in health insurance coverage. *Pediatrics* 117(6):1972-1978.

Stanwyck, C. A., M. S. Kolasa, and K. M. Shaw. 2004. Immunization requirements for childcare programs: Are they enough? *American Journal of Preventive Medicine* 27(2):161-163.

Szilagyi, P. G., S. Schaffer, L. Shone, R. Barth, S. G. Humiston, M. Sandler, and L. E. Rodewald. 2002. Reducing geographic, racial, and ethnic disparities in childhood immunization rates by using reminder/recall interventions in urban primary care practices. *Pediatrics* 110(5):e58.

U.S. Census Bureau. 2007. *Historic health insurance tables.* http://www.census.gov/hhes/www/hlthins/historic/hihistt4.xls (accessed August 27, 2009).

Vallabhaneni, S., G. E. Macalino, S. E. Reinert, B. Schwartzapfel, F. A. Wolf, and J. D. Rich. 2004. Prisoners' attitudes toward hepatitis B vaccination. *Preventive Medicine* 38(6):828-833.

Vellinga, A., P. Van Damme, and A. Meheus. 1999. Hepatitis B and C in institutions for individuals with intellectual disability. *Journal of Intellectual Disability Research* 43(Pt 6):445-453.

Villano, S. A., D. Vlahov, K. E. Nelson, S. Cohn, and D. L. Thomas. 1999. Persistence of viremia and the importance of long-term follow-up after acute hepatitis C infection. *Hepatology* 29(3):908-914.

Vogt, M., T. Lang, G. Frosner, C. Klingler, A. F. Sendl, A. Zeller, B. Wiebecke, B. Langer, H. Meisner, and J. Hess. 1999. Prevalence and clinical outcome of hepatitis C infection in children who underwent cardiac surgery before the implementation of blood-donor screening. *New England Journal of Medicine* 341(12):866-870.

Ward, J. W. 2008. Time for renewed commitment to viral hepatitis prevention. *American Journal of Public Health* 98(5):779-781.

Weiner, A. J., X. Paliard, M. J. Selby, A. Medina-Selby, D. Coit, S. Nguyen, J. Kansopon, C. L. Arian, P. Ng, J. Tucker, C. T. Lee, N. K. Polakos, J. Han, S. Wong, H. H. Lu, S. Rosenberg, K. M. Brasky, D. Chien, G. Kuo, and M. Houghton. 2001. Intrahepatic genetic inoculation of hepatitis C virus RNA confers cross-protective immunity. *Journal of Virology* 75(15):7142-7148.

Westrick, S. C., S. Watcharadamrongkun, J. K. Mount, and M. L. Breland. 2009. Community pharmacy involvement in vaccine distribution and administration. *Vaccine* 27(21): 2858-2863.

WHO (World Health Organization). 2006. *Preventing mother-to-child transmission of hepatitis B: Operational field guidelines of delivery of the birth dose of hepatitis B vaccine* Manila: World Health Organization Western Pacific Region.

———. 2009. *Table: Threshold values for intervention cost-effectiveness by region.* http://www.who.int/choice/costs/CER_levels/en/index.html (accessed November 4, 2009).

Williams, I. T., K. Boaz, and K. P. Openo. 2005. *Missed opportunities for hepatitis B vaccination in correctional settings, sexually transmitted disease (STD) clinics, and drug treatment programs [abstract 1031].* Paper presented at the 43rd Annual Meeting of the Infectious Diseases Society of America, San Francisco, CA.

Workowski, K., and S. Berman. 2006. Sexually transmitted diseases: Treatment guidelines, 2006. *Morbidity and Mortality Weekly Report* 55(RR-11):1-94.

Yawn, B. P., L. Edmonson, L. Huber, G. A. Poland, R. M. Jacobson, and S. J. Jacobsen. 1998. The impact of a simulated immunization registry on perceived childhood immunization status. *American Journal of Managed Care* 4(2):185-192.

Zimet, G. D., J. Maehr, N. A. Constantine, and A. English. 2008. School-entry vaccination requirements: A position statement of the society for adolescent medicine. *Journal of Adolescent Health* 42(3):310-311.

5

Viral Hepatitis Services

Hepatitis B virus (HBV) and hepatitis C virus (HCV) infections cause substantial morbidity and mortality despite being preventable and treatable. Deficiencies in the implementation of established guidelines for the prevention, diagnosis, and medical management of chronic HBV and HCV infections perpetuate personal and economic burdens. This chapter reviews the current status of services to prevent and manage chronic hepatitis B and chronic hepatitis C. It then discusses the general components of viral hepatitis services. The chapter ends with an assessment of gaps in existing services, including a description of some models for services and committee recommendations to improve viral hepatitis prevention and management and to fill research needs. Services for the general US population are considered first and then services for special populations and service venues that have unique opportunities for interventions. Hepatitis B immunization is covered in Chapter 4 and so is not discussed in detail here.

The recommendations offered by the committee here are presented in the context of the current health-care system in the United States. The committee believes strongly that if the system changes as a result of health-care reform efforts, viral hepatitis services should have high priority in components of the reformed system that deal with prevention, chronic disease, and primary-care delivery. The committee's recommendations regarding viral hepatitis services are summarized in Box 5-1.

> **BOX 5-1**
> **Summary of Recommendations Regarding**
> **Viral Hepatitis Services**
>
> **General Population**
> - 5-1. Federally funded health-insurance programs—such as Medicare, Medicaid, and the Federal Employees Health Benefits Program—should incorporate guidelines for risk-factor screening for hepatitis B and hepatitis C as a required core component of preventive care so that at-risk people receive serologic testing for hepatitis B virus and hepatitis C virus and chronically infected patients receive appropriate medical management.
>
> **Foreign-Born Populations**
> - 5-2. The Centers for Disease Control and Prevention, in conjunction with other federal agencies and state agencies, should provide resources for the expansion of community-based programs that provide hepatitis B screening, testing, and vaccination services that target foreign-born populations.
>
> **Illicit Drug Users**
> - 5-3. Federal, state, and local agencies should expand programs to reduce the risk of hepatitis C virus infection through injection-drug use by providing comprehensive hepatitis C virus prevention programs. At a minimum, the programs should include access to sterile needle syringes and drug-preparation equipment because the shared use of these materials has been shown to lead to transmission of hepatitis C virus.
> - 5-4. Federal and state governments should expand services to reduce the harm caused by chronic hepatitis B and hepatitis C. The services should include testing to detect infection, counseling to reduce alcohol use and secondary transmission, hepatitis B vaccination, and referral for or provision of medical management.

CURRENT STATUS

Health services related to viral hepatitis prevention, screening, and medical management are both limited and fragmented among entities at the federal, state, and local levels. Numerous federal agencies administer or fund some viral hepatitis–related services, including the Centers for Disease Control and Prevention (CDC), the Health Resources and Services

- 5-5. Innovative, effective, multicomponent hepatitis C virus prevention strategies for injection drug users and non-injection-drug users should be developed and evaluated to achieve greater control of hepatitis C virus transmission.

Pregnant Women
- 5-6. The Centers for Disease Control and Prevention should provide additional resources and guidance to perinatal hepatitis B prevention program coordinators to expand and enhance the capacity to identify chronically infected pregnant women and provide case-management services, including referral for appropriate medical management.
- 5-7. The National Institutes of Health should support a study of the effectiveness and safety of peripartum antiviral therapy to reduce and possibly eliminate perinatal hepatitis B virus transmission from women at high risk for perinatal transmission.

Incarcerated Populations
- 5-8. The Centers for Disease Control and Prevention and the Department of Justice should create an initiative to foster partnerships between health departments and corrections systems to ensure the availability of comprehensive viral hepatitis services for incarcerated people.

Community Health Facilities
- 5-9. The Health Resources and Services Administration should provide adequate resources to federally funded community health facilities for provision of comprehensive viral-hepatitis services.

High Impact Settings
- 5-10. The Health Resources and Services Administration and the Centers for Disease Control and Prevention should provide resources and guidance to integrate comprehensive viral hepatitis services into settings that serve high-risk populations such as STD clinics, sites for HIV services and care, homeless shelters, and mobile health units.

Administration (HRSA), the Office of Minority Health, the Agency for Healthcare Quality and Research, the Centers for Medicare and Medicaid Services (CMS), the Substance Abuse and Mental Health Services Administration (SAMHSA), and the National Institutes of Health. Because there is no coordinated federal strategy for HBV and HCV prevention and control, those efforts are uneven in their application and funding. States, communities, and nongovernment organizations (NGOs) also provide viral hepatitis services, often with funding from federal agencies.

Most viral hepatitis–related activities in CDC are administered by the Division of Viral Hepatitis (DVH), which is part of the National Center for HIV/AIDS, Viral Hepatitis, Sexually Transmitted Disease, and Tuberculosis Prevention (NCHHSTP). The activities of the DVH, shown in Box 5-2, include surveillance and epidemiologic studies and clinical and laboratory research related to viral hepatitis. It supports viral hepatitis programs at the national, state, and community levels; disseminates hepatitis-related information to the public; and develops guidelines for prevention and control. In FY 2008, the DVH received $17.6 million, 2% of the NCHHSTP

BOX 5-2
Mission Statement of Centers for Disease Control and Prevention Division of Viral Hepatitis

The Division of Viral Hepatitis (DVH) is the Public Health Service component that provides the scientific and programmatic foundation for the prevention, control, and elimination of hepatitis virus infections in the United States, and assists the international public health community in these activities.

To achieve its mission, DVH:

1. conducts surveillance and special studies to determine the epidemiology and disease burden associated with acute and chronic infections and liver disease associated with hepatitis viruses;
2. conducts epidemiologic and laboratory studies, including outbreak investigations, to determine risk factors for transmission of infections with hepatitis viruses, define the natural history and pathogenesis of these infections, and determine their health impact;
3. conducts epidemiologic, clinical, laboratory, behavioral, and health communications research to develop and evaluate methods and strategies for the prevention of infections with hepatitis viruses and their acute and chronic disease consequences;
4. develops, implements, communicates and evaluates recommendations and standards for the prevention and control of infections and liver disease associated with hepatitis viruses;
5. provides technical and programmatic leadership and assistance to state and local health departments, non-governmental organizations and the international community to develop, implement and evaluate programs to prevent infections with hepatitis viruses and their consequences, including immunization to prevent hepatitis A

budget (Ward, 2008a). In contrast, domestic HIV activities received 69%, sexually transmitted diseases (STDs) received 15%, and tuberculosis received 14% of the NCHHSTP FY 2008 budget. In FY 2009, the amount of NCHHSTP funding received by the DVH was not much greater, at $18.3 million (NASTAD, 2009) (personal communication, J. Efird, CDC, July 9, 2009). That low level of funding for the DVH has been relatively flat for the last 5 years.

HRSA, part of the US Department of Health and Human Services (HHS), is charged with increasing access to health care for people who are medically underserved. Several HRSA programs provide some direct services for viral hepatitis, including the Bureau of Primary Health Care, the

---

and eliminate transmission of hepatitis B virus infection, the prevention and control of hepatitis C virus infection through counseling and testing and the prevention of transmission of bloodborne virus infections, including hepatitis viruses, through improved medical practices to reduce the frequency of unsafe injections and the improvement of the safety of blood transfusions;

6. provides the leadership and coordination required to integrate viral hepatitis prevention and control activities into other prevention programs conducted by CDC, other Federal agencies and health care providers;
7. conducts laboratory, clinical and epidemiologic studies to develop and evaluate methods for the diagnosis of infections with hepatitis viruses;
8. identifies and characterizes agents and host factors associated with hepatitis and acute and chronic liver disease;
9. provides epidemic aid, epidemiologic and laboratory consultation, reference diagnostic services and technical assistance to state and local health departments, other Federal agencies, other components of CDC, and national and international health organizations;
10. disseminates information through health communications materials, tools and programs, scientific publications and presentations;
11. provides training opportunities for Epidemic Intelligence Service Officers and others in CDC sponsored programs, including postgraduate students, post-doctoral fellows, and other public health and laboratory scientists; and
12. serves as a WHO Collaborating Center for Reference and Research on Viral Hepatitis.

SOURCE: CDC, 2009a.

Healthcare Systems Bureau, the HIV/AIDS Bureau, the Maternal and Child Health Bureau, the Office of Minority Health and Health Disparities, the Office of Planning and Evaluation, the Office of Rural Health Policy, and the Center for Quality (Raggio Ashley, 2009). In addition, viral hepatitis education and training activities are administered by the Bureau of Health Professions. HRSA funding supports federally qualified health centers that serve migrant, rural, tribal, and homeless populations. It also provides funding for Ryan White Care Act services and maternal and child health programs, such as Title V and Healthy Start, which provides some hepatitis B vaccination, testing, and counseling for HBV and HCV infections. Many people in HRSA-funded programs are foreign-born, including people from countries that have a high prevalence of hepatitis B or have behavior risk factors for HBV and HCV infection.

CMS, also a part of DHHS, provides health insurance through Medicare and Medicaid programs. Medicare covers people 65 years old or older, people under 65 years old who have specified disabilities, and people who have end-stage renal disease. Hepatitis B vaccination and its administration costs are covered by Part B of Medicare for people at high or intermediate risk for HBV infection (Rogers, 2009). People at low risk for HBV infection can receive the vaccine under Part D with a copayment that depends on their income level. Medicare will cover laboratory testing for HBV and HCV and treatment for chronic hepatitis B or hepatitis C. Medicaid is a state-administered program available to low-income individuals and families who fit into an eligibility group that is recognized by federal and state law. Eligibility for Medicaid and coverage for viral hepatitis services vary from state to state.

State and local (county and city) health departments obtain funds for viral hepatitis prevention and control activities from a variety of sources, including CDC, HRSA, SAMHSA, states, counties, cities, and private foundations. CDC funding supports adult viral hepatitis prevention coordinator (AVHPC) positions in 49 states and five cities (Ward, 2008a). The total funding level is about $5 million per year, and the average award is $90,000. CDC also funds perinatal hepatitis B coordinators in 64 states, cities, and territories at a total program cost of $7.5 million per year (CDC, 2009d). Funding for the AVHPC and perinatal hepatitis B coordinator positions covers only the coordinators' salaries but not programmatic activities. CDC provides viral hepatitis program support—about $900,000 per year—in the form of grants for viral hepatitis training and education at the state and local levels.

A number of states have developed viral hepatitis prevention plans. At the committee's request, the Institute of Medicine asked CDC to survey the 55 AVHPCs about the status of their jurisdiction's plans (CDC, 2009g). All coordinators responded to the questionnaire. Of the 55, 32 (58.2%) indicated that their states had a viral hepatitis prevention plan in place, half of which were completed in the last 5 years. Just over half of the plans include all the components in Table 5-1. All plans address hepatitis C prevention, and two-thirds (65.6%) address hepatitis B prevention. About 78% of the plans include hepatitis B vaccinations whether or not other hepatitis B prevention services are included. Some coordinators indicated that the CDC Section 317 vaccination initiative resulted in substantial progress toward implementing hepatitis B vaccination services in their jurisdictions. The medical management component is included in the smallest percentage of plans (62.5%) and just one-quarter of those plans have acted on this component. Overall, the coordinator survey revealed that over 40% of jurisdictions do not have plans; of the states that do have plans, only half have all the components, and only 20.7% of these reported that they had made progress in all the components. The primary barrier to plan implementation was financial constraints on overall funding and staffing (96.9%).

A number of NGOs have been established to address the prevention and control of HBV and HCV infections. Most of them focus on advocacy efforts, such as raising public awareness about viral hepatitis and encouraging people, especially in high-risk populations, to be vaccinated for hepatitis B, to undergo risk-factor screening for hepatitis B and hepatitis C, and to determine whether laboratory testing and medical management are needed. Many organizations target specific populations. For example, the Jade Ribbon Campaign targets Asians and Pacific Islanders to reduce the

TABLE 5-1 Summary of Adult Viral Hepatitis Prevention Coordinators Survey

Jurisdiction Plan's Program Components	Percentage of Jurisdictions with Plans That Included Component	Percentage of Jurisdictions with Plan Components That Have Been Acted On
Public education	96.6%	83.9%
Surveillance	90.6%	64.5%
Training for health-service, human-service providers	87.5%	90.3%
Advocacy, community planning	84.4%	Not reported
Counseling, testing, referral	81.3%	83.9%
Vaccination	78.1%	90.3%
Medical management	62.5%	25.8%

NOTES: All 55 adult viral hepatitis prevention coordinators completed the survey; 23 of the 55 jurisdictions do not have a viral hepatitis plan.
SOURCE: CDC, 2009f.

prevalence of chronic HBV infection and HBV-related liver cancer (Asian Liver Center, 2009). The Harm Reduction Coalition is an example of an organization that develops and disseminates hepatitis C information among illicit-drug users (Harm Reduction Coalition, 2009). Information regarding the activities and programs supported by NGOs are presented primarily in Chapter 3.

Health services provided by federal agencies, state and local governments, and NGOs do not form part of a coordinated national campaign. Existing efforts at interagency information exchange, intermittent meetings to share plans and results, and joint administration of funds for some grants are not sufficient for the scale of the health burden presented by hepatitis B and hepatitis C. The lack of an accountable entity to lead a coordinated national effort has led to missed opportunities for prevention and identification of and treatment for chronic HBV and HCV infections.

COMPONENTS OF VIRAL HEPATITIS SERVICES

The committee has identified five core functions for *comprehensive* viral hepatitis services—(1) community outreach, (2) prevention, (3) identification of infected persons, (4) social and peer support, and (5) medical management (Box 5-3). Community outreach and immunization for primary prevention are discussed in depth in Chapters 3 and 4, respectively. Identification of infected persons, harm reduction, and medical management are reviewed below.

Identification of Infected Persons

There are two goals for identifying people chronically infected with HBV and HCV: to prevent transmission to close contacts (for example, through sharing of needles and other paraphernalia and through household and sexual contacts) and to reduce the risk of chronic liver disease through medical treatment and support. The identification of HBV-infected and HCV-infected people requires engagement of at-risk people and activism by the health-care–provider community. As discussed in Chapter 3, culturally relevant, accessible, and trusted sources of communication are required to increase awareness and promote use of appropriate services. Health-care and social-service providers, particularly primary-care providers, should be knowledgeable about chronic HBV and HCV infection and identify patients who are at risk because of their behavior or previous potential exposure to HBV or HCV. Programs and venues that serve at-risk populations—such as foreign-born people from HBV-endemic countries, the uninsured and underinsured, illicit-drug users, and homeless people—should also be knowl-

> **BOX 5-3**
> **Components of Comprehensive Viral Hepatitis Services**
>
> **Community Outreach**
> - Community-awareness programs
> - Provider-awareness programs
>
> **Prevention**
> - Vaccination
> - Harm reduction
> - Needle-exchange programs
>   - Drug and alcohol treatment services
>   - Vaccination of hepatitis B virus-susceptible contacts
>
> **Identification of Infected Persons**
> - Risk-factor screening
> - Laboratory testing
>
> **Social and Peer Support**
> - Positive prevention services
> - Education and referral to other related services and care
>
> **Medical Management**
> - Assessment for and provision of long-term monitoring for viral hepatitis and selection of appropriate persons for treatment (in accordance with American Association for the Study of Liver Diseases guidelines)
> - Psychiatric and other mental-health care
> - Adherence support

edgeable about viral hepatitis and should have mechanisms for identifying infected people and referring them to followup medical management.

The committee has defined a two-step process for identifying infected people:

1. *Risk-factor screening.* Risk-factor screening is the process of determining whether a person is at risk for being chronically infected or becoming infected with HBV or HCV. Risk factors include being born in a country where the disease is prevalent, and behavior such as illicit-drug use and having multiple sexual partners.

2. *Serologic testing.* Serologic testing is laboratory testing of blood specimens for biomarker confirmation of HBV or HCV infection.

Risk-Factor Screening

Hepatitis B Risk-Factor Screening CDC has identified risk factors for becoming infected or chronically infected with HBV (see Box 5-4). As discussed in Chapter 3, improved provider awareness about risk factors is critical for ensuring that people at risk for chronic HBV infection are identified and that those at risk for becoming infected with HBV are vaccinated. Providers should review patients' backgrounds (for example, country of birth) and discuss relevant behaviors to determine what services they need.

Figure 5-1 illustrates the pathway of services and care for people depending on their risk factors identified. People who have HIV infection or other sexually transmitted infections, men who have sex with men, injection-drug users (IDUs), and institutionalized and incarcerated persons

---

BOX 5-4
Summary of CDC At-Risk Populations for Hepatitis B Virus Infection

- Persons born in geographic regions that have HBsAg prevalence of at least 2%
- Infants born to infected mothers
- Household contacts of persons who have chronic HBV infection
- Sex partners of infected persons
- Injection-drug users
- Sexually active persons who are not in long-term, mutually monogamous relationships (for example, more than one sex partner during previous 6 months)
- Men who have sex with men
- Health-care and public-safety workers at risk for occupational exposure to blood or blood-contaminated body fluids
- Residents and staff of facilities for developmentally disabled persons
- Persons who have chronic liver disease
- Hemodialysis patients
- Travelers to countries that have intermediate or high prevalence of HBV infection

SOURCE: Mast et al., 2005, 2006.

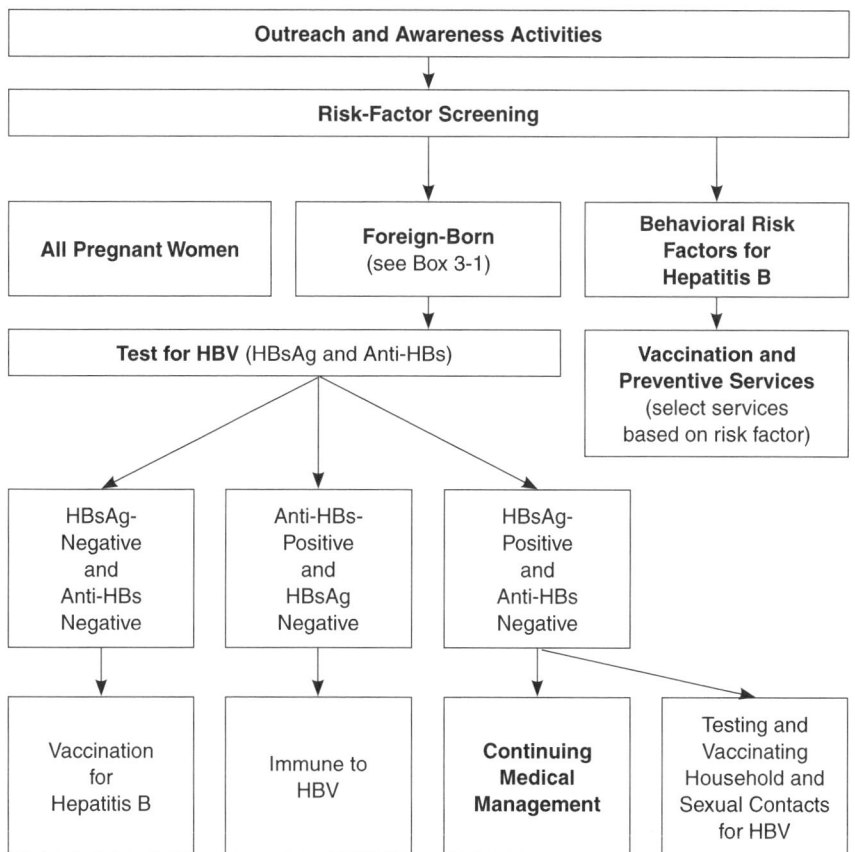

FIGURE 5-1 Hepatitis B services model.
Abbreviations: HBV, hepatitis B virus; HBsAg, hepatitis B surface antigen; anti-HBs, antibody to hepatitis B surface antigen.

are at increased risk for HBV infection. CDC recommends that all those populations be tested and given a first dose of vaccine at the time of testing. However, the committee believes that an acceptable alternative is hepatitis B vaccination without testing for all the populations except HIV-infected persons. This approach may facilitate increased vaccination rates. All persons found to have risk factors for HBV infection should receive counseling about prevention.

Hepatitis C Risk-Factor Screening CDC has identified risk factors for people at risk for being infected with HCV or becoming infected with HCV (see Box 5-5). Risk-factor screening has been tested by using question-

> **BOX 5-5**
> **Summary of CDC At-Risk Populations for Hepatitis C Virus Infection**
>
> - Persons who have ever injected illegal drugs, including those who injected only once many years ago
> - Recipients of clotting-factor concentrates made before 1987
> - Recipients of blood transfusions or solid-organ transplants before July 1992
> - Patients who have ever received long-term hemodialysis treatment
> - Persons who have known exposures to HCV, such as
>   — Health-care workers after needlesticks involving HCV-positive blood
>   — Recipients of blood or organs from donors who later tested HCV-positive
> - All persons who have HIV infection
> - Patients who have signs or symptoms of liver disease (for example, abnormal liver-enzyme tests)
> - Children born to HCV-positive mothers (to avoid detecting maternal antibody, these children should not be tested before the age of 18 months)
>
> Abbreviation: HCV, hepatitis C virus.
> SOURCE: CDC, 2001.

naires to assess a person's potential exposure to HCV infection. It has been found to correlate with infection status and is an effective mechanism for identifying candidates for testing (Armstrong et al., 2006; McGinn et al., 2008; Zuniga et al., 2006). Armstrong et al. (2006) reported that 85% of HCV-infected people could be identified on the basis of three risk factors: injection-drug use, blood transfusion before 1992, and abnormal serum alanine aminotransferase levels. Additional studies have also found that questioning patients about exposures to known risk factors for hepatitis C is predictive of HCV infection in US veterans (Zuniga et al., 2006). People who are current or past users of illicit drugs may not fit the stereotype of an IDU, so all patients should be questioned about any past episode of illicit-drug injection. It has also been suggested that people who have tattoos and body piercings should be tested for HCV (Carey, 2003). Researchers who were evaluating hepatitis C incidence along the Texas–Mexico border found tattooing to be an independent risk factor for infection in their majority-Hispanic population (Hand and Vasquez, 2005). However, it is unclear whether tattooing and body piercing are risk factors for infection or surrogates for other etiologic factors. As mentioned in Chapter 1, there is a high prevalence of HCV infection in Egypt, so Egyptian immigrants to the United States should be considered for serologic testing.

The issue of risk-factor screening and testing for HCV is controversial. In 1998, the US Public Health Service (USPHS) recommended a process of screening persons for HCV risk factors followed by laboratory testing for those potentially exposed to HCV (CDC, 1998). The 1998 USPHS recommendation to screen for risk factors among adults in the general population and to test those at risk was endorsed by a number of organizations, including the American Association for the Study of Liver Diseases (AASLD), the Infectious Diseases Society of America, and the American College of Physicians (Alter et al., 2004; Ghany et al., 2009). CDC recommends that all patients be evaluated for risk factors for HCV infection (Alter et al., 2004). In 2004, a separate group, the US Preventive Services Task Force (USPSTF), concluded that there was no direct evidence of the benefit of serologic testing for HCV infection in the general adult population and that there were inadequate data for determining accurately the benefits and risks associated with serological testing for HCV infection in otherwise healthy asymptomatic at-risk adults (Chou et al., 2004). As outcomes of treatment for chronic HCV infection improve, the controversy regarding screening and testing may diminish. An example of how improvements in treatment can change the value of identifying infected people can be seen in the advances in treatment for HIV. As effective antiretroviral therapies emerged, recommendations for screening and testing were expanded (Myers et al., 2009; Paltiel et al., 2005; Sanders et al., 2005).

Serologic Testing for Hepatitis B Virus and Hepatitis C Virus

Serologic tests to detect a history of exposure or to ascertain infection or immune status with respect to HBV and HCV use virus-specific antigens and antibodies, recombinant immunoblot assays (RIBAs), and viral nucleic acid (DNA and RNA) tests.

Rapid HBV and HCV detection tests are not available in the United States although they are available in other countries (Randrianirina et al., 2008). Rapid tests for HBsAg are available in developing countries and have high sensitivity and specificity (Randrianirina et al., 2008). Rapid testing in HIV interventions has been demonstrated to add substantial value in engaging hard-to-reach populations (Begley et al., 2008; Bowles et al., 2008; Clark et al., 2008; Kassler et al., 1997; Keenan and Keenan, 2001; Liang et al., 2005; Molitor et al., 1999; Reynolds et al., 2008; Schulden et al., 2008; Shrestha et al., 2008; Smith et al., 2006; Spielberg et al., 2001, 2003, 2005; Sullivan et al., 2004). The availability of rapid tests in the

> **BOX 5-6**
> **Hepatitis B Virus-Specific Antigens and Antibodies Used for Testing**
>
> **Hepatitis B surface antigen (HBsAg):** A protein on the surface of hepatitis B virus; it can be detected at high levels in serum during acute or chronic HBV infection. The presence of HBsAg indicates that a person is infected and infectious. The body normally produces antibodies to HBsAg as part of the normal immune response to infection. HBsAg is the antigen used to make hepatitis B vaccine.
>
> **Hepatitis B surface antibody (anti-HBs):** The presence of anti-HBs is generally interpreted as indicating recovery and immunity from HBV infection. Anti-HBs also develops in a person who has been successfully vaccinated against hepatitis B.
>
> **Total hepatitis B core antibody (anti-HBc):** This appears at the onset of symptoms in acute hepatitis B and generally persists for life. The presence of anti-HBc indicates previous or current infection with HBV in an undefined time frame.
>
> **IgM antibody to hepatitis B core antigen (IgM anti-HBc):** Positivity indicates recent infection with HBV (less than 6 months). Its presence indicates acute infection.
>
> SOURCE: CDC, 2009c.

United States could enhance HBV and HCV detection and help to close gaps in care, particularly in hard-to-reach populations.

Hepatitis B Virus Laboratory Testing Serologic markers can be used to identify the different phases of HBV infection (Box 5-6). The preferred laboratory test for detecting current HBV infection is for hepatitis B surface antigen (HBsAg), and the principal test for detecting recovery from HBV infection is for anti-HB surface antibody (anti-HBs). An alternative is to test initially for anti-HB core antibody (anti-HBc)—which is present during acute, chronic, and resolved HBV infection—and, if the result is positive, to conduct followup testing for HBsAg and anti-HBs. HBV markers can be misinterpreted by clinicians, and this can lead to clinical errors in patient evaluations, counseling, or treatment. For example, anti-HBc and anti-HBs can be misinterpreted as indicators of active infection (Weinbaum, 2008).

TABLE 5-2 Interpretation of Hepatitis B Serologic Diagnostic Test Results

Antigen or Antibody Test	Result	Interpretation
HBsAg Anti-HBc Anti-HBs	All negative	Susceptible
HBsAg Anti-HBc Anti-HBs	Negative Positive Positive	Immune because of natural infection
HBsAg Anti-HBc Anti-HBs	Negative Negative Positive	Immune because of hepatitis B vaccination
HBsAg Anti-HBc IgM anti-HBc Anti-HBs	Positive Positive Positive Negative	Acutely infected
HBsAg Anti-HBc IgM anti-HBc Anti-HBs	Positive Positive Negative Negative	Chronically infected
HBsAg Anti-HBc Anti-HBs	Negative Positive Negative	Interpretation unclear; could be due to • Resolved infection • False-positive anti-HBc test • Low-level chronic infection • Resolving acute infection

Abbreviations: HBsAg, hepatitis B surface antigen; anti-HBc, total hepatitis B core antibody; anti-HBs, hepatitis B surface antibody; IgM anti-HBc, IgM antibody to hepatitis B core antigen.
SOURCE: CDC, 2009c.

Clinicians also may not know which tests to order to test for chronic vs acute viral HBV infection. Table 5-2 provides guidance on the interpretation of hepatitis B serologic test results.

Cost-effectiveness data on the use of laboratory testing in particular at-risk populations are available. As mentioned above, people born in foreign countries that have high rates of HBV (2% or more) are at the highest risk for chronic HBV infection and constitute the largest pool of undiagnosed persons (see Box 3-1). Laboratory testing of adult Asian and Pacific Islanders for HBV infection (10% prevalence of chronic HBV infection), monitoring and treating people who are found to be chronically infected, and ring vaccination of their close contacts have been shown to be cost-effective (Hutton et al., 2007). That suggests that foreign-born persons from countries that have chronic HBV rates of 2% or greater should be screened for HBV infection. If they are negative for HBV seromarkers, they should be offered vaccination.

Other populations to be tested for HBV include IDUs, pregnant women, infants born to HBsAg-positive mothers, household contacts and sex partners of HBV-infected persons, men who have sex with men, and people infected with HIV. People scheduled for immunosuppressive therapy should also be tested for HBV infection because studies have clearly shown that persons who are HBsAg-positive have a risk of 20–50% of developing flares of hepatitis when undergoing cancer chemotherapy (Lok et al., 1991; Yeo and Johnson, 2006; Yeo et al., 2000). Reactivations have also been reported to occur with other types of immunosuppressives, notably anti–tumor-necrosis factor therapy for rheumatoid arthritis and inflammatory bowel disease (Esteve et al., 2004; Ostuni et al., 2003). Most flares of hepatitis in HBsAg-positive persons in this setting are asymptomatic, but icteric flares, hepatic decompensation, and death have been reported (Lok et al., 1991; Yeo et al., 2000). It has also been demonstrated that lamivudine prophylaxis can cause a substantial reduction in the incidence and severity of hepatitis flares in HBsAg-positive persons who are undergoing cancer chemotherapy (Hsu et al., 2008; Lau et al., 2002, 2003; Li et al., 2006; Rossi et al., 2001). Therefore, all persons scheduled to undergo cancer chemotherapy or immunosuppressive treatments should be screened for hepatitis B risk factors, and followup testing for HBsAg should be performed if warranted. Persons who are HBsAg-positive should be treated as recommended by established practice guidelines (Lok and McMahon, 2009).

Hepatitis C Virus Laboratory Testing Persons at risk for hepatitis C should be tested for antibodies to HCV with a licensed enzyme immunoassay (EIA), which has a high sensitivity (Alter et al., 2003). As with all screening tests, the predictive value of a positive test varies with the population prevalence, which for HCV is lowest in volunteer blood donors and highest in IDUs. False-negative EIA tests may occur in immunosuppressed populations, such as patients on hemodialysis or infected with HIV (Rahnavardi et al., 2008; Thio et al., 2000). In those settings, EIA-negative persons suspected of having HCV infection should also be tested for HCV RNA (Ghany et al., 2009). Table 5-3 provides guidance on the interpretation of hepatitis C test results.

HCV EIA-positive results should be confirmed with a second test, ideally before the information is presented to the patient to minimize the unnecessary harm of a false-positive result. There are two separate goals of confirming a positive EIA: to make sure that the antibodies detected in the EIA were truly to HCV and not cross-reactive and to assess persons with antibodies to HCV to ascertain whether HCV infection is current or cleared spontaneously. The likelihood that a positive HCV EIA represents antibodies to HCV (as opposed to cross-reactive antibodies) depends on the strength of the EIA reaction. Values that exceed a particular threshold (for example, 3.8 for tests commonly used in the United States) are likely to be true HCV infections and unlikely to be false-positive (Alter et al., 2003; Pawlotsky et al., 1998). Thus, some laboratories report the ratio of the test result to the cutoff value, and ratios above that threshold can be assumed to represent HCV antibodies. Another way to establish whether a positive EIA reflects HCV antibodies is to run a supplemental antibody test, such as a RIBA recombinant immunoblot assay. By separating the antigens that are grouped in the screening EIA, the supplemental antibody test provides better specificity (Damen et al., 1995). However, supplemental antibody testing does not achieve the second goal of determining whether a person has HCV infection. Thus, most authorities recommend use of HCV-RNA testing as the next step after detection of HCV antibodies with EIA in all settings in which HCV testing is done in at-risk persons (Alter et al., 2003; Ghany et al., 2009). A positive result in both EIA and RNA tests means that a person needs further counseling and medical evaluation for chronic or acute HCV infection.

HCV-RNA testing is more expensive than antibody testing with EIA and may require more sophisticated laboratory capability and a longer reporting interval (Alter et al., 2003). Thus, although all reasonable efforts should be made to confirm positive EIA HCV results before presenting them, HCV-RNA testing may not be feasible in some settings. Lack of available HCV-RNA testing should not be an impediment to EIA testing, but counseling must reflect the uncertainty and the urgency of followup in another venue for further assessment.

Laboratory testing of at-risk populations to identify HCV-infected people has been found to be cost-effective when combined with proper medical-management and harm-reduction strategies (Tramarin et al., 2008). In particular, studies have found that HCV laboratory testing among current and former IDUs is cost-effective. A 2006 study of former IDUs in a prison in the United Kingdom found that laboratory testing and later treatment of inmates cost £16,514 (about $25,000) per quality adjusted life year (Castelnuovo et al., 2006). A 2008 study in Italy found that laboratory testing (followed by appropriate medical management) of IDUs resulted in a substantial difference in the incidence of premature death. In contrast, HCV laboratory testing for people who are in the hospital for surgery but have no other risk factors is unlikely to be cost-effective (Tramarin et al., 2008).

TABLE 5-3 Interpretation of Hepatitis C Virus Diagnostic Test Results

If HCV Test Result Is:			Interpretation	Action
Anti-HCV Screening Test (EIA or CIA)	Anti-HCV Supplemental Test: RIBA	Anti-HCV Supplemental Test: HCV RNA	HCV Status	Additional Testing or Evaluation Required
Positive	Not done	Not done	Not known	HCV RNA; RIBA if RNA negative
Positive	Not done	Negative	Probably not currently HCV infected; further testing required[a]	Obtain RIBA; if RIBA positive, repeat RNA
Positive (high s/co ratio)	Not done	Not done	Antibody probably true positive; need to distinguish past from current infection	HCV RNA
Positive	Negative	Not done	False positive anti-HCV	None
Positive	Positive	Not done	Past or current HCV infection	HCV RNA; if RNA positive, evaluate for liver disease
Positive	Positive	Negative	Probable past HCV infection with recovery[a]	Repeat HCV RNA to rule out active infection[a]

Positive	Positive or not done	Positive	Current acute or chronic HCV infection	Evaluate for chronic infection and liver disease
Positive	Indeterminate	Not done	Not known; possible false-positive anti-HCV or recovery from past HCV infection	Test for HCV RNA or repeat anti-HCV testing
Positive	Indeterminate	Positive	Current acute or chronic HCV infection	Evaluate for chronic infection and liver disease
Positive	Indeterminate	Negative	Probably not currently infected;[a] possible false-positive anti-HCV or recovery from past HCV infection	Repeat HCV RNA or repeat anti-HCV testing

[a] A single negative HCV-RNA result cannot determine infection status, inasmuch as a person might have intermittent viremia.

Abbreviations: anti-HCV, antibody to HCV; EIA, enzyme immunoassay; CIA, enhanced chemiluminescence immunoassay; RIBA, recombinant immunoblot assay; RNA, ribonucleic acid; s/co ratio, signal-to-cutoff ratio.

SOURCE: Adapted from Ghany et al., 2009. Diagnosis, management, and treatment of Hepatitis C: An update. *Hepatology* 49(4):1335-1374. Copyright 2009. Reprinted with permission of John Wiley & Sons, Inc.; CDC, 2009e.

Prevention

Vaccination

A vaccine for hepatitis B has been available since the 1980s. Research to develop a vaccine for hepatitis C continues although it is unlikely that a vaccine will be developed and licensed in the near future. Given the complexity of the issues surrounding vaccination of children and adults, this report devotes a separate chapter (Chapter 4) to immunization.

Harm Reduction

Harm reduction refers to programs and policies that seek to reduce the medical, social, and economic harms associated with illicit-drug use (IHRA, 2009). Support for abstinence is an element of harm reduction but is not a requirement for participation in harm-reduction programs. Harm reduction focuses on providing information about safer practices (for example, how to inject without exposing oneself to contaminated blood), providing materials for engaging in safer practices (such as needle syringes and condoms), and offering hepatitis B vaccination. Because harm reduction does not condemn illicit-drug use and instead seeks practical solutions to mitigate its harmful consequences, these programs can be controversial (Des Jarlais et al., 2009).

Medical Management

Evidence-based practice guidelines for both chronic hepatitis B and chronic hepatitis C have been published by the American Association for the Study of Liver Diseases (AASLD) and other organizations (Ghany et al., 2009; Lok and McMahon, 2009). The guidelines are updated regularly to reflect advances in care and should be referred to as the basis of appropriate medical management. For the purposes of this report, the committee specifies that the goals of medical management of chronically infected people are to decrease the risk of developing cirrhosis, to prevent hepatic decompensation, to decrease the risk of hepatocellular carcinoma in people chronically infected with HBV or HCV, and to effect secondary prevention of virus transmission.

The AASLD guidelines include recommendations for selection of patients who have chronic hepatitis B or hepatitis C for referral to specialists and for treatment with medications (Ghany et al., 2009; Lok and McMahon, 2009). Persons who are identified as HBsAg-positive should have a history taken and a physical examination performed by a primary-care provider with an emphasis on symptoms and signs of liver disease

(Lok and McMahon, 2009). Initial laboratory evaluation should include a full liver panel, complete blood count (CBC), and hepatitis B e antigen (HBeAg), anti-HB e antibody (anti-HBe), and HBV DNA tests. Further management will depend on the results. Persons who are HBeAg-positive and have increased alanine aminotransferase (ALT) should be referred for evaluation for possible liver biopsy and treatment. Likewise, persons who are HBeAg-negative and anti-HBe-positive, have increased HBV DNA (over 2,000 IU/mL), and have increased ALT should be referred to a specialist. People who have normal ALT, are HBeAg-negative and anti-HBe-positive, and have HBV DNA below 2,000 IU/mL can be followed with ALT and aspartate aminotransferase (AST) tests every 6 months by a primary care provider. If ALT increases above the normal limit, HBV DNA should be tested again; if it is above 2,000 IU/mL, the patient should be referred to a specialist. If a patient is HBeAg-positive and has normal ALT (that is, in the immune tolerant phase), tests for ALT, AST, HBeAg, and anti-HBe should be repeated every 6 months. If ALT rises above the normal range, the patient should be referred to a specialist. In patients who have increased ALT and HBV DNA, liver biopsy is often appropriate to determine the best candidates for treatment because it is recommended that patients who have more than mild inflammation and fibrosis on biopsy receive treatment, and laboratory tests are often unable to distinguish degrees of liver involvement (Lok and McMahon, 2004; NIH, 2008). In addition, any patient who has stigmata of liver disease—ascites, enlarged spleen, jaundice, or encephalopathy—or a platelet count below 100,000 (which is a sign of possible splenomegaly) should be referred immediately to a specialist. The AASLD provides hepatitis B–specific treatment guidelines, including how to select appropriate candidates for treatment, guidance on which antiviral medications to use, and how to address antiviral resistance (Lok and McMahon, 2009). All chronically HBV-infected patients, regardless of their ALT and HBV DNA status, must be followed on a regular basis, every 3–12 months depending on the activity of their disease.

Persons who are identified as anti-HCV-positive and who have HCV RNA present in their serum may initially be evaluated by a primary care provider (Ghany et al., 2009). The primary care provider should take a history and perform a physical examination with emphasis on symptoms and signs of liver disease. The initial laboratory evaluation should include a full liver panel, CBC, and HCV genotype tests. Patients found to have signs or symptoms of liver disease or a low platelet count (below 100,000) should be referred to a specialist who has experience in managing persons with advanced hepatitis C. Patients who are infected with HCV genotype 2 or 3 and who are interested in receiving treatment can be referred immediately for treatment consideration. A primary care provider should discuss with a patient who is infected with HCV genotype 1 the possibility of receiving treatment and should emphasize that the treatment is successful in only about 50% of cases and that the side effects can be severe. For genotype 1 patients, it may be preferable first to do a liver biopsy to determine the degree of liver involvement and scarring before making a decision about whether treatment should be considered sooner rather than later. The AASLD provides hepatitis C–specific treatment guidelines, including how to select appropriate candidates for treatment and guidance on which antiviral medications to use (Ghany et al., 2009). Patients who do not want immediate referral or treatment should be followed every 6 months with a full liver panel and yearly CBC tests. Finally, primary care providers should counsel patients to abstain from, or at least limit, alcohol consumption because heavy alcohol use is the greatest contributor to the rate of progressive liver fibrosis. Patients who have a history of heavy alcohol intake should receive counseling.

Studies have found racial and ethnic disparities in the evaluation of and treatment for HCV infection (Butt et al., 2007; Rousseau et al., 2008). One study of veterans reported similar rates of referral and liver biopsy for HCV-infected persons of various racial populations but found that blacks were less likely than whites to have complete laboratory evaluations, including viral genotyping, and to receive antiviral treatment (Rousseau et al., 2008). Because patient characteristics that are associated with not responding to treatment generally are associated with not receiving treatment, it is difficult to ascertain from available research findings the degree to which lower uptake into treatment represents discrimination against minority populations or appropriate implementation of treatment guidelines. For example, in another study of veterans, less treatment was received by minority-groups members and by persons who were older, who had a history of drug and alcohol use, or who had comorbid illnesses (Butt et al., 2007).

Chronic HCV infection has been found to be an important cause of liver-related death in Alaska Natives (Wise et al., 2008). The federal government is responsible by treaty laws to provide medical care at no cost to American Indians and Alaska Natives, but the amount spent per person is far less than that spent for Medicare and Medicaid recipients or for incarcerated persons, and is not enough to pay for treatment for HCV infection in many tribal health-care systems. There is evidence that not all patients who initiate therapy complete it. Over 80% of participants in clinical trials completed the HCV antiviral therapy. However, researchers found that in a large national cohort of veterans less than one-fourth of the patients who began treatment for chronic hepatitis C completed a 48-week course. The major predictors of treatment noncompletion were pretreatment anemia and depression (Butt et al., 2009). Treatment completion rates appear to vary among ethnic and racial populations. For example, a study found that Hispanic patients were more likely to be candidates for treatment but were less likely to initiate it; they were also more likely to discontinue treatment early, and discontinuation of treatment was associated with alcohol use (Cheung et al., 2005).

The risk of developing hepatocellular carcinoma (HCC) is a serious concern for patients who are infected with HBV or HCV, and providers should initiate regular monitoring for HCC (Bruix and Sherman, 2005). Patients who have chronic HBV infection and are at the highest risk for HCC include those who have first-degree relatives who developed HCC, persons who have cirrhosis, men 40 years old and older, and women 50 years old and older. Of patients who have chronic HCV infection, only those who have cirrhosis or advanced liver fibrosis (that is, bridging fibrosis) should be monitored for HCC. Monitoring of patients at high risk for HCC should be performed every 6 months.

Studies have found ethnic disparities in HCC treatment rates and mortality (Davila and El-Serag, 2006; Siegel et al., 2008; Sonnenday et al., 2007). Blacks and Hispanics had significantly higher HCC-related mortality than other racial and ethnic populations. Even after adjustment for stage of HCC and other demographic characteristics, blacks were 40% less likely than whites to receive local or surgical therapy. Another study found that blacks and Hispanics were 24–27% less likely than whites to receive surgical therapy (Sonnenday et al., 2007). A study that looked at liver transplants necessitated by HCC found that in 1998–2002, black and Asian patients were significantly less likely than white patients to receive a liver transplant (Siegel et al., 2008). Once researchers controlled for receipt of treatment, the difference in mortality in black patients was no longer significant (Davila and El-Serag, 2006). Those data on racial and ethnic disparities in the outcomes of and treatments for chronic hepatitis underscore the need for additional research to understand the biologic and societal basis of the disparities. They also indicate the urgency of new policies that ensure that optimal medical care is given to all without regard to race or ethnicity.

The economic costs of chronic hepatitis B and hepatitis C are high. In 2004, the average annual medical-care costs of chronic HBV infection and its complications per infected person in the United States were as follows: chronic HBV infection, $761; compensated cirrhosis, $227; decompensated cirrhosis, $11,459; liver transplantation, $86,552; transplantation care more than 12 months after transplantation, $12,560; and hepatocellular carcinoma, $7,533 (Lee et al., 2004). Medication costs were the largest proportion of the chronic HBV infection and compensated cirrhosis states and hospitalization costs made up the largest proportion of the other health states. In the same year, Chesson et al. (2004) estimated the annual net cost per case of chronic liver disease at $32,837 in the United States.

Although treatment costs are high, some studies have found that treatment can be cost-effective. In particular, several studies compared the costs of various treatments for chronic HBV infection (for example, interferon, pegylated interferon, lamivudine, and adefovir) and found them to be cost-effective (Kanwal et al., 2005; Rajendra and Wong, 2007). Treatments for HCV infection with interferon or pegylated interferon plus ribavirin have also been shown to be cost-effective (Campos et al., 2007; Lidgren et al., 2007; Rajendra and Wong, 2007; Salomon et al., 2003).

There is evidence that people's ability to pay affects whether they seek and receive appropriate medical care for chronic hepatitis B and hepatitis C. For example, among people who tested positive for HCV antibody at public STD clinics in San Diego and an HIV test-site screening program, the presence or absence of health insurance was strongly associated with whether later medical care was received for HCV (Mark et al., 2007).

MAJOR GAPS IN SERVICES

The lack of comprehensive case management (that is, initial clinical evaluation and laboratory testing, regularly scheduled clinical and laboratory monitoring, appropriate referral and treatment, and monitoring for HCC) for people who have chronic hepatitis B or hepatitis C and who do not have access to private health insurance and care is an important gap in control of chronic viral hepatitis. The committee believes that people who are living with chronic HBV or HCV infection should receive the health-care services outlined in Box 5-3. The Ryan White Care program for people who are living with HIV/AIDS is a federal approach that could be replicated to fill the void in health-care services for patients who have HBV or HCV infection. The committee recognizes that uncertainties in funding and health-care reform may make implementation of such a program challenging.

General Population

Various factors can lead to difficulties in accessing screening, prevention, testing, and care related to viral hepatitis. Obstacles to obtaining such services may be limitations in private or public insurance coverage and cost-sharing, lack of access to public health insurance, lack of public funding to support implementation of state viral hepatitis plans, lack of hepatitis awareness and health literacy, inadequacy of sites or practice settings where health-care services are received, transportation needs, social stigmas, fear of legal prosecution related to drug use and immigration, and such cultural factors as religious beliefs, beliefs about biologic products, health perceptions, and language. Among those, however, the most important barriers to receipt of existing services are inadequacy of health-insurance coverage and lack of money to pay for services.

Having insurance, either privately or publicly funded, has a positive association with laboratory testing for HBV infection, and those who have private insurance have the highest testing rates. For example, Choe et al. (2006) reported a strong relation between having ever been tested for HBV and insurance coverage in Vietnamese American men in Seattle, Washington. In their study, 70% of privately insured people and 51% of people insured by the Washington State Basic Health Insurance Plan were ever tested for HBV. As discussed in Chapter 4, health insurance must provide strong coverage for immunization, counseling services, medical treatment, and prescription drugs, or the insurance's cost-sharing features will prevent use of services. High deductibles (amounts to be paid out of pocket before coverage begins) or benefit limits are common in insurance policies that are provided by medium and small employers or in-network plans (which provide different coverage in network from out of network). That is not the case with more comprehensive insurance coverage typically seen in integrated delivery systems and health maintenance organizations (HMOs). As of 2007, 21% of workers who had employer-sponsored health insurance were covered under HMOs (Claxton et al., 2007). In publicly funded venues—where services for the poor or special risk populations, such as STD clinics, or for IDUs are provided—inadequacies in funding for hepatitis-related services may limit testing or other services (Boutwell et al., 2005; Brown et al., 2007; Heseltine and McFarlane, 2007; McIntyre et al., 2008).

The current fragmentation of viral hepatitis services involving vaccination, risk-factor screening, laboratory testing, and medical management is a major obstacle to the effective delivery of needed services and makes compliance more difficult. The lack of coordination between services can inhibit use by requiring people to travel to multiple sites to obtain care, impairs the development of trusting relationships among multiple providers, and taxes a health system's ability to transfer information where and when it is needed for good clinical care. Studies have examined program integration for HIV, STD, and viral hepatitis services and found that integration brings more at-risk people into the system (Birkhead et al., 2007; Gilbert et al., 2005; Gunn et al., 2007; Hennessy et al., 2007; Kresina et al., 2008; Stopka et al., 2007; Zimmerman et al., 2007).

One important consequence of the fragmentation of viral-hepatitis services is inconsistency in referral of people who have chronic viral hepatitis for appropriate medical care. That gap reflects deficiencies primary-care providers' knowledge, and it can be substantial when there are barriers, such as physical barriers (that is, screening and testing services in a different location from medical-management services), economic barriers, and cultural barriers. As discussed below, the Department of Veterans Affairs (VA) is notable for having bridged the gap integrating health services.

The VA Medical Center in Minnesota developed a hospital-based model that could serve as a template for health-care providers in integrated delivery systems, accountable care organizations, and HMOs (Groom et al., 2008). The medical center established a method to screen patients for HCV risk factors, to initiate appropriate viral testing, to counsel patients, and to refer them to a dedicated hepatitis clinic for medical evaluations, liver biopsies, and appropriate antiviral therapy. In addition, it traced the outcome of therapy and continued to follow those who did not respond. VA performed risk-assessment screening of 36,422 patients for HCV infection (Groom et al., 2008). The screening identified 12,485 patients (34%) who had risk indications for anti-HCV testing. Anti-HCV antibodies were identified in 681 (5.4% of those at risk) and HCV RNA was detected in 520 (4.2% of those at risk and 76% of those who were anti-HCV positive). Of those who tested positive for HCV RNA, 430 (83%) were referred to the hepatitis clinic, of whom 382 (73%) attended. A relatively large percentage of patients (45%) were evaluated in the clinic and underwent liver biopsy. On the basis of the extent of fibrosis on biopsy, 124 patients received antiviral therapy—32% of the patients referred to the clinic and 24% of those who had viremia. A sustained virologic response occurred in 37% of the treated patients. Thus, 46 patients could be considered cured, and 17 had stage 3 or 4 fibrosis, which could potentially result in end-stage liver disease and possibly HCC.

Closed systems, such as HMOs, and integrated delivery systems have the potential to replicate the VA model. Those sources of health care share the VA advantages of control of the various providers and care settings, comprehensive coverage that reduces financial barriers to compliance, administrative and information systems to track and share information, team-based processes of care, and the ability to enforce standards of performance.

The federal government is the largest purchaser of health insurance nationally, with about 8 million people covered through the Federal Employees Health Benefits Program and those covered through Medicare, Medicaid, and the Children's Health Insurance Program. Given its tremendous purchasing power, the federal government is well positioned to be the leader in the development and enforcement of guidelines to ensure that the people for whom it provides health care have access to risk-factor screening, serologic testing for HBV and HCV, and appropriate medical management.

Recommendation 5-1. Federally funded health-insurance programs—such as Medicare, Medicaid, and the Federal Employees Health Benefits Program—should incorporate guidelines for risk-factor screening for hepatitis B and hepatitis C as a required core component of preventive care so that at-risk people receive serologic testing for hepatitis B virus and hepatitis C virus and chronically infected patients receive appropriate medical management.

The committee has included recommendations regarding coverage of vaccination for infants, children, and adults in Chapter 4.

Foreign-Born People

There are over 37 million foreign-born residents in the United States; they represent about 12% of the nation's population (U.S. Census Bureau, 2008). Of the foreign-born population, 27% were born in Asia, 4% in Africa, and roughly 7% in other regions that have intermediate or high HBV endemicity (see Box 3-1). Nearly half the US foreign-born population (6% of the total population) originated in HBV-endemic countries (U.S. Census Bureau, 2008), and 40,000–45,000 legal immigrants from these countries enter the United States each year (U.S. Department of Homeland Security, 2009; Weinbaum, 2008). It is increasingly urgent that culturally appropriate programs provide hepatitis B screening and related services to this high-risk population.

Efforts to deliver hepatitis B–related services to the foreign-born population have been sparse. At the federal level, there are limited and fragmented resources to track and fund such services. On the local and regional levels, some culturally tailored community-based or faith-based screening programs target foreign-born people, such as those involving Asian and Pacific Islander populations in San Francisco, Maryland, and New York City (CDC, 2006; Chao et al., 2009a; Hsu et al., 2007). However, few of the independent programs have been replicated in other communities of at-risk foreign-born populations, so many regions in the United States that have at-risk foreign-born populations lack community-based hepatitis B screening (Rein et al., 2009). Few HBV screening programs are designed for other high-risk foreign-born populations, including Africans, Middle Easterners, eastern Europeans, and others from HBV-endemic regions. It is unknown whether the model programs developed for Asians and Pacific Islanders could be adapted for some of those populations or whether new culturally tailored programs would need to be created.

The key to eliminating HBV transmission is identification of people who are living with chronic HBV infection. As described in Chapter 3, there is a pervasive ignorance about hepatitis B among Asians and Pacific Islanders, and it can be assumed that other foreign-born populations in the United States are similarly uninformed about HBV risks, prevention, testing, and management. That contributes to the observation that up to two-thirds of those who are chronically infected with HBV are unaware of their infection status (Lin et al., 2007). The lack of awareness in foreign-born populations from HBV-endemic countries is compounded by gaps in knowledge and preventive practice among health-care providers, particularly if they are serving a large number of foreign-born, high-risk patients (see Chapter 3).

Cultural and institutional impediments are particularly important for the foreign-born. For example, culture-specific stigmas may be attached to a diagnosis of chronic hepatitis B. In China, there is discrimination against people who are chronically infected with HBV, and such people reportedly have been expelled from schools, fired from jobs, and shunned by other community members despite the recent passage of national antidiscrimination laws (China Digital Times, 2009). Such social stigma and discrimination may contribute to the reluctance of immigrants from HBV-endemic countries to undergo HBsAg testing or to seek medical attention for a positive test result after settling in the United States.

Institutional barriers include administrative procedures and the absence of culturally responsive support services. For example, a recent survey of hospitals in the San Francisco Bay area—a region where 29% of the population is foreign-born—found that fewer than half routinely collect information on patients' birthplaces (Gomez et al., 2003). The collection of information on the birthplace of patients' parents is even rarer—but relevant for risk assessment. English-language proficiency and cultural preferences of foreign-born patients may pose additional challenges to institutions that are not prepared to work with these patient factors. Non-English-speaking patients report that physicians are intolerant and impatient toward them and fail to use interpreter services, even when available, to facilitate communication (Barr and Wanat, 2005; Giordano and Cooper, 2009; Giordano et al., 2009). As a result of patient–physician language discordance and impaired communication, such patients have poorer comprehension of medical conditions, testing, and treatment; have low compliance; and are more likely to miss followup appointments (Giordano and Cooper, 2009; Giordano et al., 2009; Jacobs et al., 2006; Manson, 1988; Zickmund et al., 2004).

There is a need for evidence-based strategies and programs to disseminate information about hepatitis B transmission, infection, and treatment to culturally and demographically diverse populations. A community-based participatory research approach, in which communities are actively engaged in equal partnership with scientists, is needed to ensure that the programs are acceptable, accessible, and sustainable in the communities where they are based. Such programs should also be flexible and scalable so that other communities can tailor them to their own needs. The committee believes that these tasks are best accomplished with the approach outlined in Recommendations 3-1 and 3-2 in Chapter 3. The community-based approach as outlined in Recommendation 3-2 would be strengthened by additional resources to provide screening, testing, and vaccination services. Therefore, the committee offers the following recommendation:

> **Recommendation 5-2.** The Centers for Disease Control and Prevention, in conjunction with other federal agencies and state agencies, should provide resources for the expansion of community-based programs that provide hepatitis B screening, testing, and vaccination services that target foreign-born populations.

Illicit-Drug Users

Preventing bloodborne infectious diseases, particularly hepatitis C, in illicit-drug users is an important public-health challenge. Hepatitis C incidence in IDUs has been reported to be 2–40 per 100 person-years (PY) of observation, with most rates in the range of 15–30 per 100 PY (Maher et al., 2006; Mathei et al., 2005; van den Berg et al., 2007b). HCV prevalence in IDUs is typically 35–70%, depending on geographic location and duration of exposure to injection-drug use (Hagan et al., 2008). The early years after onset of drug injection are high-risk periods when HCV seroconversion rates are particularly high (Maher et al., 2006).

Non-injection-drug users (NIDUs) who sniff or snort heroin, cocaine, and other drugs also have a high risk of HCV infection. A meta-analysis of 26 studies showed that HCV prevalence in NIDUs was 2–35%, with a median of 14% (Scheinmann et al., 2007). Whether drug practices, sexual exposures, or both are the sources of HCV transmission is unclear (Scheinmann et al., 2007). Low rates of HCV seroconversion have been reported in NIDUs—0.4–2.7 per 100 PY—rates that are similar to those observed in sex partners of HCV-RNA–positive persons (1.2 per 100 PY) (Fuller et al., 2004; Neaigus et al., 2007; Rooney and Gilson, 1998). Studies have shown that HCV RNA can be detected on the surface of crack pipes, so it is biologically plausible that drug-use practices are a route of transmission in these people (Fischer et al., 2008). Research is needed to explicate the etiology of HCV infection in NIDUs so that effective prevention strategies can be designed.

To understand the development and opportunities for control of this hyperendemic state of HCV infection in IDUs, it is important to consider multiple features of the disease agent, the human host, and the environment that determine the occurrence of infection (Lillienfeld and Lillienfeld, 1980). HCV is efficiently transmitted via bloodborne exposure, and several studies have shown that transmission can occur via the shared use of syringes, drug cookers, and filtration cotton (Hagan et al., 2001; Hahn et al., 2002; Thorpe et al., 2002). It takes only a very small amount of infectious blood on injection equipment to result in infection. Awareness of risk of HCV infection associated with the shared use of cookers and cotton is not widespread, and about 40% of HCV transmission may be attributable to the sharing of these items (Hagan et al., 2010). Injection often takes place in settings that are chaotic, rushed, or otherwise not conducive to safe practices, thereby increasing the risk of disease transmission (Rhodes and Treloar, 2008). The persistence of moderate levels of unsafe injection behaviors seems to be sufficient to maintain relatively high rates of new infections (Thiede et al., 2007). The high prevalence of infectious carriers also means that there is a high probability that one or more IDUs present in the injection setting may be capable of transmitting HCV.

HBV infection rates in both IDUs and NIDUs are high. Seroincidence in IDUs has been reported to be 10–12% per year (Hagan et al., 1999; Ruan et al., 2007). A study that looked at evidence of past or present HBV infections found rates of 37% in IDUs and 19% in NIDUs (Kuo et al., 2004). HBV transmission in these populations generally occurs as a result of drug-related and sexual exposures to infected people. A study of more than 800 young IDUs (up to 30 years old) found low hepatitis B vaccination coverage (22%) and a high prevalence of HBV infection (21%) (Lum et al., 2008).

Although drug use is associated with many serious acute and chronic medical conditions, health-care utilization among drug users is low compared with persons who do not use illicit drugs (Chitwood et al., 1999; Contoreggi et al., 1998; O'Toole et al., 2007, 2008). Health care for both IDUs and NIDUs is sporadic and generally received in hospital emergency rooms, correction facilities, and STD clinics (Chitwood et al., 1999; Huckans et al., 2005). Given this population's limited access to health care and services, it is important to have prevention and care services in settings that IDUs and NIDUs are likely to frequent or to develop programs that will draw them into care.

Program Venues

Because of its similarity to HIV in transmission routes, public-health practitioners expected that strategies that were working for HIV would work similarly in the case of HCV. The two major public-health interventions that have been shown to reduce HIV risk in IDUs are drug-treatment programs and syringe-exchange programs (SEPs) (Des Jarlais et al., 1996; Metzger et al., 1998).

Drug-treatment programs offer few services related to hepatitis B and hepatitis C and are constrained by lack of funding (Stanley, 1999). A nationwide study of drug-treatment clinics found that although most clinics educated patients about the importance of testing for HCV, only 7% tested all clients for HCV and 22% tested none (Astone et al., 2003; Strauss et al., 2002, 2004).

Starting in the 1980s with the introduction of HIV into IDU populations, there were mass awareness and safe-injection campaigns that resulted in substantial reductions in syringe-sharing (Des Jarlais and Semaan, 2008). In the United States, SEPs are now available in 31 states, the District of Columbia, and Puerto Rico (Des Jarlais et al., 2009). Several characteristics support the use of SEPs as sites of care for and prevention of hepatitis B and hepatitis C. SEPs, in addition to providing safe injection materials and counseling services, are key access points for screening and referral to followup medical care (Des Jarlais et al., 2009). SEPs appear to attract and retain high-risk injectors, in particular those at highest risk for HIV or HCV seroconversion (Hagan et al., 2001; Schechter et al., 1999). SEPs can be referral pathways to other programs. Demand for drug treatment is high among exchange users and SEPs are important venues for drug-treatment referral (Kidorf et al., 2009; Strauss et al., 2003a). About 92% of US SEPs offer referrals to substance-abuse treatment programs (Des Jarlais et al., 2009), and 33% offer on-site medical care (Des Jarlais et al., 2009), although the services offered vary and there is great geographic variability in their distribution. Syringe coverage rates—the number of syringes available via SEPs per 100 injections—are also highly variable, ranging between 0.03 and 20 per 100 injections, and there are vast regions of the United States where SEPs are not available (Tempalski et al., 2008). Those factors limit the impact of the programs for HCV control (Tempalski et al., 2007, 2008). In addition, SEPs have not been as successful in reducing the shared use of other injection equipment, such as cookers and cottons, as they have been in reducing syringe-sharing (Hagan and Thiede, 2000).

Prevention Strategies

Several strategies to reduce HCV transmission in IDUs have been evaluated. A number of studies have examined opiate-substitution treatment and HCV seroconversion (summarized in Table 5-4). Results of those studies suggest that retention in drug treatment is likely to be protective against HCV seroconversion (Dolan et al., 2005; Rezza et al., 1996; Smyth et al., 2000; Thiede et al., 2000). Retention in drug treatment may also be associated with personal characteristics that are related to lower risk of HCV infection, but in any case it appears that risk is reduced in persons who do remain in treatment. It is plausible for drug treatment to reduce the risk of HCV infection inasmuch as it reduces the frequency of injection, and some IDUs stop injecting altogether. One limitation of drug-treatment programs is that only a relatively small proportion of IDUs (about one-sixth) are in treatment at any given time. In addition, the studies were limited to opiate-substitution programs; cocaine injectors and other non-opiate injectors may not experience similar benefits.

TABLE 5-4 Studies of Association Between Opiate Substitution Treatment and Hepatitis C Virus Seroconversion

Reference	Location	Design	Results
Rezza et al., 1996	Italy	Case-control	MMTP protective against HCV seroconversion (OR, 0.34; 95% CI, 0.1–1.1)
Crofts et al., 1997	Melbourne, Australia	Cohort	HCV incidence in people Continuously in MMTP: 36.9/100 PY (95% CI 19.1-70.9) Interrupted MMTP: 14.2/100 PY (95% CI 6.3-31.6) No MMTP: 21.4 (95% CI 8.0-57.0)
Thiede et al., 2000	Seattle, WA	Cohort in MMTP at enrollment	Reduced incidence in those who continued treatment vs those who left treatment (adjusted OR, 0.4; 95% CI, 0–4.2)
Patrick et al., 2001	Vancouver, Canada	Cohort	Cumulative HCV incidence 25% in those in MMTP vs 42% in others ($p = 0.20$)
Smyth et al., 2003	Dublin, Ireland	Cohort	Lower incidence in those in MMTP over 3 months vs others (52 vs. 75 per 100 PY; $p = 0.06$)
Dolan et al., 2005	Sydney, Australia	Cohort of incarcerated IDUs	Lowest incidence in those in continuous MMTP (8/100 PY) vs. those in for less than 5 months (23/100 PY) ($p = 0.01$)
Maher et al., 2006	Sydney, Australia	Cohort	Being in treatment during the follow-up period had no effect on HCV seroconversion (OR = 0.83, 95% CI 0.51-1.35)

Abbreviations: CI, confidence interval; HCV, hepatitis C virus; IDU, injection-drug user; MMTP, methadone maintenance therapy program; NS, not significant; OR, odds ratio; PY, person-years.

Research results suggest that multicomponent risk reduction may be needed to control HCV in active injectors. Some studies have shown that the incidence of HCV infection continues to be high in IDUs who participate in SEPs (Hagan et al., 1999; Holtzman et al., 2009; Mansson et al., 2000; Patrick et al., 2001). However, other studies have found associations between SEPs and reductions in HCV infection rates. A case-control study showed that use of a SEP in Tacoma, Washington, was associated with an 88% lower risk of HCV infection and an 82% lower risk of HBV infection (Hagan et al., 1995). A study in Amsterdam showed that IDUs who had "full participation in harm reduction"—they obtained all syringes from a syringe exchange or received at least 60 mg of methadone per day—had substantially and significantly lower rates of HCV seroconversion: fewer than 5 per 100 PY versus more than 25 per 100 PY in others who did not participate fully (van den Berg et al., 2007a).

A recent study of long-term IDUs who remained HIV- and HCV-seronegative showed that they relied on a number of strategies to avoid infection, including maintaining a regular supply of syringes and drug-preparation equipment, managing their addiction by entering drug treatment as needed to reduce their dosage, and maintaining social support to provide stability (Mateu-Gelabert et al., 2007). Drug users who are successful in avoiding infection have developed strategies to maintain control over their chaotic lives. It is clear that HCV prevention is more challenging than HIV prevention for IDUs and will require greater efforts and resources (Hagan et al., 2008).

Research related to the practice of disinfecting syringes with bleach indicates that it has no effect on HCV seroconversion (Hagan and Thiede, 2003; Kapadia et al., 2002). Development of new disinfecting agents that are effective in drug-injection settings may contribute to prevention of HCV infection in IDUs.

Other potentially useful prevention strategies focus on HCV education, testing, and counseling. A large multicity randomized controlled trial of young HIV-negative and HCV-negative IDUs showed that participation in a six-session peer-education training program led to significant reductions in unsafe injections (Garfein et al., 2007). A randomized controlled trial of a similar intervention for HCV-positive young injectors also showed reductions in behavior that may transmit HCV (Latka et al., 2008).

Recommendations

Given the large set of factors that favor HCV transmission in IDUs, it is not surprising that interventions that address individual aspects of risk have not been shown to reduce incidence in individual injectors. In light of the biology of HCV transmission—exposure to very small doses of in-

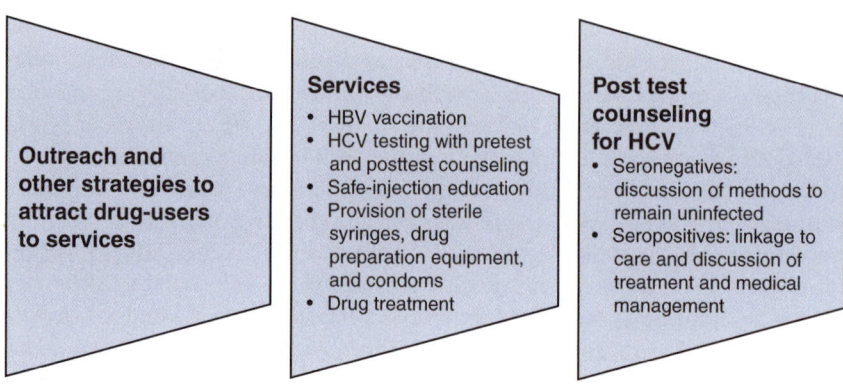

FIGURE 5-2 Essential viral hepatitis services for illicit-drug users.
Abbreviations: HBV, hepatitis B virus; HCV, hepatitis C virus.

fectious blood on injection equipment can result in infection—methods to promote safe injection can be considered essential for HCV control. Safe-injection strategies require access to sterile syringes and other equipment and education to promote adoption and maintenance of safe behavior. HCV testing and counseling to increase awareness of infection status will also support safe practices. Access to sterile syringes and other equipment can be increased through a combination of SEPs, pharmacy sales, and other methods, such as the use of syringe-vending machines (Islam et al., 2008; McDonald, 2009; Moatti et al., 2001). Drug treatment will reduce injection frequency and assist a modest proportion of injectors to achieve abstinence. Research has shown that none of those approaches by itself is sufficient to eliminate HCV transmission. Because HCV prevention is a function of multiple factors—safe-injection strategies, education, testing, and drug treatment—an integrated program that includes all these essential elements is more likely to be effective in preventing hepatitis C (see Figure 5-2).

> Recommendation 5-3. Federal, state, and local agencies should expand programs to reduce the risk of hepatitis C virus infection through injection-drug use by providing comprehensive hepatitis C virus prevention programs. At a minimum, the programs should include access to sterile needle syringes and drug-preparation equipment because the shared use of these materials has been shown to lead to transmission of hepatitis C virus.

> Recommendation 5-4. Federal and state governments should expand services to reduce the harm caused by chronic hepatitis B and hepati-

tis C. The services should include testing to detect infection, counseling to reduce alcohol use and secondary transmission, hepatitis B vaccination, and referral for or provision of medical management.

On the basis of current knowledge of the etiology and prevention of HCV in IDUs, prevention strategies should include access to sterile injection equipment, safe-injection education, HCV testing and counseling, and access to drug-treatment programs. Programs should include education about safe drug use (avoiding the shared use of implements to administer drugs by smoking or inhalation) and reduction in sex-related risks, and all participants in the programs should be offered the hepatitis B vaccine. The programs should be studied to elucidate the etiology of HCV infection in IDUs and to guide the design of prevention programs. As mentioned above, studies have shown that the first few years after onset of injection-drug use constitute a high-risk period in which the rate of HCV infection can exceed 40%. Preventing the transition from non-injection-drug use to injection-drug use will probably avert many HCV infections. The committee therefore offers the following research recommendation.

Recommendation 5-5. Innovative, effective, multicomponent hepatitis C virus prevention strategies for injection-drug users and non-injection-drug users should be developed and evaluated to achieve greater control of hepatitis C virus transmission. In particular,
- Hepatitis C prevention programs for persons who smoke or sniff heroin, cocaine, and other drugs should be developed and tested.
- Programs to prevent the transition from noninjection use of illicit drugs to injection should be developed and implemented.

Pregnant Women

The Advisory Committee on Immunization Practices has recommended routine screening of all pregnant women for HBsAg since 1988 (see Chapter 4). The value and benefits of routine screening of pregnant women for HBsAg were reaffirmed by the USPSTF in 2009 (U.S. Preventive Services Task Force, 2009). Today, 27 states have maternal HBsAg-screening laws, and 24 have specific maternal-HBsAg regulations that require health providers to report all cases of positive HBsAg blood tests to the local health department (CDC, 2007).

More than 95% of pregnant women in the United States are tested prenatally for HBsAg (Mast et al., 2005). States and large metropolitan areas are eligible to receive federal funding to support perinatal hepatitis B prevention programs through CDC's National Center for Immunization and Respiratory Disease (Jacques-Carroll et al., 2007). The programs are administered by state and local public-health departments and vary in reach and intensity. As mentioned in Chapter 2, many programs simply provide surveillance, and others provide comprehensive case management that even includes client home visits by local coordinators. That variability accounts for the wide variation (17–59%) in rates of vaccination of household contacts of HBsAg-positive pregnant women (Euler et al., 2003a).

Adequately funded perinatal hepatitis B programs are effective. Among women enrolled in such programs for case management, the rate of administration of the birth dose of hepatitis B vaccine and HBIG was as high as 94%, with a three-dose completion rate of 71% (Jacques-Carroll, 2008). Perinatal hepatitis B programs identify twice as many household and sexual contacts per infant as was reported to the national database, with high rates of programmatic compliance in households of foreign-born people (Euler et al., 2003a). Most US programs are understaffed and underfunded, however, making adequate case management difficult. This gap has a two-fold effect in that chronically infected women do not receive the appropriate medical management and referral and perinatal transmission continues to occur. CDC estimates that only 50% of HBsAg-positive pregnant women are identified for case management (CDC, 2005). It has been estimated that failure of perinatal HBV-prevention efforts result in about 1,000 cases of chronic HBV infection in newborns each year (Ward, 2008b).

Hepatitis B Medical Management of Pregnant Women

An estimated 20,000 infants a year are born to women who test positive for HBV (Euler et al., 2003b). Those women require followup services to ensure that they are knowledgeable about risks posed by their chronic infection and that they receive appropriate referral for long-term medical management. Their close contacts at home should be tested for HBV infection, those who are uninfected should be vaccinated, and medical referral should be provided to those found to have chronic HBV infection. Cases among household contacts are not uncommon when this risk group is pursued aggressively for testing. Data reported by Euler et al. (2003a) showed that 7–35% of household contacts of HBsAg-positive pregnant women were HBsAg-positive.

Deficiencies in health-care providers' knowledge or appropriate followup of HBsAg-positive pregnant women are noteworthy and require special emphasis in HBV prevention and control strategies. Obstetricians' knowledge and preventive practices are suboptimal. In a 1997 study of San Francisco obstetricians, over 90% of respondents acknowledged the public-health importance of HBV infection and believed that HBV education was feasible, but only 53% of the responding obstetricians offered

HBV information to their patients (Zola et al., 1997). In a more recent California study of obstetrical practices in 2008, only 62% referred patients who had new diagnoses of HBV to internists or specialists for followup of their chronic HBV infection (Chao et al., 2009b).

Hepatitis B services for foreign-born pregnant women are in need of improved resources that are more culturally and linguistically appropriate. Some 73% of HBsAg-positive pregnant women in the United States were born in East Asia or Southeast Asia (Din, 2009). Among them, Asian and Pacific Islanders, who account for only 5.7% of all births in the United States (CDC, 2009b), account for over two-thirds of births to mothers who have chronic HBV infection. CDC-funded perinatal HBV prevention coordinators are responsible for educating HBsAg-positive mothers and for referring them for appropriate medical management. The coordinators are restricted in their ability to fulfill that responsibility in culturally relevant ways, because of inadequate training and resources (Chao et al., 2009a). To strengthen the capacity and capabilities of the perinatal-HBV coordinators, the committee offers the following recommendation:

Recommendation 5-6. The Centers for Disease Control and Prevention should provide additional resources and guidance to perinatal hepatitis B prevention program coordinators to expand and enhance the capacity to identify chronically infected pregnant women and provide case-management services, including referral for appropriate medical management.

Preventing Perinatal Transmission

Practice guidelines and additional recommendations focused on vaccination to prevent perinatal transmission are detailed in Chapter 4. There is a need to fund research to guide the effective use of antiviral medications late in pregnancy to prevent maternofetal HBV transmission, particularly by high-risk pregnant women who are positive for HBeAg or who have high HBV loads. Results of a few small studies have suggested that the use of lamivudine in the last trimester of pregnancy reduces the rate of perinatal transmission from mothers with high HBV DNA (Li et al., 2003; van Nunen et al., 2000; van Zonneveld et al., 2003). Xu et al. (2009) reported the results of a small randomized, double-blind, placebo-controlled trial involving 155 participants divided into treatment groups; the purpose of the trial was to see whether lamivudine given during late pregnancy could reduce perinatal transmission of HBV. Results suggested that lamivudine in late pregnancy was safe and could reduce HBV transmission from mothers who had high viral loads to their infants who also received HBIG passive immunization. However, the study was small, and large randomized, double-blind, placebo-controlled trials are needed to evaluate the efficacy and safety of oral hepatitis B antiviral therapy in eliminating perinatal HBV transmission from women at high risk for perinatal transmission. Although an increasing number of effective HBV antiviral suppressive medications have become available for the management of chronic HBV infection, very little research has been done on the use of these medications during the last trimester of pregnancy to eliminate the risk of perinatal transmission, particularly in the high-risk population of women who test positive for HBeAg or have a high HBV load.

Recommendation 5-7. The National Institutes of Health should support a study of the effectiveness and safety of peripartum antiviral therapy to reduce and possibly eliminate perinatal hepatitis B virus transmission from women at high risk for perinatal transmission.

Correctional Settings

Incarcerated populations have higher rates of both HBV infection and HCV infection than the general population. Correctional facilities present a unique opportunity to bring viral hepatitis services to at-risk populations. The period of incarceration is opportune for education about hepatitis B and hepatitis C (see Chapter 3). Inmate peer-education programs have been particularly effective for HIV/AIDS education and have also been used for hepatitis education (Simmons, 2004), but relatively few prison systems provide such programs (Collica, 2007).

Correctional facilities include both jails and prisons. Jails are operated by county and local jurisdictions and house people who have been arrested and are awaiting trial, people who have been convicted of misdemeanor crimes, and people who have been convicted of felony crimes with short-term sentences (usually less than one year). The length of stay in jail can be a short as a few hours or longer than a year. Prisons are operated by states and the federal government. They house people who have been convicted of felony crimes with sentences generally of one year or longer. A few states have combined systems that include both jail and prison inmates.

The prevalence of chronic HBV infection in correctional settings (prisons and jails) is estimated to be 1–4%, and that of chronic HCV infection has been reported to vary from 12% to 35% (Boutwell et al., 2005; Weinbaum et al., 2003). The high prevalence in this population is not primarily a result of incarceration but rather indicative of people who engage in risky behavior and were in risky settings before incarceration.

Hennessey et al. (2009) looked at HBV-infection and HCV-infection prevalence in jail inmates. They found evidence of past HBV infections in 31% of Asian inmates, 21% of black inmates, 14% of white inmates, and

11% of Hispanic inmates. Asian inmates had the highest percentage of chronic HBV infection (4.7%), and Hispanic inmates had the second highest percentage (3.6%). White inmates had the highest prevalence of HCV infection (24%). People who had previously been incarcerated had higher HCV prevalence in all age groups.

Correctional systems are constitutionally required to provide necessary health care to inmates that is consistent with the community standard of care. Screening of all incarcerated people for risk factors can identify those for whom blood tests for infection are indicated, and the high prevalence of HCV infection in prisons justifies such screening so that appropriate treatment can be provided to inmates whose blood tests are positive. Although screening, testing, and treatment could impose an economic burden (Spaulding et al., 2006), a number of correctional systems have successfully implemented medical management programs for viral hepatitis (Allen et al., 2003; Chew et al., 2009; Farley et al., 2005; Maru et al., 2008; Sabbatani et al., 2006; Sterling et al., 2004).

Hepatitis B vaccination in prisons is highly cost-effective; it was estimated in 2002 to cost $415 per HBV infection averted (Pisu et al., 2002). When made available, vaccinations in prisons have high uptake rates. Texas and Michigan inmate vaccination uptake rates have been reportedly been 60–80% (Vallabhaneni et al., 2004). Vallabhaneni et al. (2004) found that 93% of 153 male inmates who were asked said that they would agree to hepatitis B vaccination while incarcerated. Such prevention interventions save society money because they reduce postincarceration morbidity and mortality (Pisu et al., 2002). However, prison budgets have often not been sufficient to provide hepatitis B vaccinations, or other HBV and HCV services.

To capitalize on inmate readiness to participate in hepatitis prevention and control activities, correctional systems and public-health departments need to collaborate to provide targeted testing, appropriate standard-of-care medical management during incarceration, and followup medical services after release into the community. However, there are several barriers to such collaboration. Health departments and correctional facilities do not always exchange health information, and it can be difficult to track prisoners once they are released. State registries for hepatitis B and hepatitis C cases are needed so that incarcerated persons with these diseases can be quickly identified and properly managed once returned into local communities. The primary barrier to such collaboration is funding (McIntyre et al., 2008). Most correctional systems do not initiate treatment for chronic HCV infection unless an incarcerated person has sufficient time remaining on his or her sentence to complete treatment, which generally takes 6–12 months (Spaulding et al., 2006).

Obstacles to collaboration between correctional systems and government health institutions can be overcome. For example, in New York State, an effort known as the Hepatitis C Continuity Program, which has been in place since 2006, involves collaboration among the state Department of Correctional Services, the state Department of Health, the state Division of Parole, the New York City Health and Hospitals Corporation, medical centers throughout the state, and manufacturers of medications for hepatitis C (Klein et al., 2007). Such collaborative programs should serve as a model nationally.

Recommendation 5-8. The Centers for Disease Control and Prevention and the Department of Justice should create an initiative to foster partnerships between health departments and corrections systems to ensure the availability of comprehensive viral hepatitis services for incarcerated people.

The initiative should include at least the following:

- All incarcerated people should be offered screening and testing for hepatitis B and hepatitis C.
- All susceptible incarcerated people should be offered hepatitis B vaccine.
- Educational programs, including peer education, should include emphasis on hepatitis B and hepatitis C.
- Systems should be developed to ensure the continuity of medical management for hepatitis B and hepatitis C once infected persons are released from incarceration.

Community Health Facilities

There is a great deal of variation in the types of viral hepatitis services available within the United States. Several states—including Florida, California, Massachusetts, and Texas—have attempted to introduce some hepatitis services into publicly funded settings because of a lack of adequate federal funding for hepatitis B and hepatitis C services. Florida has been offering laboratory testing and vaccination through county health departments since 1999 by using a Hepatitis Prevention Program established and funded by the state legislature (Baldy et al., 2007). The program has expanded services and coordination between the county health departments, the Bureau of HIV/AIDS, the Bureau of Epidemiology, the Bureau of Immunization, and the Bureau of Tuberculosis and Refugee Health. Texas funded a program from 2000 to 2005 to support statewide HCV counseling and testing among high-risk adults (Heseltine and McFarlane, 2007). The program also included a Web-based data-tracking system for monitoring hepatitis C testing and counseling across the state. Of the almost 40,000 tests performed, 23.2% were HCV-positive. Because funding was inadequate, the number of tests administered dropped from almost 12,000 in 2003 to about 1,200 in 2004. As is apparent in the examples above, a state-by-state approach of providing publicly funded viral-hepatitis screening, testing, and care leads to wide variability in the type and quality of services available in different regions and leaves many regions in need without the necessary services.

As mentioned earlier in this chapter, the Health Resources and Services Administration (HRSA) administers grant programs across the country to deliver care to uninsured or underinsured people in community health centers, migrant health centers, homeless programs, and public-housing primary-care programs. The role of federally funded community health facilities is to provide critical and timely access to comprehensive primary-care services to medically underserved communities. Data from HRSA's Health Center Program's Uniform Data System showed that those facilities served about 16.1 million patients in 2007 at over 7,000 service sites. Of the patients seeking care, 91% were below the poverty level, 39% were uninsured, 930,589 were homeless, and 826,977 were migrant or seasonal farm workers. The facilities also serve a high percentage of foreign-born people (for example, refugee and immigrants). Such facilities often provide the only health-care services available to disadvantaged populations, particularly in rural areas. Although 20% of the US population lives in rural areas, just 11% of the nation's physicians work there. People who live in rural areas tend to have lower incomes and lower rates of health insurance, and they are in poorer health than their urban counterparts (Ricketts, 2000). Community health centers are the sole source of primary care in many rural areas (Regan et al., 2003; Ricketts, 2000; Rust et al., 2009; Wright, 2009). For people who reside in urban areas, the barriers to health care are related principally to health insurance, transportation, and information about affordable care (Ahmed et al., 2001).

About one-third of patients who seek care at community health facilities are uninsured, and uninsured patients who seek care at these facilities are likely to use them as a medical home for primary care (Carlson et al., 2001). For the most part, the types of services sought at these facilities are similar to those sought by the general population and consist principally of primary care (Henning et al., 2008). Patients at community health facilities are also more likely to discuss health-promotion strategies than patients in other primary-care settings (Carlson et al., 2001). The availability of these facilities has also been shown to decrease the hospitalization rates in the areas that they service (Probst et al., 2009).

The committee did not find published information on viral-hepatitis services in community health facilities, but several studies have looked at the quality of care for other chronic conditions and for preventive services, such as immunizations. Those studies have found that despite serving disadvantaged populations, community health centers are able to offer high-quality preventive and chronic health-care services at costs comparable with those of facilities used by the general population (Appel et al., 2006; Carlson et al., 2001; Christman et al., 2004; Eisert et al., 2008; Falik et al., 2001; Hicks et al., 2006). Community health facilities have also been found to mitigate racial and ethnic disparities in health-care delivery and services (Appel et al., 2006; Christman et al., 2004; Eisert et al., 2008).

HRSA has oversight over its grantees and has the authority to implement health-care interventions on a national scale. HRSA facilities are well positioned to develop and implement a national strategy to expand viral-hepatitis services to medically underserved and often at-risk populations. HRSA has no centralized viral-hepatitis prevention or control program and is unable to determine the burden of hepatitis B and hepatitis C infections in the patients served in its programs (Raggio Ashley, 2009). Many community health facilities already offer some viral-hepatitis services that include prevention (such as immunizations), screening, testing and medical management. However, there is little published information about these programs.

Although there are no HRSA programs at a national level that focus on viral hepatitis, there are programs for other health concerns that could be used as models. For example, the Health Disparities Collaborative is a national effort to eliminate health disparities and improve health-care delivery in HRSA service-delivery organizations, including community health facilities. The initiative includes intervention to improve health-care delivery processes and chronic health conditions, such as asthma and diabetes (Chin et al., 2004; HRSA, 2009b). It has improved the quality of care in community health facilities for specific conditions (Landon et al., 2007). Viral hepatitis is not one of the diseases included in the program, but this type of program could be expanded to include viral-hepatitis services.

HRSA's Uniform Data Systems (UDS) tracks a variety of information at the national, state, and individual-grantee levels, such as community health centers, migrant health centers, health-care programs for the homeless, and public-housing primary-care programs. The information collected includes patient demographics, services, staffing, clinical indicators, use rates, and associated costs (HRSA, 2009a). Such data systems could potentially be modified to include collection of data on viral-hepatitis services.

On the basis of those findings, the committee offers the following recommendation to expand the provision of viral hepatitis services:

Recommendation 5-9. The Health Resources and Services Administration should provide adequate resources to federally funded community health facilities for provision of comprehensive viral-hepatitis services.

Targeting Settings That Serve At-Risk Populations

Integrating viral hepatitis services in a broad array of settings creates more opportunities to identify at-risk clients and to get them other services that they need (Hoffman et al., 2004). STD/HIV clinics, shelter-based programs, and mobile health units are settings that serve populations that are at risk for hepatitis B and hepatitis C.

STD–HIV Clinics

Clinical venues that provide screening, identification, and care for people at risk for or infected with STDs and HIV present critical opportunities to provide similar viral hepatitis services. CDC has estimated that almost 30% of people who have received a diagnosis of acute hepatitis B have previously been treated for an STD (Goldstein et al., 2002). Among HIV-infected people, rates of chronic hepatitis B are about 6–14%, and rates of chronic hepatitis C about 33% (Alter, 2006; Sherman et al., 2002; Sulkowski, 2008; Thio et al., 2002). In 2001, the National Alliance of State and Territorial AIDS Directors recommended that state health programs integrate HIV, STD, and viral hepatitis prevention services and that programs offer hepatitis A and hepatitis B vaccination; counseling and testing for HIV, STDs, hepatitis B, and hepatitis C; and partner services and referrals to additional prevention and health-care services (NASTAD, 2001). CDC's 2006 STD *Treatment Guidelines* recommend that all unvaccinated persons attending STD clinics receive the hepatitis B vaccine (Workowski and Berman, 2006). The concept of integrating hepatitis B vaccination into STD clinics has been accepted and needs to be expanded to all STD clinic venues.

Some progress has been made in the integration of viral hepatitis services into health-care settings, such as STD or HIV clinics, that serve high-risk populations. A study by Gilbert et al. (2005) showed that many STD clinics have effectively introduced a policy and a plan for hepatitis B prevention; 55% of STD clinics had come to consider hepatitis B vaccination a program responsibility, and 78% had established a vaccination program. From 1997 to 2001, there was a marked increase in the proportion of clinics that offered hepatitis B vaccine (from 61% to 82%), provided hepatitis B educational materials (from 49% to 84%), and accessed federal vaccination programs (from 48% to 84%). In areas where a state STD program had distributed a hepatitis B prevention plan, 88% of STD clinics offered hepatitis B vaccination compared with 50% in areas where a prevention plan had not been developed. The main obstacles cited were the lack of resources for services and low patient compliance. The need for and effect of hepatitis B vaccination was underscored in a study of an urban STD clinic in San Diego that began to offer risk-factor screening, laboratory testing, and immunizations services in 1998 (Gunn et al., 2007); the program included risk-factor screening of 21,631 people and found that about 69% of patients offered the hepatitis B vaccine accepted it.

A study of risk factors for hepatitis C and laboratory testing of people who sought care at an STD clinic found that 4.9% of the 3,367 attendees who were tested for HCV infection were positive (Gunn et al., 2003). Almost 85% of those who tested positive learned of their infection for the first time through this screening process.

Subiadur et al. (2007) found that viral hepatitis prevention services can be incorporated into a busy STD clinic if staff and resources are available. Similarly, an evaluation of Texas's HCV program found that staff did not find it difficult to integrate hepatitis C services if sufficient resources were available, such as access to laboratory testing and adequate staffing levels (Heseltine and McFarlane, 2007).

Integrating viral hepatitis services into existing programs increases the opportunity for people to identify other unmet health needs or conditions. A study that assessed the integration of viral hepatitis services (vaccination and screening) into a New York City STD clinic found that the services attracted at-risk people to the clinic and that they benefited from the other services offered (Hennessy et al., 2007). Of 8,778 people in the STD clinic who received hepatitis services, 279 (3%) were self-reported IDUs and 161 (58% of these) reported that the availability of hepatitis services was the primary reason for their clinic visit. Among the 161, 12 new STDs and two HIV infections were diagnosed. IDUs made up only a small proportion of those who attended STD clinics in this demonstration project, but it seems clear that some IDUs will seek hepatitis services if they are offered without charge.

As with STD clinics, there are data that indicate that viral hepatitis prevention and care can be integrated into HIV clinics. The USPHS guidelines for management of opportunistic infections in HIV-infected persons include guidance for detection and management of chronic viral hepatitis (CDC, 2002). The guidelines call for testing of all HIV-infected persons for chronic hepatitis B and hepatitis C and for provision of hepatitis A and hepatitis B vaccination to those who are susceptible. In addition, there are guidelines for medical treatment of those who are chronically infected. There are data that suggest that a much lower proportion of patients actually receive treatment for chronic viral hepatitis. A study of 845 HIV–HCV coinfected patients who attended the Johns Hopkins HIV Clinic in Baltimore found 277 were referred for hepatitis C care. Of those patients referred to care, only 185 of these came for more than one appointment, 125 completed a pretreatment assessment, and 29 started HCV treatment (Mehta et al., 2006).

Shelter-Based Programs

People who are temporarily or consistently homeless are at increased risk for infectious diseases, including hepatitis B and hepatitis C, because of poor living conditions, poor access to health care, high prevalence of drug use, sexual contact with multiple partners, and sharing of personal-hygiene equipment, such as razors (Badiaga et al., 2008; Boyce et al., 2009). The prevalence of HIV, HBV, and HCV among drug-involved street sex workers in Miami, Florida, was 22.4%, 53.4%, and 29.7%, respectively; and 42% of participants were homeless (Inciardi et al., 2006). Homeless adolescents and runaways are at particular risk because they are less likely than their peers to be vaccinated for HBV and to have access to health care and are more likely to engage in risky behaviors, such as drug use and sex work (Sneller et al., 2008).

The current literature suggests that public-health programs for the homeless should address issues related to unsafe sex, drug abuse, homelessness, and other lifestyle factors that contribute to adverse health outcomes. Reaching that population is difficult, and appropriate street-based and shelter-based interventions are potentially effective in doing so. Collaboration among providers of services to the homeless will be needed to provide counseling, education, testing, and such interventions as condom distribution, syringe-access programs, and vaccination against HBV (Badiaga et al., 2008; Boyce et al., 2009; Inciardi et al., 2006; Rosenheck et al., 2003; Roy et al., 2007; Sneller et al., 2008). All homeless persons should be offered the hepatitis B vaccine. A study of vaccination of homeless adults found that reducing HBV-related disease through vaccinations in this population is cost-effective and is associated with substantial improvements in quality of life (Greengold et al., 2009).

Mobile Health Units

Community-based mobile services, such as the use of mobile health vans, can mitigate some access issues. Programs that use mobile health-care vans have been successful in providing HIV prevention and testing services to at-risk people who might not seek health-care services in other settings. Street outreach programs have been successful in reaching marginalized populations in HIV/AIDS prevention programs (Valentine and Wright-De Aguero, 1996). Kahn et al. (2003) found that mobile vans are a feasible approach to community-based STD screening and treatment, are accepted by the community, and are capable of identifying people who have STDs. A study of polysubstance abuse and HIV/STD risk behaviors in men who have sex with men used a mobile van as the service access point and found that polysubstance users had high rates of uninsurance (21%) and that 96%

were first-time users of mobile health-van services (Mimiaga et al., 2008). Mobile vans have some drawbacks. Shrestha et al. (2008) reviewed the cost effectiveness of clinic-based versus mobile outreach efforts to identify HIV cases. They found that the cost of providing a new HIV diagnosis was considerably higher in the outreach settings than in the clinic (Clark et al., 2008). However, a clinic setting is effective only if clients are drawn to the facility. Hence, innovative approaches of this type should be considered for hard-to-reach populations.

Recommendation

Integration of viral hepatitis services into venues such as STD-HIV clinics, shelters, and mobile health units, is likely to have long-term benefits because most of the people who use these types of clinics engage in high-risk behaviors or are in high-risk settings. Therefore, the committee offers the following recommendation:

Recommendation 5-10. The Health Resources and Services Administration and the Centers for Disease Control and Prevention should provide resources and guidance to integrate comprehensive viral hepatitis services into settings that serve high-risk populations such as STD clinics, sites for HIV services and care, homeless shelters, and mobile health units.

REFERENCES

Ahmed, S. M., J. P. Lemkau, N. Nealeigh, and B. Mann. 2001. Barriers to healthcare access in a non-elderly urban poor American population. *Health & Social Care in the Community* 9(6):445-453.

Allen, S. A., A. C. Spaulding, A. M. Osei, L. E. Taylor, A. M. Cabral, and J. D. Rich. 2003. Treatment of chronic hepatitis C in a state correctional facility. *Annals of Internal Medicine* 138(3):187-190.

Alter, M. J. 2006. Epidemiology of viral hepatitis and HIV co-infection. *Journal of Hepatology* 44(Suppl 1):S6-S9.

Alter, M. J., W. L. Kuhnert, and L. Finelli. 2003. Guidelines for laboratory testing and result reporting of antibody to hepatitis C virus. Centers for Disease Control and Prevention. *Morbidity and Morality Weekly: Recommendations and Reports* 52(RR-3):1-13, 15; quiz CE11-CE14.

Alter, M. J., L. B. Seeff, B. R. Bacon, D. L. Thomas, M. O. Rigsby, and A. M. Di Bisceglie. 2004. Testing for hepatitis C virus infection should be routine for persons at increased risk for infection. *Annals of Internal Medicine* 141(9):715-717.

Appel, A., R. Everhart, P. S. Mehler, and T. D. MacKenzie. 2006. Lack of ethnic disparities in adult immunization rates among underserved older patients in an urban public health system. *Medical Care* 44(11):1054-1058.

Armstrong, G. L., A. Wasley, E. P. Simard, G. M. McQuillan, W. L. Kuhnert, and M. J. Alter. 2006. The prevalence of hepatitis C virus infection in the United States, 1999 through 2002. *Annals of Internal Medicine* 144(10):705-714.
Asian Liver Center. 2009. *Jade Ribbon Campaign.* http://liver.stanford.edu/Outreach/JRC.html (accessed August 29, 2009).
Astone, J., S. M. Strauss, Z. P. Vassilev, and D. C. Des Jarlais. 2003. Provision of hepatitis C education in a nationwide sample of drug treatment programs. *Journal of Drug Education* 33(1):107-117.
Badiaga, S., D. Raoult, and P. Brouqui. 2008. Preventing and controlling emerging and re-emerging transmissible diseases in the homeless. *Emerging Infectious Diseases* 14(9): 1353-1359.
Baldy, L. M., C. Urbas, J. L. Harris, T. S. Jones, and P. E. Reichert. 2007. Establishing a viral hepatitis prevention and control program: Florida's experience. *Public Health Reports* 122(Suppl 2):24-30.
Barr, D. A., and S. F. Wanat. 2005. Listening to patients: Cultural and linguistic barriers to health care access. *Family Medicine* 37(3):199-204.
Begley, E. B., A. M. Oster, B. Song, L. Lesondak, K. Voorhees, M. Esquivel, R. L. Merrick, J. Carrel, D. Sebesta, J. Vergeront, D. Shrestha, and J. D. Heffelfinger. 2008. Incorporating rapid HIV testing into partner counseling and referral services. *Public Health Reports* 123(Suppl 3):126-135.
Birkhead, G. S., S. J. Klein, A. R. Candelas, D. A. O'Connell, J. R. Rothman, I. S. Feldman, D. S. Tsui, R. A. Cotroneo, and C. A. Flanigan. 2007. Integrating multiple programme and policy approaches to hepatitis C prevention and care for injection drug users: A comprehensive approach. *International Journal of Drug Policy* 18(5):417-425.
Boutwell, A. E., S. A. Allen, and J. D. Rich. 2005. Opportunities to address the hepatitis C epidemic in the correctional setting. *Clinical Infectious Diseases* 40(s5):S367-S372.
Bowles, K. E., H. A. Clark, E. Tai, P. S. Sullivan, B. Song, J. Tsang, C. A. Dietz, J. Mir, A. Mares-DelGrasso, C. Calhoun, D. Aguirre, C. Emerson, and J. D. Heffelfinger. 2008. Implementing rapid HIV testing in outreach and community settings: Results from an advancing HIV prevention demonstration project conducted in seven U.S. Cities. *Public Health Reports* 123(Suppl 3):78-85.
Boyce, D. E., A. D. Tice, F. V. Ona, K. T. Akinaka, and H. Lusk. 2009. Viral hepatitis in a homeless shelter in Hawai'i. *Hawaii Medical Journal* 68(5):113-115.
Brown, L. S., S. Kritz, R. J. Goldsmith, E. J. Bini, J. Robinson, D. Alderson, and J. Rotrosen. 2007. Health services for HIV/AIDS, HCV, and sexually transmitted infections in substance abuse treatment programs. *Public Health Reports* 122(4):441-451.
Bruix, J., and M. Sherman. 2005. Management of hepatocellular carcinoma. *Hepatology* 42(5):1208-1236.
Butt, A. A., A. C. Justice, M. Skanderson, M. O. Rigsby, C. B. Good, and C. K. Kwoh. 2007. Rate and predictors of treatment prescription for hepatitis C. *Gut* 56(3):385-389.
Butt, A. A., K. A. McGinnis, M. Skanderson, and A. C. Justice. 2009. Hepatitis C treatment completion rates in routine clinical care. *Liver International* 1478-3223.
Campos, N. G., J. A. Salomon, J. C. Servoss, D. P. Nunes, J. H. Samet, K. A. Freedberg, and S. J. Goldie. 2007. Cost-effectiveness of treatment for hepatitis C in an urban cohort co-infected with HIV. *American Journal of Medicine* 120(3):272-279.
Carey, W. 2003. Tests and screening strategies for the diagnosis of hepatitis C. *Cleveland Clinic Journal of Medicine* 70(Suppl 4):S7-S13.
Carlson, B. L., J. Eden, D. O'Connor, and J. Regan. 2001. Primary care of patients without insurance by community health centers. *Journal of Ambulatory Care Management* 24(2):47-59.

Castelnuovo, E., J. Thompson-Coon, M. Pitt, M. Cramp, U. Siebert, A. Price, and K. Stein. 2006. The cost-effectiveness of testing for hepatitis C in former injecting drug users. *Health Technology Assessment* 10(32): III-IV, IX-XII, 1-93.

CDC (Centers for Disease Control and Prevention). 1998. Recommendations for prevention and control of hepatitis C virus (HCV) infection and HCV-related chronic disease. Centers for Disease Control and Prevention. *Morbidity and Morality Weekly: Recommendations and Reports* 47(RR-19):1-39.

———. 2001. *National hepatitis C prevention strategy: A comprehensive strategy for the prevention and control of hepatitis C virus infection and its consequences.* Atlanta, GA: CDC. http://www.cdc.gov/hepatitis/HCV/Strategy/PDFs/NatHepCPrevStrategy.pdf (accessed August 21, 2009)

———. 2002. 2001 USPHS/IDSA guidelines for the prevention of opportunistic infections in persons infected with human immunodeficiency virus. *Infectious Diseases in Obstetrics and Gynecology* 10(1):3-64.

———. 2005. A comprehensive immunization strategy to eliminate transmission of hepatitis B virus in the United States. Part 1: Immunization of infants, children, and adolescents. *Morbidity and Mortality Weekly Report* 54(RR16):1-23.

———. 2006. Screening for chronic hepatitis B among Asian/Pacific Islander populations—New York City, 2005. *Morbidity and Mortality Weekly Report* 55(18):505-509.

———. 2007. *National immunization survey: Hepatitis B vaccine birth-dose rates.* http://www.cdc.gov/Hepatitis/Partners/PeriHepBCoord.htm (accessed June 28, 2009).

———. 2009a. *About the Division of Viral Hepatitis.* http://www.cdc.gov/hepatitis/AboutUs.htm (accessed August 21, 2009).

———. 2009b. Births: Final data for 2006. *National Vital Statistics Reports* 57(7). http://www.cdc.gov/nchs/data/nvsr/nvsr57/nvsr57_07.pdf (accessed August 21, 2009).

———. 2009c. *Interpretation of hepatitis B serologic test results.* http://www.cdc.gov/hepatitis/HBV/PDFs/SerologicChartv8.pdf (accessed August 21, 2009).

———. 2009d. *Perinatal hepatitis B coordinator list.* http://www.cdc.gov/vaccines/vpd-vac/hepb/perinatal-contacts.htm (accessed August 18, 2009).

———. 2009e. *Reference for the interpretation of hepatitis C virus (HCV) test results.* http://www.cdc.gov/hepatitis/HCV/PDFs/hcv_graph.pdf (accessed August 21, 2009).

———. 2009f. *Report on the status of state viral hepatitis plans for the Institute of Medicine executive summary of responses (n=55).* National Hepatitis TA Center, New York State Department of Health.

———. 2009g. Status of state electronic disease surveillance systems—United States, 2007. *Morbidity and Mortality Weekly Report* 58(29):804-807.

Chao, S. D., E. T. Chang, and S. K. So. 2009a. Eliminating the threat of chronic hepatitis B in the Asian and Pacific Islander community: A call to action. *Asian Pacific Journal of Cancer Prevention* 10(3):497-512.

Chao, S. D., C. Cheung, A. Yue, and S. K. So. 2009b. *Low hepatitis B knowledge among perinatal healthcare providers serving county with nation's highest rate of births to mothers chronically infected with hepatitis B.* Paper presented at Poster presentation at the 13th International Symposium on Viral Hepatitis and Liver Disease, Washington, DC. March 20-24, 2009.

Chesson, H. W., J. M. Blandford, T. L. Gift, G. Tao, and K. L. Irwin. 2004. The estimated direct medical cost of sexually transmitted diseases among American youth, 2000. *Perspectives on Sexual and Reproductive Health* 36(1):11-19.

Cheung, R. C., S. Currie, H. Shen, S. B. Ho, E. J. Bini, B. S. Anand, N. Brau, and T. L. Wright. 2005. Chronic hepatitis C in latinos: Natural history, treatment eligibility, acceptance, and outcomes. *American Journal of Gastroenterology* 100(10):2186-2193.

Chew, K. W., S. A. Allen, L. E. Taylor, J. D. Rich, and E. Feller. 2009. Treatment outcomes with pegylated interferon and ribavirin for male prisoners with chronic hepatitis C. *Journal of Clinical Gastroenterology* 43(7):686-691.

Chin, M. H., S. Cook, M. L. Drum, L. Jin, M. Guillen, C. A. Humikowski, J. Koppert, J. F. Harrison, S. Lippold, and C. T. Schaefer. 2004. Improving diabetes care in midwest community health centers with the health disparities collaborative. *Diabetes Care* 27(1):2-8.

China Digital Times. 2009. *China news tagged with: hepatitis B*. http://chinadigitaltimes.net/china/hepatitis-b/ (accessed August 21, 2009).

Chitwood, D. D., D. C. McBride, M. T. French, and M. Comerford. 1999. Health care need and utilization: A preliminary comparison of injection drug users, other illicit drug users, and nonusers. *Substance Use and Misuse* 34(4-5):727-746.

Choe, J. H., V. M. Taylor, Y. Yasui, N. Burke, T. Nguyen, E. Acorda, and J. C. Jackson. 2006. Health care access and sociodemographic factors associated with hepatitis B testing in Vietnamese American men. *Journal of Immigrant and Minority Health* 8(3):193-201.

Chou, R., E. C. Clark, and M. Helfand. 2004. Screening for hepatitis C virus infection: A review of the evidence for the U.S. Preventive Services Task Force. *Annals of Internal Medicine* 140(6):465-479.

Christman, L. K., R. Abdulla, P. B. Jacobsen, A. B. Cantor, D. Y. Mayhew, K. S. Thompson, J. P. Krischer, and R. G. Roetzheim. 2004. Colorectal cancer screening among a sample of community health center attendees. *Journal of Health Care for the Poor and Underserved* 15(2):281-293.

Clark, H. A., K. E. Bowles, B. Song, and J. D. Heffelfinger. 2008. Implementation of rapid HIV testing programs in community and outreach settings: Perspectives from staff at eight community-based organizations in seven U.S. Cities. *Public Health Reports* 123(Suppl 3):86-93.

Claxton, G., B. DiJulio, B. Finder, E. Becker, S. Hawkins, J. Pickreign, H. Whitmore, and J. Gabel. 2007. *Kaiser and the Health Research and Education Trust survey of employer-sponsored health benefits, 1999-2007*. Chicago, IL.

Collica, K. 2007. The prevalence of HIV peer programming in American prisons: An opportunity wasted. *Journal of Correctional Health Care* 13:278.

Contoreggi, C., V. E. Rexroad, and W. R. Lange. 1998. Current management of infectious complications in the injecting drug user. *Journal of Substance Abuse Treatment* 15(2):95-106.

Crofts, N., R. Louie, and B. Loff. 1997. The next plague: Stigmatization and discrimination related to hepatitis C virus infection in Australia. *Health and Human Rights* 2(2):87-97.

Damen, M., H. Zaaijer, H. Cuypers, H. Vrielink, C. Poel, H. Reesink, and P. Lelie. 1995. Reliability of the third-generation recombinant immunoblot assay for hepatitis C virus. *Transfusion* 35(9):745-749.

Davila, J. A., and H. B. El-Serag. 2006. Racial differences in survival of hepatocellular carcinoma in the United States: A population-based study. *Clinical Gastroentorology and Hepatology* 4(1):104-110; quiz 104-105.

Des Jarlais, D. C., and S. Semaan. 2008. HIV prevention for injecting drug users: The first 25 years and counting. *Psychosomatic Medicine* 70(5):606-611.

Des Jarlais, D. C., M. Marmor, D. Paone, S. Titus, Q. Shi, T. Perlis, B. Jose, and S. R. Friedman. 1996. HIV incidence among injecting drug users in New York city syringe-exchange programmes. *Lancet* 348(9033):987-991.

Des Jarlais, D. C., C. McKnight, C. Goldblatt, and D. Purchase. 2009. Doing harm reduction better: Syringe exchange in the United States. *Addiction* 104(9):1441-1446.

Din, E. 2009. *Estimating the number of births to hepatitis B surface antigen-positive women in select US states, 2004.* Paper presented at 13th International Symposium of Viral Hepatitis and Liver Disease, Washington, DC. March 20-24, 2009.

Dolan, K. A., J. Shearer, B. White, J. Zhou, J. Kaldor, and A. D. Wodak. 2005. Four-year follow-up of imprisoned male heroin users and methadone treatment: Mortality, re-incarceration and hepatitis C infection. *Addiction* 100(6):820-828.

Eisert, S. L., P. S. Mehler, and P. A. Gabow. 2008. Can America's urban safety net systems be a solution to unequal treatment? *Journal of Urban Health* 85(5):766-778.

Esteve, M., C. Saro, F. Gonzalez-Huix, F. Suarez, M. Forne, and J. M. Viver. 2004. Chronic hepatitis B reactivation following infliximab therapy in Crohn's disease patients: Need for primary prophylaxis. *Gut* 53(9):1363-1365.

Euler, G. L., J. Copeland, and W. W. Williams. 2003a. Impact of four urban perinatal hepatitis B prevention programs on screening and vaccination of infants and household members. *American Journal of Epidemiology* 157(8):747-753.

Euler, G. L., J. R. Copeland, M. C. Rangel, and W. W. Williams. 2003b. Antibody response to postexposure prophylaxis in infants born to hepatitis B surface antigen-positive women. *Pediatric Infectious Disease Journal* 22(2):123-129.

Falik, M., J. Needleman, B. L. Wells, and J. Korb. 2001. Ambulatory care sensitive hospitalizations and emergency visits: Experiences of Medicaid patients using federally qualified health centers. *Medical Care* 39(6):551-561.

Farley, J., S. Vasdev, B. Fischer, E. Haydon, J. Rehm, and T. A. Farley. 2005. Feasibility and outcome of HCV treatment in a Canadian federal prison population. *American Journal of Public Health* 95(10):1737-1739.

Fischer, B., J. Powis, M. Firestone Cruz, K. Rudzinski, and J. Rehm. 2008. Hepatitis C virus transmission among oral crack users: Viral detection on crack paraphernalia. *European Journal of Gastroenterology and Hepatology* 20(1):29-32.

Fuller, C. M., D. C. Ompad, S. Galea, Y. Wu, B. Koblin, and D. Vlahov. 2004. Hepatitis C incidence—a comparison between injection and noninjection drug users in New York city. *Journal of Urban Health* 81(1):20-24.

Garfein, R. S., E. T. Golub, A. E. Greenberg, H. Hagan, D. L. Hanson, S. M. Hudson, F. Kapadia, M. H. Latka, L. J. Ouellet, D. W. Purcell, S. A. Strathdee, and H. Thiede. 2007. A peer-education intervention to reduce injection risk behaviors for HIV and hepatitis C virus infection in young injection drug users. *AIDS* 21(14):1923-1932.

Ghany, M. G., D. B. Strader, D. L. Thomas, and L. Seeff. 2009. Diagnosis, management, and treatment of hepatitis C: An update. *Hepatology* 49(4):1335-1374.

Gilbert, L. K., J. Bulger, K. Scanlon, K. Ford, D. Bergmire-Sweat, and C. Weinbaum. 2005. Integrating hepatitis B prevention into sexually transmitted disease services: U.S. sexually transmitted disease program and clinic trends—1997 and 2001. *Sexually Transmitted Diseases* 32(6):346-350.

Giordano, C., and C. Cooper. 2009. The influence of race and language on chronic hepatitis C virus infection management. *European Journal of Gastroenterology and Hepatology* 21(2):131-136.

Giordano, C., E. F. Druyts, G. Garber, and C. Cooper. 2009. Evaluation of immigration status, race and language barriers on chronic hepatitis C virus infection management and treatment outcomes. *European Journal of Gastroenterology and Hepatology* 21(9):963-968.

Goldstein, S. T., M. J. Alter, I. T. Williams, L. A. Moyer, F. N. Judson, K. Mottram, M. Fleenor, P. L. Ryder, and H. S. Margolis. 2002. Incidence and risk factors for acute hepatitis B in the United States, 1982-1998: Implications for vaccination programs. *Journal of Infectious Diseases* 185(6):713-719.

Gomez, S. L., G. M. Le, D. W. West, W. A. Satariano, and L. O'Connor. 2003. Hospital policy and practice regarding the collection of data on race, ethnicity, and birthplace. *American Journal of Public Health* 93(10):1685-1688.

Greengold, B., A. Nyamathi, G. Kominski, D. Wiley, M. A. Lewis, F. Hodge, M. Singer, and B. Spiegel. 2009. Cost-effectiveness analysis of behavioral interventions to improve vaccination compliance in homeless adults. *Vaccine* 27(5):718-725.

Groom, H., E. Dieperink, D. B. Nelson, J. Garrard, J. R. Johnson, S. L. Ewing, H. Stockley, J. Durfee, Y. Jonk, M. L. Willenbring, and S. B. Ho. 2008. Outcomes of a hepatitis C screening program at a large urban VA medical center. *Journal of Clinical Gastroenterology* 42(1):97-106.

Gunn, R. A., M. A. Lee, P. J. Murray, R. A. Gilchick, and H. S. Margolis. 2007. Hepatitis B vaccination of men who have sex with men attending an urban STD clinic: Impact of an ongoing vaccination program, 1998-2003. *Sexually Transmitted Diseases* 34(9):663-668.

Gunn, R. A., P. J. Murray, C. H. Brennan, D. B. Callahan, M. J. Alter, and H. S. Margolis. 2003. Evaluation of screening criteria to identify persons with hepatitis C virus infection among sexually transmitted disease clinic clients: Results from the San Diego viral hepatitis integration project. *Sexually Transmitted Diseases* 30(4):340-344.

Hagan, H., and H. Thiede. 2000. Changes in injection risk behavior associated with participation in the Seattle needle-exchange program. *Journal of Urban Health* 77(3):369-382.

———. 2003. Does bleach disinfection of syringes help prevent hepatitis C virus transmission? *Epidemiology* 14(5):628-629; author reply 629.

Hagan, H., D. C. Jarlais, S. R. Friedman, D. Purchase, and M. J. Alter. 1995. Reduced risk of hepatitis B and hepatitis C among injection drug users in the Tacoma syringe exchange program. *American Journal of Public Health* 85(11):1531-1537.

Hagan, H., J. P. McGough, H. Thiede, N. S. Weiss, S. Hopkins, and E. R. Alexander. 1999. Syringe exchange and risk of infection with hepatitis B and C viruses. *American Journal of Epidemiology* 149(3):203-213.

Hagan, H., E. R. Pouget, D. C. Des Jarlais, and C. Lelutiu-Weinberger. 2008. Meta-regression of hepatitis C virus infection in relation to time since onset of illicit drug injection: The influence of time and place. *American Journal of Epidemiology* 168(10):1099-1109.

Hagan, H., E. R. Pouget, I. T. Williams, R. L. Garfein, S. A. Strathdee, S. M. Hudson, M. Latka, and L. Ouellet. 2010. Attribution of HCV seroconversion risk in young injection drug users in five U.S. cities. *Journal of Infectious Diseases* 201(3):328-385.

Hagan, H., H. Thiede, N. S. Weiss, S. G. Hopkins, J. S. Duchin, and E. R. Alexander. 2001. Sharing of drug preparation equipment as a risk factor for hepatitis C. *American Journal of Public Health* 91(1):42-46.

Hahn, J. A., K. Page-Shafer, P. J. Lum, P. Bourgois, E. Stein, J. L. Evans, M. P. Busch, L. H. Tobler, B. Phelps, and A. R. Moss. 2002. Hepatitis C virus seroconversion among young injection drug users: Relationships and risks. *Journal of Infectious Diseases* 186(11):1558-1564.

Hand, W. L., and Y. Vasquez. 2005. Risk factors for hepatitis C on the Texas–Mexico border. *American Journal of Gastroenterology* 100:2180–2185.

Harm Reduction Coalition. 2009. *Hepatitis C*. http://www.harmreduction.org/article.php?list=type&type=50 (accessed August 21, 2009).

Hennessey, K. A., A. A. Kim, V. Griffin, N. T. Collins, C. M. Weinbaum, and K. Sabin. 2009. Prevalence of infection with hepatitis B and C viruses and co-infection with HIV in three jails: A case for viral hepatitis prevention in jails in the United States. *Journal of Urban Health* 86(1):93-105.

Hennessy, R. R., I. B. Weisfuse, and K. Schlanger. 2007. Does integrating viral hepatitis services into a public STD clinic attract injection drug users for care? *Public Health Reports* 122(Suppl 2):31-35.

Henning, G. F., M. Graybill, and J. George. 2008. Reason for visit: Is migrant health care that different? *Journal of Rural Health* 24(2):219-220.

Heseltine, G., and J. McFarlane. 2007. Texas statewide hepatitis C counseling and testing, 2000-2005. *Public Health Reports* 122(Suppl 2):6-11.

Hicks, L. S., A. J. O'Malley, T. A. Lieu, T. Keegan, N. L. Cook, B. J. McNeil, B. E. Landon, and E. Guadagnoli. 2006. The quality of chronic disease care in U.S. community health centers. *Health Affairs* 25(6):1712-1723.

Hoffman, H. L., C. A. Castro-Donlan, V. M. Johnson, and D. R. Church. 2004. The Massachusetts HIV, hepatitis, addiction services integration (HHASI) experience: Responding to the comprehensive needs of individuals with co-occurring risks and conditions. *Public Health Reports* 119(1):25-31.

Holtzman, D., V. Barry, L. J. Ouellet, D. C. Jarlais, D. Vlahov, E. T. Golub, S. M. Hudson, and R. S. Garfein. 2009. The influence of needle exchange programs on injection risk behaviors and infection with hepatitis C virus among young injection drug users in select cities in the United States, 1994-2004. *Preventive Medicine* 49(1):68-73.

HRSA (Health Resources and Services Administration). 2009a. *The health center program: Uniform data system (UDS).* http://bphc.hrsa.gov/uds/ (accessed November, 13, 2009).

———. 2009b. *Quality healthcare collaboration.* http://www.healthdisparities.net/hdc/html/collaborativesOverview.aspx (accessed November 12, 2009).

Hsu, C., C. A. Hsiung, I. J. Su, W. S. Hwang, M. C. Wang, S. F. Lin, T. H. Lin, H. H. Hsiao, J. H. Young, M. C. Chang, Y. M. Liao, C. C. Li, H. B. Wu, H. F. Tien, T. Y. Chao, T. W. Liu, A. L. Cheng, and P. J. Chen. 2008. A revisit of prophylactic lamivudine for chemotherapy-associated hepatitis B reactivation in non-Hodgkin's lymphoma: A randomized trial. *Hepatology* 47(3):844-853.

Hsu, C. E., L. C. Liu, H. S. Juon, Y. W. Chiu, J. Bawa, U. Tillman, M. Li, J. Miller, and M. Wang. 2007. Reducing liver cancer disparities: A community-based hepatitis-B prevention program for Asian-American communities. *Journal of the National Medical Association* 99(8):900-907.

Huckans, M. S., A. D. Blackwell, T. A. Harms, D. W. Indest, and P. Hauser. 2005. Integrated hepatitis C virus treatment: Addressing comorbid substance use disorders and HIV infection. *AIDS* 19(Suppl 3):S106-S115.

Hutton, D. W., D. Tan, S. K. So, and M. L. Brandeau. 2007. Cost-effectiveness of screening and vaccinating Asian and Pacific Islander adults for hepatitis B. *Annals of Internal Medicine* 147(7):460-469.

IHRA (International Harm Reduction Association). 2009. *What is harm reduction?* http://www.ihra.net/Whatisharmreduction (accessed September 14, 2009).

Inciardi, J. A., H. L. Surratt, and S. P. Kurtz. 2006. HIV, HBV, and HCV infections among drug-involved, inner-city, street sex workers in Miami, Florida. *AIDS Behav* 10(2):139-147.

Islam, M., A. Wodak, and K. M. Conigrave. 2008. The effectiveness and safety of syringe vending machines as a component of needle syringe programmes in community settings. *International Journal on Drug Policy* 19(6):436-441.

Jacobs, E., A. H. Chen, L. S. Karliner, N. Agger-Gupta, and S. Mutha. 2006. The need for more research on language barriers in health care: A proposed research agenda. *Milbank Quarterly* 84(1):111-133.

Jacques-Carroll, L. 2008. *Essentials of perinatal hepatitis B prevention: A training series for coordinators and case managers—assessment and evaluation.* http://www2.cdc.gov/vaccines/ed/hepbtraining (accessed June 28, 2009).

Jacques-Carroll, L., E. E. Mast, and S. Wang. 2007. *Managing a perinatal hepatitis B prevention program: A guide to life as a program coordinator.* http://www.cdc.gov/Hepatitis/Partners/PeriHepBCoord.htm (accessed August 18, 2009).

Kahn, R. H., K. E. Moseley, J. N. Thilges, G. Johnson, and T. A. Farley. 2003. Community-based screening and treatment for STDs: Results from a mobile clinic initiative. *Sexually Transmitted Diseases* 30(8):654-658.

Kanwal, F., I. M. Gralnek, P. Martin, G. S. Dulai, M. Farid, and B. M. Spiegel. 2005. Treatment alternatives for chronic hepatitis B virus infection: A cost-effectiveness analysis. *Annals of Internal Medicine* 142(10):821-831.

Kapadia, F., D. Vlahov, D. C. Des Jarlais, S. A. Strathdee, L. Ouellet, P. Kerndt, E. E. Morse, I. Williams, and R. S. Garfein. 2002. Does bleach disinfection of syringes protect against hepatitis C infection among young adult injection drug users? *Epidemiology* 13(6):738-741.

Kassler, W. J., B. A. Dillon, C. Haley, W. K. Jones, and A. Goldman. 1997. On-site, rapid HIV testing with same-day results and counseling. *AIDS* 11(8):1045-1051.

Keenan, P. A., and J. M. Keenan. 2001. Rapid HIV testing in urban outreach: A strategy for improving posttest counseling rates. *AIDS Education and Prevention* 13(6):541-550.

Kidorf, M., V. L. King, K. Neufeld, J. Peirce, K. Kolodner, and R. K. Brooner. 2009. Improving substance abuse treatment enrollment in community syringe exchangers. *Addiction* 104(5):786-795.

Klein, S. J., L. N. Wright, G. S. Birkhead, B. A. Mojica, L. C. Klopf, L. A. Klein, E. L. Tanner, I. S. Feldman, and E. J. Fraley. 2007. Promoting HCV treatment completion for prison inmates: New York state's hepatitis C continuity program. *Public Health Reports* 122(Suppl 2):83-88.

Kresina, T. F., R. D. Bruce, R. Lubran, and H. W. Clark. 2008. Integration of viral hepatitis services into opioid treatment programs. *Journal of Opioid Management* 4(6):369-381.

Kuo, I., S. G. Sherman, D. L. Thomas, and S. A. Strathdee. 2004. Hepatitis B virus infection and vaccination among young injection and non-injection drug users: Missed opportunities to prevent infection. *Drug and Alcohol Dependence* 73(1):69-78.

Landon, B. E., L. S. Hicks, A. J. O'Malley, T. A. Lieu, T. Keegan, B. J. McNeil, and E. Guadagnoli. 2007. Improving the management of chronic disease at community health centers. *New England Journal of Medicine* 356(9):921-934.

Latka, M. H., H. Hagan, F. Kapadia, E. T. Golub, S. Bonner, J. V. Campbell, M. H. Coady, R. S. Garfein, M. Pu, D. L. Thomas, T. K. Thiel, and S. A. Strathdee. 2008. A randomized intervention trial to reduce the lending of used injection equipment among injection drug users infected with hepatitis C. *American Journal of Public Health* 98(5):853-861.

Lau, G. K., M. L. He, D. Y. Fong, A. Bartholomeusz, W. Y. Au, A. K. Lie, S. Locarnini, and R. Liang. 2002. Preemptive use of lamivudine reduces hepatitis B exacerbation after allogeneic hematopoietic cell transplantation. *Hepatology* 36(3):702-709.

Lau, G. K., H. H. Yiu, D. Y. Fong, H. C. Cheng, W. Y. Au, L. S. Lai, M. Cheung, H. Y. Zhang, A. Lie, R. Ngan, and R. Liang. 2003. Early is superior to deferred preemptive lamivudine therapy for hepatitis B patients undergoing chemotherapy. *Gastroenterology* 125(6):1742-1749.

Lee, T. A., D. L. Veenstra, U. H. Iloeje, and S. D. Sullivan. 2004. Cost of chronic hepatitis B infection in the United States. *Journal of Clinical Gastroenterology* 38(10 Suppl 3):S144-S147.

Li, X. M., Y. B. Yang, H. Y. Hou, Z. J. Shi, H. M. Shen, B. Q. Teng, A. M. Li, M. F. Shi, and L. Zou. 2003. Interruption of HBV intrauterine transmission: A clinical study. *World Journal of Gastroenterology* 9(7):1501-1503.

Li, Y.-H., Y.-F. He, W.-Q. Jiang, F.-H. Wang, X.-B. Lin, L. Zhang, Z.-J. Xia, X.-F. Sun, H.-Q. Huang, T.-Y. Lin, Y.-J. He, and Z.-Z. Guan. 2006. Lamivudine prophylaxis reduces the incidence and severity of hepatitis in hepatitis B virus carriers who receive chemotherapy for lymphoma. *Cancer* 106(6):1320-1325.

Liang, T. S., E. Erbelding, C. A. Jacob, H. Wicker, C. Christmyer, S. Brunson, D. Richardson, and J. M. Ellen. 2005. Rapid HIV testing of clients of a mobile STD/HIV clinic. *AIDS Patient Care and STDs* 19(4):253-257.

Lidgren, M., A. Hollander, O. Weiland, and B. Jonsson. 2007. Productivity improvements in hepatitis C treatment: Impact on efficacy, cost, cost-effectiveness and quality of life. *Scandinavian Journal of Gastroenterology* 42(7):867-877.

Lillienfeld, A. M., and D. E. Lillienfeld. 1980. *Foundations of epidemiology*. New York: Oxford University Press.

Lin, S. Y., E. T. Chang, and S. K. So. 2007. Why we should routinely screen Asian American adults for hepatitis B: A cross-sectional study of Asians in California. *Hepatology* 46(4):1034-1040.

Lok, A. S., and B. J. McMahon. 2004. Chronic hepatitis B: Update of recommendations. *Hepatology* 39(3):857-861.

———. 2009. Chronic hepatitis B: Update 2009. *Hepatology* 50(3):661-662.

Lok, A. S., R. H. Liang, E. K. Chiu, K. L. Wong, T. K. Chan, and D. Todd. 1991. Reactivation of hepatitis B virus replication in patients receiving cytotoxic therapy. Report of a prospective study. *Gastroenterology* 100(1):182-188.

Lum, P. J., J. A. Hahn, K. P. Shafer, J. L. Evans, P. J. Davidson, E. Stein, and A. R. Moss. 2008. Hepatitis B virus infection and immunization status in a new generation of injection drug users in San Francisco. *Journal of Viral Hepatitis* 15(3):229-236.

Maher, L., B. Jalaludin, K. G. Chant, R. Jayasuriya, T. Sladden, J. M. Kaldor, and P. L. Sargent. 2006. Incidence and risk factors for hepatitis C seroconversion in injecting drug users in Australia. *Addiction* 101(10):1499-1508.

Manson, A. 1988. Language concordance as a determinant of patient compliance and emergency room use in patients with asthma. *Medical Care* 26(12):1119-1128.

Mansson, A. S., T. Moestrup, E. Nordenfelt, and A. Widell. 2000. Continued transmission of hepatitis B and C viruses, but no transmission of human immunodeficiency virus among intravenous drug users participating in a syringe/needle exchange program. *Scandinavian Journal of Infectious Diseases* 32(3):253-258.

Mark, K. E., P. J. Murray, D. B. Callahan, and R. A. Gunn. 2007. Medical care and alcohol use after testing hepatitis C antibody positive at STD clinic and HIV test site screening programs. *Public Health Reports* 122(1):37-43.

Maru, D. S., R. D. Bruce, S. Basu, and F. L. Altice. 2008. Clinical outcomes of hepatitis C treatment in a prison setting: Feasibility and effectiveness for challenging treatment populations. *Clinical Infectious Diseases* 47(7):952-961.

Mast, E. E., H. S. Margolis, A. E. Fiore, E. W. Brink, S. T. Goldstein, S. A. Wang, L. A. Moyer, B. P. Bell, and M. J. Alter. 2005. A comprehensive immunization strategy to eliminate transmission of hepatitis B virus infection in the United States: Recommendations of the advisory committee on immunization practices (ACIP) part 1: Immunization of infants, children, and adolescents. *Morbidity and Morality Weekly: Recommendations and Reports* 54(RR-16):1-31.

Mast, E. E., C. M. Weinbaum, A. E. Fiore, M. J. Alter, B. P. Bell, L. Finelli, L. E. Rodewald, J. M. Douglas, Jr., R. S. Janssen, and J. W. Ward. 2006. A comprehensive immunization strategy to eliminate transmission of hepatitis B virus infection in the United States: Recommendations of the advisory committee on immunization practices (ACIP) part II: Immunization of adults. *Morbidity and Morality Weekly: Recommendations and Reports* 55(RR-16):1-33.

Mateu-Gelabert, P., C. Treloar, V. A. Calatayud, M. Sandoval, J. C. V. Zurián, L. Maher, T. Rhodes, and S. R. Friedman. 2007. How can hepatitis C be prevented in the long term? *International Journal of Drug Policy* 18(5):338-340.

Mathei, C., G. Robaeys, P. van Damme, F. Buntinx, and R. Verrando. 2005. Prevalence of hepatitis C in drug users in Flanders: Determinants and geographic differences. *Epidemiology and Infection* 133(1):127-136.

McDonald, D. 2009. The evaluation of a trial of syringe vending machines in Canberra, Australia. *International Journal on Drug Policy* 20(4):336-339.

McGinn, T., N. O'Connor-Moore, D. Alfandre, D. Gardenier, and J. Wisnivesky. 2008. Validation of a hepatitis C screening tool in primary care. *Archives of Internal Medicine* 168(18):2009-2013.

McIntyre, A. F., A. Studzinski, H. A. Beidinger, and C. Rabins. 2008. STD, HIV/AIDS, and hepatitis services in Illinois county jails. *Sexually Transmitted Diseases* 36(2 Suppl): S37-S40.

Mehta, S. H., G. M. Lucas, L. B. Mirel, M. Torbenson, Y. Higgins, R. D. Moore, D. L. Thomas, and M. S. Sulkowski. 2006. Limited effectiveness of antiviral treatment for hepatitis C in an urban HIV clinic. *AIDS* 20(18):2361-2369.

Metzger, D. S., H. Navaline, and G. E. Woody. 1998. Drug abuse treatment as AIDS prevention. *Public Health Reports* 113(Suppl 1):97-106.

Mimiaga, M. J., S. L. Reisner, R. Vanderwarker, M. J. Gaucher, C. A. O'Connor, M. S. Medeiros, and S. A. Safren. 2008. Polysubstance use and HIV/STD risk behavior among Massachusetts men who have sex with men accessing department of public health mobile van services: Implications for intervention development. *AIDS Patient Care and STDs* 22(9):745-751.

Moatti, J. P., D. Vlahov, I. Feroni, V. Perrin, and Y. Obadia. 2001. Multiple access to sterile syringes for injection drug users: Vending machines, needle exchange programs and legal pharmacy sales in Marseille, France. *European Addiction Research* 7(1):40-45.

Molitor, F., R. A. Bell, S. R. Truax, J. D. Ruiz, and R. K. Sun. 1999. Predictors of failure to return for HIV test result and counseling by test site type. *AIDS Education and Prevention* 11(1):1-13.

Myers, J. J., C. Modica, M. S. Dufour, C. Bernstein, and K. McNamara. 2009. Routine rapid HIV screening in six community health centers serving populations at risk. *Journal of General Internal Medicine* 24(12):1269-1274.

NASTAD (National Alliance of State and Territorial AIDS Directors). 2001. Integrating viral hepatitis into HIV/AIDS/STD programs. *HIV Prevention Bulletin* September.

———. 2009. *Fact sheet describing need for FY2010 appropriations for hepatitis prevention.* National Alliance for State and Territorial AIDS Directors.

Neaigus, A., V. A. Gyarmathy, M. Zhao, M. Miller, S. R. Friedman, and D. C. Des Jarlais. 2007. Sexual and other noninjection risks for HBV and HCV seroconversions among noninjecting heroin users. *Journal of Infectious Diseases* 195(7):1052-1061.

NIH (National Institutes of Health). 2008. *NIH consensus development conference statement on the management of Hepatitis B.* http://consensus.nih.gov/2008/hebB%20 draft%20statement%20102208_FINAL.pdf (accessed August 21, 2009).

Ostuni, P., C. Botsios, L. Punzi, P. Sfriso, and S. Todesco. 2003. Hepatitis B reactivation in a chronic hepatitis B surface antigen carrier with rheumatoid arthritis treated with infliximab and low dose methotrexate. *Annals of the Rheumatic Diseases* 62(7):686-687.

O'Toole, T. P., R. A. Pollini, D. E. Ford, and G. Bigelow. 2008. The health encounter as a treatable moment for homeless substance-using adults: The role of homelessness, health seeking behavior, readiness for behavior change and motivation for treatment. *Addictive Behaviors* 33(9):1239-1243.

O'Toole, T. P., R. Pollini, P. Gray, T. Jones, G. Bigelow, and D. E. Ford. 2007. Factors identifying high-frequency and low-frequency health service utilization among substance-using adults. *Journal of Substance Abuse Treatment* 33(1):51-59.

Paltiel, A. D., M. C. Weinstein, A. D. Kimmel, G. R. Seage, 3rd, E. Losina, H. Zhang, K. A. Freedberg, and R. P. Walensky. 2005. Expanded screening for HIV in the United States—an analysis of cost-effectiveness. *New England Journal of Medicine* 352(6):586-595.

Patrick, D. M., M. W. Tyndall, P. G. Cornelisse, K. Li, C. H. Sherlock, M. L. Rekart, S. A. Strathdee, S. L. Currie, M. T. Schechter, and M. V. O'Shaughnessy. 2001. Incidence of hepatitis C virus infection among injection drug users during an outbreak of HIV infection. *Canadian Medical Association Journal* 165(7):889-895.

Pawlotsky, J.-M., I. Lonjon, C. Hezode, B. Raynard, F. Darthuy, J. Remire, C.-J. Soussy, and D. Dhumeaux. 1998. What strategy should be used for diagnosis of hepatitis C virus infection in clinical laboratories? *Hepatology* 27(6):1700-1702.

Pisu, M., M. I. Meltzer, and R. Lyerla. 2002. Cost-effectiveness of hepatitis B vaccination of prison inmates. *Vaccine* 21(3-4):312-321.

Probst, J., J. Laditka, and S. Laditka. 2009. Association between community health center and rural health clinic presence and county-level hospitalization rates for ambulatory care sensitive conditions: An analysis across eight US states. *BMC Health Services Research* 9(1):134.

Raggio Ashley, T. P. 2009. *Community health centers, the federal perspective: Hepatitis B and C activities at HRSA*. Presentation to the committee, March 3, 2009.

Rahnavardi, M., S. M. Hosseini Moghaddam, and S. M. Alavian. 2008. Hepatitis C in hemodialysis patients: Current global magnitude, natural history, diagnostic difficulties, and preventive measures. *American Journal of Nephrology* 28(4):628-640.

Rajendra, A., and J. B. Wong. 2007. Economics of chronic hepatitis B and hepatitis C. *Journal of Hepatology* 47(4):608-617.

Randrianirina, F., J. F. Carod, E. Ratsima, J. B. Chretien, V. Richard, and A. Talarmin. 2008. Evaluation of the performance of four rapid tests for detection of hepatitis B surface antigen in Antananarivo, Madagascar. *Journal of Virological Methods* 151(2):294-297.

Regan, J., A. H. Schempf, J. Yoon, and R. M. Politzer. 2003. The role of federally funded health centers in serving the rural population. *Journal of Rural Health* 19(2):117-124; discussion 115-116.

Rein, D. B., S. B. Lesesne, P. J. Leese, and C. M. Weinbaum. 2009. Community-based hepatitis B screening programs in the United States in 2008. *Journal of Viral Hepatitis* 17(1):28-33.

Reynolds, G. L., D. G. Fisher, L. E. Napper, K. A. Marsh, C. Willey, and R. Brooks. 2008. Results from a multiple morbidities testing program offering rapid HIV testing bundled with hepatitis and sexually transmitted infection testing. *Public Health Reports* 123(Suppl 3):63-69.

Rezza, G., L. Sagliocca, M. Zaccarelli, M. Nespoli, M. Siconolfi, and C. Baldassarre. 1996. Incidence rate and risk factors for HCV seroconversion among injecting drug users in an area with low HIV seroprevalence. *Scandinavian Journal of Infectious Diseases* 28(1):27-29.

Rhodes, T., and C. Treloar. 2008. The social production of hepatitis C risk among injecting drug users: A qualitative synthesis. *Addiction* 103(10):1593-1603.

Ricketts, T. C. 2000. The changing nature of rural health care. *Annual Review of Public Health* 21(1):639-657.

Rogers, W. 2009. *Viral hepatitis prevention polices and programs, Centers for Medicare and Medicaid services*. Presentation to the committee, March 3, 2009.

Rooney, G., and R. J. Gilson. 1998. Sexual transmission of hepatitis C virus infection. *Sexually Transmitted Infections* 74(6):399-404.

Rosenheck, R. A., S. G. Resnick, and J. P. Morrissey. 2003. Closing service system gaps for homeless clients with a dual diagnosis: Integrated teams and interagency cooperation. *Journal of Mental Health Policy and Economics* 6(2):77-87.

Rossi, G., A. Pelizzari, M. Motta, and M. Puoti. 2001. Primary prophylaxis with lamivudine of hepatitis B virus reactivation in chronic HBsAg carriers with lymphoid malignancies treated with chemotherapy. *British Journal of Haematology* 115(1):58-62.

Rousseau, C. M., G. N. Ioannou, J. A. Todd-Stenberg, K. L. Sloan, M. F. Larson, C. W. Forsberg, and J. A. Dominitz. 2008. Racial differences in the evaluation and treatment of hepatitis C among veterans: A retrospective cohort study. *American Journal of Public Health* 98(5):846-852.

Roy, E., E. Nonn, N. Haley, and J. Cox. 2007. Hepatitis C meanings and preventive strategies among street-involved young injection drug users in Montreal. *International Journal on Drug Policy* 18(5):397-405.

Ruan, Y., G. Qin, L. Yin, K. Chen, H. Z. Qian, C. Hao, S. Liang, J. Zhu, H. Xing, K. Hong, and Y. Shao. 2007. Incidence of HIV, hepatitis C and hepatitis B viruses among injection drug users in southwestern China: A 3-year follow-up study. *AIDS* 21(Suppl 8):S39-S46.

Rust, G., P. Baltrus, J. Ye, E. Daniels, A. Quarshie, P. Boumbulian, and H. Strothers. 2009. Presence of a community health center and uninsured emergency department visit rates in rural counties. *Journal of Rural Health* 25(1):8-16.

Sabbatani, S., R. Giuliani, and R. Manfredi. 2006. Combined pegylated interferon and ribavirin for the management of chronic hepatitis C in a prison setting. *Brazilian Journal of Infectious Diseases* 10(4):274-278.

Salomon, J. A., M. C. Weinstein, J. K. Hammitt, and S. J. Goldie. 2003. Cost-effectiveness of treatment for chronic hepatitis C infection in an evolving patient population. *Journal of the American Medical Association* 290(2):228-237.

Sanders, G. D., A. M. Bayoumi, V. Sundaram, S. P. Bilir, C. P. Neukermans, C. E. Rydzak, L. R. Douglass, L. C. Lazzeroni, M. Holodniy, and D. K. Owens. 2005. Cost-effectiveness of screening for HIV in the era of highly active antiretroviral therapy. *New England Journal of Medicine* 352(6):570-585.

Schechter, M. T., S. A. Strathdee, P. G. Cornelisse, S. Currie, D. M. Patrick, M. L. Rekart, and M. V. O'Shaughnessy. 1999. Do needle exchange programmes increase the spread of HIV among injection drug users?: An investigation of the Vancouver outbreak. *AIDS* 13(6):F45-F51.

Scheinmann, R., H. Hagan, C. Lelutiu-Weinberger, R. Stern, D. C. Des Jarlais, P. L. Flom, and S. Strauss. 2007. Non-injection drug use and hepatitis C virus: A systematic review. *Drug and Alcohol Dependence* 89(1):1-12.

Schulden, J. D., B. Song, A. Barros, A. Mares-DelGrasso, C. W. Martin, R. Ramirez, L. C. Smith, D. P. Wheeler, A. M. Oster, P. S. Sullivan, and J. D. Heffelfinger. 2008. Rapid HIV testing in transgender communities by community-based organizations in three cities. *Public Health Reports* 123(Suppl 3):101-114.

Sherman, K. E., S. D. Rouster, R. T. Chung, and N. Rajicic. 2002. Hepatitis C virus prevalence among patients infected with human immunodeficiency virus: A cross sectional analysis of the US adult AIDS clinical trials group. *Clinical Infectious Diseases* 34(6):831-837.

Shrestha, R. K., H. A. Clark, S. L. Sansom, B. Song, H. Buckendahl, C. B. Calhoun, A. B. Hutchinson, and J. D. Heffelfinger. 2008. Cost-effectiveness of finding new HIV diagnoses using rapid HIV testing in community-based organizations. *Public Health Reports* 123(Suppl 3):94-100.

Siegel, A. B., R. B. McBride, H. B. El-Serag, D. L. Hershman, R. S. Brown, Jr., J. F. Renz, J. Emond, and A. I. Neugut. 2008. Racial disparities in utilization of liver transplantation for hepatocellular carcinoma in the United States, 1998-2002. *American Journal of Gastroenterology* 103(1):120-127.

Simmons, T. M. 2004. Inmate peer education programs: 101. *Infectious Diseases in Corrections Report*. December 2004.

Smith, L. V., E. T. Rudy, M. Javanbakht, A. Uniyal, L. S. Sy, T. Horton, and P. R. Kerndt. 2006. Client satisfaction with rapid HIV testing: Comparison between an urban sexually transmitted disease clinic and a community-based testing center. *AIDS Patient Care and STDs* 20(10):693-700.

Smyth, B. P., E. Keenan, and J. J. O'Connor. 2000. Assessment of hepatitis C infection in injecting drug users attending an addiction treatment clinic. *Irish Journal of Medical Science* 169(2):129-132.

Smyth, B. P., J. J. O'Connor, J. Barry, and E. Keenan. 2003. Retrospective cohort study examining incidence of HIV and hepatitis C infection among injecting drug users in Dublin. *Journal of Epidemiology and Community Health* 57(4):310-311.

Sneller, V. P., D. B. Fishbein, C. M. Weinbaum, A. Lombard, P. Murray, J. A. McLaurin, and L. Friedman. 2008. Vaccinating adolescents in high-risk settings: Lessons learned from experiences with hepatitis B vaccine. *Pediatrics* 121(Suppl 1):S55-S62.

Sonnenday, C. J., J. B. Dimick, R. D. Schulick, and M. A. Choti. 2007. Racial and geographic disparities in the utilization of surgical therapy for hepatocellular carcinoma. *Journal of Gastrointestinal Surgery* 11(12):1636-1646; discussion 1646.

Spaulding, A. C., C. M. Weinbaum, D. T.-Y. Lau, R. Sterling, L. B. Seeff, H. S. Margolis, and J. H. Hoofnagle. 2006. A framework for management of hepatitis C in prisons. *Annals of Internal Medicine* 144(10):762-769.

Spielberg, F., B. M. Branson, G. M. Goldbaum, D. Lockhart, A. Kurth, C. L. Celum, A. Rossini, C. W. Critchlow, and R. W. Wood. 2003. Overcoming barriers to HIV testing: Preferences for new strategies among clients of a needle exchange, a sexually transmitted disease clinic, and sex venues for men who have sex with men. *Journal of Acquired Immune Deficiency Syndromes* 32(3):318-327.

Spielberg, F., B. M. Branson, G. M. Goldbaum, D. Lockhart, A. Kurth, A. Rossini, and R. W. Wood. 2005. Choosing HIV counseling and testing strategies for outreach settings: A randomized trial. *Journal of Acquired Immune Deficiency Syndromes* 38(3):348-355.

Spielberg, F., A. Kurth, P. M. Gorbach, and G. Goldbaum. 2001. Moving from apprehension to action: HIV counseling and testing preferences in three at-risk populations. *AIDS Education and Prevention* 13(6):524-540.

Stanley, A. H. 1999. Primary care and addiction treatment: Lessons learned from building bridges across traditions. *Journal of Addictive Diseases* 18(2):65-82.

Sterling, R. K., C. M. Hofmann, V. A. Luketic, A. J. Sanyal, M. J. Contos, A. S. Mills, and M. L. Shiffman. 2004. Treatment of chronic hepatitis C virus in the Virginia Department of Corrections: Can compliance overcome racial differences to response? *American Journal of Gastroenterology* 99(5):866-872.

Stopka, T. J., C. Marshall, R. N. Bluthenthal, D. S. Webb, and S. R. Truax. 2007. HCV and HIV counseling and testing integration in California: An innovative approach to increase HIV counseling and testing rates. *Public Health Reports* 122(Suppl 2):68-73.

Strauss, S. M., J. M. Astone, D. D. Jarlais, and H. Hagan. 2004. A comparison of HCV antibody testing in drug-free and methadone maintenance treatment programs in the United States. *Drug and Alcohol Dependence* 73(3):227-236.

Strauss, S. M., J. M. Astone, Z. P. Vassilev, D. C. Des Jarlais, and H. Hagan. 2003. Gaps in the drug-free and methadone treatment program response to Hepatitis C. *Journal of Substance Abuse Treatment* 24(4):291-297.

Strauss, S. M., G. P. Falkin, Z. Vassilev, D. C. Des Jarlais, and J. Astone. 2002. A nationwide survey of hepatitis C services provided by drug treatment programs. *Journal of Substance Abuse Treatment* 22(2):55-62.

Subiadur, J., J. L. Harris, and C. A. Rietmeijer. 2007. Integrating viral hepatitis prevention services into an urban STD clinic: Denver, Colorado. *Public Health Reports* 122(Suppl 2):12-17.

Sulkowski, M., S. 2008. Viral hepatitis and HIV coinfection. *Journal of Hepatology* 48(2): 353-367.

Sullivan, P. S., A. Lansky, and A. Drake. 2004. Failure to return for HIV test results among persons at high risk for HIV infection: Results from a multistate interview project. *Journal of Acquired Immune Deficiency Syndromes* 35(5):511-518.

Tempalski, B., H. L. Cooper, S. R. Friedman, D. C. Des Jarlais, J. Brady, and K. Gostnell. 2008. Correlates of syringe coverage for heroin injection in 35 large metropolitan areas in the US in which heroin is the dominant injected drug. *International Journal on Drug Policy* 19(Suppl 1):S47-S58.

Tempalski, B., P. L. Flom, S. R. Friedman, D. C. Des Jarlais, J. J. Friedman, C. McKnight, and R. Friedman. 2007. Social and political factors predicting the presence of syringe exchange programs in 96 US metropolitan areas. *American Journal of Public Health* 97(3):437-447.

Thiede, H., H. Hagan, and C. S. Murrill. 2000. Methadone treatment and HIV and hepatitis B and C risk reduction among injectors in the Seattle area. *Journal of Urban Health* 77(3):331-345.

Thiede, H., H. Hagan, J. V. Campbell, S. A. Strathdee, S. L. Bailey, S. M. Hudson, F. Kapadia, and R. S. Garfein. 2007. Prevalence and correlates of indirect sharing practices among young adult injection drug users in five U.S. Cities. *Drug and Alcohol Dependence* 91(Suppl 1):S39-S47.

Thio, C. L., K. R. Nolt, J. Astemborski, D. Vlahov, K. E. Nelson, and D. L. Thomas. 2000. Screening for hepatitis C virus in human immunodeficiency virus-infected individuals. *Journal of Clinical Microbiology* 38(2):575-577.

Thio, C. L., E. C. Seaberg, R. Skolasky, Jr., J. Phair, B. Visscher, A. Munoz, and D. L. Thomas. 2002. HIV-1, hepatitis B virus, and risk of liver-related mortality in the multicenter cohort study (MACS). *Lancet* 360(9349):1921-1926.

Thorpe, L. E., L. J. Ouellet, R. Hershow, S. L. Bailey, I. T. Williams, J. Williamson, E. R. Monterroso, and R. S. Garfein. 2002. Risk of hepatitis C virus infection among young adult injection drug users who share injection equipment. *American Journal of Epidemiology* 155(7):645-653.

Tramarin, A., N. Gennaro, F. A. Compostella, C. Gallo, L. J. Wendelaar Bonga, and M. J. Postma. 2008. HCV screening to enable early treatment of hepatitis C: A mathematical model to analyse costs and outcomes in two populations. *Current Pharmaceutical Design* 14(17):1655-1660.

U.S. Census Bureau. 2008. *2007 American community survey*. http://factfinder.census.gov/servlet/STTable?_bm=y&-qr_name=ACS_2008_3YR_G00_S0502&-geo_id=01000US&-ds_name=ACS_2008_3YR_G00_&-_lang=en&-format=&-CONTEXT=st (accessed August 20, 2009).

U.S. Department of Homeland Security. 2009. *Yearbook of immigration statistics: 2008. Table 3: Persons obtaining legal permanent resident status by region and country of birth: Fiscal years 1999 to 2008.* http://www.dhs.gov/files/statistics/publications/yearbook.shtm (accessed August 21, 2009).

U.S. Preventive Services Task Force. 2009. Screening for hepatitis B virus infection in pregnancy: U.S. Preventive Services Task Force reaffirmation recommendation statement. *Annals of Internal Medicine* 150(12):869-873, W154.

Valentine, J., and L. Wright-De Aguero. 1996. Defining the components of street outreach for HIV prevention: The contact and the encounter. *Public Health Reports* 111(Suppl 1):69-74.

Vallabhaneni, S., G. E. Macalino, S. E. Reinert, B. Schwartzapfel, F. A. Wolf, and J. D. Rich. 2004. Prisoners' attitudes toward hepatitis B vaccination. *Preventive Medicine* 38(6):828-833.

van den Berg, C. H., C. Smit, M. Bakker, R. B. Geskus, B. Berkhout, S. Jurriaans, R. A. Coutinho, K. C. Wolthers, and M. Prins. 2007b. Major decline of hepatitis C virus incidence rate over two decades in a cohort of drug users. *European Journal of Epidemiology* 22(3):183-193.

van den Berg, C., C. Smit, G. Van Brussel, R. Coutinho, and M. Prins. 2007a. Full participation in harm reduction programmes is associated with decreased risk for human immunodeficiency virus and hepatitis C virus: Evidence from the Amsterdam cohort studies among drug users. *Addiction* 102(9):1454-1462.

van Nunen, A. B., R. A. de Man, R. A. Heijtink, H. G. Niesters, and S. W. Schalm. 2000. Lamivudine in the last 4 weeks of pregnancy to prevent perinatal transmission in highly viremic chronic hepatitis B patients. *Journal of Hepatology* 32(6):1040-1041.

van Zonneveld, M., A. B. van Nunen, H. G. Niesters, R. A. de Man, S. W. Schalm, and H. L. Janssen. 2003. Lamivudine treatment during pregnancy to prevent perinatal transmission of hepatitis B virus infection. *Journal of Viral Hepatitis* 10(4):294-297.

Ward, J. 2008a. FY 2008 domestic enacted funds. Presentation to the committee: December 4, 2008.

Ward, J. W. 2008b. Time for renewed commitment to viral hepatitis prevention. *American Journal of Public Health* 98(5):779-781.

Weinbaum, C. M. 2008. *Recommendations for identification and public health management of persons with chronic hepatitis b virus infection.* Paper presented at NIH Consensus Development Conference: Management of Hepatitis B, Natcher Conference Center, National Institutes of Health (Bethesda, MD).

Weinbaum, C., R. Lyerla, and H. S. Margolis. 2003. Prevention and control of infections with hepatitis viruses in correctional settings. Centers for Disease Control and Prevention. *Morbidity and Mortality Weekly Report Recommendations and Reports* 52(RR-1):1-36; quiz CE31-CE34.

Wise, M., S. Bialek, L. Finelli, B. P. Bell, and F. Sorvillo. 2008. Changing trends in hepatitis C-related mortality in the United States, 1995-2004. *Hepatology* 47(4):1128-1135.

Workowski, K., and S. Berman. 2006. Sexually transmitted diseases: Treatment guidelines, 2006. *Morbidity and Mortality Weekly Report* 55(RR-11):1-94.

Wright, D. B. 2009. Care in the country: A historical case study of long-term sustainability in 4 rural health centers. *American Journal of Public Health* 99(9):1612-1618.

Xu, W. M., Y. T. Cui, L. Wang, H. Yang, Z. Q. Liang, X. M. Li, S. L. Zhang, F. Y. Qiao, F. Campbell, C. N. Chang, S. Gardner, and M. Atkins. 2009. Lamivudine in late pregnancy to prevent perinatal transmission of hepatitis B virus infection: A multicentre, randomized, double-blind, placebo-controlled study. *Journal of Viral Hepatitis* 16(2):94-103.

Yeo, W., and P. J. Johnson. 2006. Diagnosis, prevention and management of hepatitis B virus reactivation during anticancer therapy. *Hepatology* 43(2):209-220.

Yeo, W., P. K. Chan, S. Zhong, W. M. Ho, J. L. Steinberg, J. S. Tam, P. Hui, N. W. Leung, B. Zee, and P. J. Johnson. 2000. Frequency of hepatitis B virus reactivation in cancer patients undergoing cytotoxic chemotherapy: A prospective study of 626 patients with identification of risk factors. *Journal of Medical Virology* 62(3):299-307.

Zickmund, S., S. L. Hillis, M. J. Barnett, L. Ippolito, and D. R. LaBrecque. 2004. Hepatitis C virus-infected patients report communication problems with physicians. *Hepatology* 39(4):999-1007.

Zimmerman, R., C. Finley, C. Rabins, and K. McMahon. 2007. Integrating viral hepatitis prevention into STD clinics in Illinois (excluding Chicago), 1999-2005. *Public Health Reports* 122(Suppl 2):18-23.

Zola, J., N. Smith, S. Goldman, and B. A. Woodruff. 1997. Attitudes and educational practices of obstetric providers regarding infant hepatitis B vaccination. *Obstetrics and Gynecology* 89(1):61-64.

Zuniga, I. A., J. J. Chen, D. S. Lane, J. Allmer, and V. E. Jimenez-Lucho. 2006. Analysis of a hepatitis C screening programme for US veterans. *Epidemiology and Infection* 134(02):249-257.

A

Committee Biographies

R. Palmer Beasley, MD (*Chair*), is the Ashbel Smith Professor and dean emeritus of the University of Texas School of Public Health at Houston. Previously, Dr. Beasley was a member of the faculty of the Department of Epidemiology at the University of Washington and the Department of Internal Medicine at the University of California, San Francisco. The focus of his research has been the hepatitis B virus. His contributions to the field include discovery of mother-to-infant transmission of the hepatitis B virus, establishing that the hepatitis B virus is the major cause of liver cancer, and a series of clinical trials that established the effectiveness and strategies for the use of hepatitis B vaccine for the prevention of perinatal transmission. Dr. Beasley has won many awards for his work, including the Charles F. Mott General Motors International Prize for Research on Cancer, the Prince Mahidol Award for Medicine (Thailand), and the Health Medal of the First Order (Taiwan). He has served on numerous national and international government advisory panels on viral hepatitis and is chair of the Association of Schools of Public Health. He also served on the National Academies Committee on the Middle East Regional Infectious Disease Research Program and Committee on the Assessment of Future Scientific Needs for Variola Virus and on the Public Health and Biotechnology Review Panel. Dr. Beasley received his MD from Harvard School of Medicine, and his MS in preventative medicine from the University of Washington.

Harvey J. Alter, MD, is chief of clinical studies and associate director for research in the Department of Transfusion Medicine at the National Institutes of Health. Dr. Alter's research interest is in viral hepatitis and the safety of the blood supply. He was a major contributor in the fight to reduce the incidence of transfusion-induced viral hepatitis, and he collaborated in the discovery of hepatitis C and described its natural history. He is a member of IOM and NAS. For his contributions, Dr. Alter has been awarded the US Pubic Health Service Distinguished Service Medal, the Landsteiner Prize, the Presidential Award of the International Society of Blood Transfusion, the James Blundell Award of the British Blood Transfusion Society, and the Distinguished Scientist Awards of both the Hepatitis B Foundation and the American Liver Foundation, and he was elected to fellowship in the American Association of Physicians. He was the corecipient of the 2000 Clinical Lasker Award and was made a master of the American College of Physicians. In 2007, he was named Distinguished NIH Investigator. Dr. Alter received his MD from the University of Rochester.

Margaret L. Brandeau, PhD, is a professor in the Department of Management Science and Engineering of Stanford University. She also holds a courtesy appointment in the Department of Medicine of the same institution. Dr. Brandeau is an operations researcher and policy analyst with extensive background in the development of applied mathematical and economic models. She has conducted research on HIV, focusing on mathematical and economic models to assess the value of different HIV and drug-abuse interventions, and on hepatitis B screening and vaccination policies. She received her PhD in engineering and economic systems from Stanford University.

Daniel R. Church, MPH, is the adult viral hepatitis prevention coordinator and an epidemiologist in the Division of Epidemiology and Immunization of the Massachusetts Department of Health. He coordinates the statewide viral hepatitis program, including disease surveillance; medical-management services; counseling and testing programs; adult vaccination programs; educational campaigns for providers, patients, and communities; and evaluation of projects. Mr. Church received his MPH in epidemiology and biostatistics from the Boston University School of Public Health.

Alison A. Evans, ScD, is an assistant professor in the Department of Epidemiology and Biostatistics of the Drexel University School of Public Health. She is also the director of public-health research in the Hepatitis B Foundation, Doylestown, PA, and is an adjunct associate member of the Fox Chase Cancer Center in Philadelphia, PA. Her research interests include the epidemiology and natural history of the hepatitis B virus and other chronic viral infections. She received her ScD in epidemiology from the Harvard School of Public Health.

Holly Hagan, PhD, MPH, is a senior research scientist in the New York University College of Nursing, deputy director of the Center for Drug Use and HIV Research, and director of the center's Interdisciplinary Research Methods Core. Previously, she was deputy director of the Institute for AIDS Research in the National Development and Research Institutes. She was a senior epidemiologist in the Department of Public Health in Seattle, WA. Her broad research interest is in the etiology and prevention of hepatitis C and other bloodborne viral infections in drug users and other high-risk populations; her work has also examined drug users' access to screening and health care. Dr. Hagan has served on several national government advisory groups, including the steering committee for the National Institutes of Health hepatitis C vaccine trial. She received her MPH in epidemiology from the University of Massachusetts at Amherst School of Public Health and her PhD in epidemiology from the University of Washington School of Public Health and Community Medicine.

Sandral Hullett, MD, MPH, is the chief executive officer and medical director of the Jefferson Health System, which consists of Cooper Green–Mercy Hospital and Jefferson Outpatient Care. Jefferson Health System's primary focus is service to the underserved populations of Jefferson County, AL. Previously, Dr. Hullett was the executive director of Family HealthCare of Alabama, which is headquartered in Eutaw, Alabama, and provided services to patients of west central Alabama. She has an interest in rural health care, including health-care planning and delivery to the underserved, underinsured, and poor; and she has extensive experience in research, clinical trials, community outreach, and teaching of direct care delivery. Dr. Hullett is a member of IOM and has served on several IOM committees, including committees that produced *America's Health Care Safety Net: Intact but Endangered*; *Quality Through Collaboration: The Future of Rural Health*; and *Measuring What Matters: Allocation, Planning, and Quality Assessment for the Ryan White CARE Act*; the Planning Committee for a Workshop on Military Medical Ethics: Issues Regarding Dual Loyalties; and the Committee on Human Rights of NAS, NAE, and IOM. She has received many awards and honors, including the Rural Practitioner of the Year Award in 1988 from the National Rural Health Association, the Clinical Recognition Award for Education and Training from the National Association of Community Health Centers in 1993, the Public Health Hero Award for Year 2000 from the University of Alabama at Birmingham School of Public Health, the National Medical Fellowship in 2001, Lifetime Achievement of Women in Health Care from Rutgers University in 2002, and the Local Legends Award from the American Medical Women's Association in February 2004. She received her MD from the Medical College of Pennsylvania and her MPH from the University of Alabama at Birmingham.

Stacene R. Maroushek, MD, PhD, MPH, is a staff pediatrician at Hennepin County Medical Center in Minneapolis, MN. She is also an assistant professor in the Division of Pediatric Infectious Diseases of the University of Minnesota. Dr. Maroushek works with immigrant pediatric patients and has published extensively on medical evaluation and screening of immigrant children for infectious diseases. She received her MD, her PhD in microbiology, and her MPH from the University of Minnesota.

Randall R. Mayer, MS, MPH, is an epidemiologist and chief of the Bureau of HIV, STD, and Hepatitis in the Iowa Department of Public Health. He provides oversight for HIV, sexually trasmitted disease (STD), and hepatitis prevention, care, and surveillance activities, including disease reporting, counseling and testing, risk-reduction programs, partner services, community planning, adult immunizations for hepatitis A and hepatitis B, HIV case management and support services, and HIV and STD drug-treatment assistance programs. While working with the Iowa Department of Public Health, Mr. Mayer has served as the HIV/AIDS/Hepatitis Program manager and as the HIV/AIDS surveillance coordinator. He received his MPH in epidemiology from the University of Minnesota and his MS in plant cell physiology from Purdue University.

Brian J. McMahon, MD, is medical director of the liver disease and hepatitis program at the Alaska Native Tribal Health Consortium and a clinical hepatologist at the Alaska Native Medical Center. He was previously employed by the Centers for Disease Control and Prevention in Alaska. Dr. McMahon has worked to reduce the rate of hepatitis B in the native Alaskan population, which went from one of the highest in the world to one of the lowest. He provides clinical care for patients who have viral hepatitis and liver disease and conducts research in population-epidemiology hepatitis and liver disease. He has served as a consultant on viral hepatitis issues to the World Health Organization and other international and national organizations. Dr. McMahon received the Assistant Secretary for Health Award for Exceptional Achievement in 1985; the Alvan R. Feinstein Memorial Award from the American College of Physicians in 2003 for the Program to Control Hepatitis B in Alaska Natives; and the 2009 Scientist of the Year from the Hepatitis B Foundation for notable contributions in clinical epidemiology regarding research on and control of hepatitis A, hepatitis B, and hepatitis C in Alaska natives. He was elected a master in the American College of Physicians. He received his MD from the University of Washington.

Martín J. Sepúlveda, MD, FACP, is IBM Fellow and vice president of integrated health services for the International Business Machines Corporation. His research interests and health-care reform initiatives include patient-centered primary care and medical homes, care management and coordination, total health management, workplace health promotion, risk-reduction program measurement, value-based health-care purchasing, and global occupational and health services delivery. He is a fellow of the IBM Corporation, the American College of Physicians, the American College of Occupational and Environmental Medicine, and the American College of Preventive Medicine. Dr. Sepúlveda was recently chosen as an IBM Fellow, IBM's highest technical achievement; was awarded honorary membership in the American Academy of Family Physicians; and received the John D. Thompson Distinguished Fellow Award from Yale University and the Distinguished Alumnus Award for Professional Achievement from the University of Iowa. His team has received numerous national and international awards in health care, health promotion, and occupational health and safety. He serves on the IOM Board on Population Health and Public Health Practice, the Board of Directors of the Employee Benefits Research Institute, the Board of Advisors to the School of Public Health of the University of Iowa, and the Board of the National Business Group on Health; and he chairs the Global Health Benefits Institute. He received his MD and MPH from Harvard University.

Samuel So, MB, BS, is a professor of surgery and the Lui Hac Minh Professor at Stanford University. He is also the director of the Asian Liver Center and director of the Multidisciplinary Liver Cancer Program at the same institution. He has published numerous studies on solid-organ transplantation and gastric and liver cancers. Dr. So is well known for his work on hepatitis B and liver-cancer education and prevention programs. Through his research, Dr. So has identified the need for a public-health approach to liver-cancer prevention in recent Asian immigrants and first- and second-generation Asians living in the United States. Those populations have not been the typical focus of US screening and prevention programs. Dr. So is listed in *The Best Doctors in America,* published by Woodward/White, Inc. For his work in education and prevention, he received the 2005 National Leadership Award from the New York University Center for the Study of Asian American Health, the 2008 American Liver Foundation Salute to Excellence Award, and the 2009 Asian Pacific Islander Heritage Award from the California Asian Pacific Islander Joint Legislative Caucus. He is a member of IOM's Board on Population Health and Public Health Practice. Dr. So received his MB and his BS in medicine and surgery from the University of Hong Kong and did postdoctoral and clinical fellowships at the University of Minnesota.

David L. Thomas, MD, MPH, is chief of the Division of Infectious Diseases, Department of Medicine, of the Johns Hopkins School of Medicine. He is also a professor in the Department of Epidemiology in the Johns Hopkins Bloomberg School of Public Health. His broad research interest is viral hepatitis, and current research projects include the progression of hepatitis C in injection-drug users, hepatitis C pathogenesis and the host genome, and antiviral therapy for HIV–hepatitis C virus coinfection. Dr. Thomas received his MD from the West Virginia School of Medicine and his MPH from the Johns Hopkins School of Hygiene and Public Health.

Lester N. Wright, MD, MPH, is the deputy commissioner and chief medical officer for the New York Department of Correctional Services. He oversees health care for some 62,000 residents in 70 facilities, who currently include about 4,500 HIV-positive patients and 8,000 who have hepatitis C virus infection. Before his employment in the New York Department of Correctional Services, Dr. Wright worked in several state and county health departments, including the Virginia Department of Health and the Delaware Public Health Division. He spent 7 years working in Africa on delivery of primary health care and health-system development. He has served on two National Academies committees: the Committee on Regulating Occupational Exposure to Tuberculosis and the Committee on the Elimination of Tuberculosis in the United States. Dr. Wright received his MD from the Loma Linda University School of Medicine and his MPH from the Harvard School of Public Health.

B

Public Meeting Agendas

FIRST MEETING-DECEMBER 4, 2008

National Academy of Sciences Building, Washington, DC

Welcome and opening statement

Palmer Beasley, Committee Chair

Charge to the committee

John Ward, Centers for Disease Control and Prevention (CDC)
Chris Taylor and Martha Saly, National Viral Hepatitis Roundtable

Presentations to the committee

Dale Hu, CDC
Broad Overview of Hepatitis B

Cindy Weinbaum, CDC
Broad Overview of Hepatitis C

Lorren Sandt, Caring Ambassadors Program
Hepatitis C: Moving Beyond the Silence

Joan Block, Hepatitis B Foundation
Hepatitis B: Time for Zero Tolerance

Public comment period

SECOND MEETING-MARCH 3, 2009

The National Academies Beckman Center, Irvine, California

Welcome and opening statement

Palmer Beasley, Committee Chair

Presentations to the committee

Gary Heseltine
Lead Consultant, Viral Hepatitis Team, Council of State and Territorial Epidemiologists
Surveillance Strengths and Weaknesses

William Rogers
Director of CMS, Physician's Regulatory Issues Team
Viral Hepatitis Prevention Policies and Programs, Centers for Medicare and Medicaid (CMS)

Tanya Pagán Raggio Ashley
Director, Office of Minority Health and Health Disparities, and Chief Medical Officer, HRSA
Community Health Centers: Health Resources and Services Administration (HRSA) Policies and Programs

Daniel Raymond
Policy Director, Harm Reduction Coalition
Hepatitis C Prevention: Harm Reduction

David Bell
Associate Director for Science and Global Activities, Division of Viral Hepatitis, Centers for Disease Control and Prevention
Global Viral Hepatitis Burden: Implications for the US and CDC Response

Mark Kane
Former Director of the Children's Vaccine Program, PATH
Global Control Programs and HBV Immunization

Question and answer period

Index

A

Acute disseminated encephalomyelitis, 32
Acute infections
    characteristics, 19
    clinical outcomes, 117, 118, 136, 137
    HBV, 1, 19, 23, 27, 34, 48, 50, 59, 70-71, 99, 117, 118, 119, 120, 121, 125, 161, 189
    HCV, 19, 28, 29, 34, 47, 49, 51, 71, 136, 137, 163, 165
    incarcerated people, 121
    injection-drug use and, 120, 137, 189
    outbreak detection and control, 48, 67, 70
    prevalence and incidence, 1, 50, 70-71, 99, 118, 119, 120, 121, 125
    screening and testing for, 47-51, 160, 161, 163, 165
    surveillance, 29, 44, 47-51, 59, 64, 67, 71
Adolescents and young adults, 7, 11, 23, 25, 31, 44, 68, 71, 93, 98, 100, 110, 112, 127, 131, 134, 191
Adult Hepatitis B Vaccine Initiative, 129
Adult viral-hepatitis prevention coordinators (AVHPC), 42-43, 57, 59, 61, 64, 70, 152-153
Adults. *See also* At-risk populations; *specific populations*
    asymptomatic infections, 47
    HBV, 11, 27, 32, 47, 93, 110, 111, 113, 117-125, 127, 128, 129, 132, 134
    HCV, 51
    vaccination, 11, 32, 93, 110, 111, 113, 117-125, 127, 128, 129, 132, 134
Advisory Committee on Immunization Practices (ACIP), 4, 9-10, 11, 55, 83, 88, 93, 100, 110-111, 112-115, 116, 125, 127, 132, 133, 134, 181
African Americans/Blacks, 1, 2, 10, 27, 29, 30, 32, 93, 116, 124, 168, 169, 184
Agency for Healthcare Quality and Research, 149
Alabama, 27 n.1, 91, 116
Alanine aminotransferase (ALT), 48, 49, 50, 53, 93, 158, 167
Alaska, 120-121, 122-123. *See also* American Indians and Alaska Natives
Alcohol consumption, 5, 14, 29, 30, 48, 84, 93, 148, 155, 168, 169, 181
Alternative-care providers, educational programs for, 86, 87, 89
American Academy of Pediatrics, 111
American Association for the Study of Liver Diseases (AASLD), 32, 155, 159, 166, 167, 168
American College of Obstetricians and Gynecologists, 84, 97

219

American College of Physicians, 159
American Indians and Alaska Natives, 29, 62, 81, 93, 129, 131, 168
Anti–tumor-necrosis factor therapy, 162
Asian American Hepatitis B Program, 92
Asians and Pacific Islanders (APIs). *See also* Foreign-born
 access to care, 56, 169
 educational programs for, 87, 92, 93, 153, 183
 health-care providers, 82
 incidence and prevalence of HBV infection, 1-2, 23, 27, 29, 81-82, 83, 93, 117-118, 153-154, 161, 183, 184-185
 knowledge and awareness of HBV, 13, 82, 89-90, 173
 liver cancer, 29, 153-154, 169
 medical management of hepatitis, 183
 risk of HBV, 90
 screening/testing, 161, 173
 surveillance, 32, 62, 68
 treatment disparities, 169
 vaccination, 10, 90, 92, 116, 117-118, 161-162
Aspartate transaminase, 49, 167
Asymptomatic infected individuals, awareness of infection, 1, 3, 24, 26, 27, 50, 51, 90
At-risk populations. *See also* Foreign-born populations; Illicit-drug users; Incarcerated populations; Men who have sex with men; Pregnant women
 access to services, 3, 56, 79
 defined, 27, 86, 156
 education programs, 4, 14, 85-86, 92-93, 95-96, 97, 98-100
 health service provider knowledge of, 80, 81-84, 89
 immunization, 4, 9, 10-11, 27, 81, 93, 113, 120-125
 knowledge and awareness of hepatitis, 3, 4, 8, 9, 34, 89-91, 93-96
 prevalence and incidence of hepatitis, 62, 81
 recommendations, 16-17
 screening and testing, 3, 4, 5, 6, 8, 9, 11, 13-14, 16, 27, 71-72, 85, 86, 97, 124-125, 148, 153, 155, 156-159, 161, 173
 services, 3, 5, 6, 13, 16-17, 56, 79, 149, 189-192
 surveillance, 2, 4, 6, 7, 61-62, 67, 68, 71-72
Awareness. *See* Knowledge and awareness of chronic hepatitis

B

Baltimore, 28, 92, 122-123, 190
Blacks. *See* African Americans/Blacks
Blood transfusions, 2, 21, 24, 28, 50, 83, 84, 151, 158
Brachial neuritis, 32
Brazil, 138
Breastfeeding, 84
Bureau of Primary Health Care, 151

C

California, 58, 81, 83, 89, 99, 120, 121, 122, 173, 174, 182, 183, 186
Cambodian Americans, 90, 92
Cancer chemotherapy, 162
Case definitions for hepatitis, 7, 48-49, 50, 51, 52-53, 54, 55, 65, 68, 69
Case management, 43, 45-46, 57-58, 62-63, 65, 68, 70, 72
Centers for Disease Control and Prevention (CDC), 2
 Adult Hepatitis B Vaccine Initiative, 129
 case definitions for hepatitis B and C, 48-49, 50, 52-53, 54, 55, 68
 Division of Viral Hepatitis, 150-151
 educational programs, 4, 8-9, 86, 87, 97, 96
 Emerging Infections Program, 43, 58, 59
 Epidemiologic Surveillance Project, 60
 estimates of hepatitis burden, 25, 26, 27, 62, 120, 182, 189
 National Immunization Program, 126
 NEDSS, 61
 NETSS, 60-61, 64
 partner services guidelines, 63
 PHIN-compliant systems, 64, 70
 prevention and control recommendations of, 30
 resource allocation for services, 5-6, 14, 15, 16-17, 26, 42, 54, 126-127, 148-150, 151, 152, 153, 175, 183, 186, 192

INDEX   221

risk factors for hepatitis, 156, 157-158, 159
screening and counseling recommendations of, 82-83, 84, 156-157, 159, 183
state cooperative agreements with, 4, 7, 42, 54, 57, 64-66, 67
surveillance initiatives, 4, 6, 7-8, 42-43, 44, 45, 50, 57, 58, 59-61, 63, 64, 65-66, 67, 68, 69, 70-71
vaccination recommendations and programs, 12, 110-111, 124-125, 126, 128-129, 134, 136, 153, 157
VFC program, 128-129, 130, 131, 134
Centers for Medicare and Medicaid Services, 129, 149. *See also* Medicaid; Medicare
Central nervous system demyelinating disorders, 32
Chicago, 28, 116, 121
Childhood Immunization Initiative, 126
Children
asymptomatic infections, 47
HBV, 23, 25, 30, 47, 116-117, 128-132
HCV, 51
information systems on, 127-128
progression of infection in, 46, 117, 118
vaccination, 4, 9, 10, 25, 30, 93, 97, 110, 111, 112, 116-117, 128-132, 134
Children's Health Insurance Program (CHIP), 128, 129-132, 172
Chinese Americans, 68, 81, 82, 86, 89, 90, 92, 174
Chronic infections. *See also* Hepatitis B; Hepatitis C; Knowledge and awareness of chronic hepatitis
age at exposure and potential for, 19, 22, 46, 51, 82-83, 113, 117, 118, 156
asymptomatic nature of, 3, 23, 24, 25, 27, 28, 47, 50, 51, 52, 53, 55, 90, 159, 162
clinical outcomes, 23; *see also* Liver cancer and liver cirrhosis
prevalence and incidence, 1, 34, 121
surveillance, 25, 44, 51-54, 59, 64, 67, 71
Clinical outcomes. *See also* Liver cancer and liver cirrhosis
age at exposure and, 19, 22, 46, 51, 82-83, 113, 117, 118, 156
knowledge of, 80, 83, 89

Coinfection
HBV and HCV, 23, 29, 30, 32
HIV and hepatitis, 23, 29, 72, 81-82, 190
Collaborative Injection Drug User Study Drug User Intervention Trial, 94, 95
Colorado, 58
Committee task
approach, 32-35
charge to committee, 30-32
Community
health centers, 16, 149, 186-189
outreach, 9, 90, 91-92, 97, 98-99, 101
screening and testing programs, 5, 13
Confidentiality safeguards, 43-44, 65
Connecticut, 55, 58, 122
Contacts. *See also* Partner services
education of, 97, 98
vaccination, 54, 57-58, 62, 93, 117, 119-120
Correctional facilities. *See also* Incarcerated populations
educational programs on viral hepatitis, 88-89, 99-100
recommendations, 16
viral hepatitis services, 6, 13, 14, 16, 149, 184-186
Counseling, 5, 14, 31, 62, 63, 84, 85, 87, 95, 124, 134, 148, 151, 152, 157, 160, 163, 168, 171, 172, 177, 179, 180, 181, 186, 189, 191

D

Deaths, preventable, by disease, 20
Denmark, 121
Department of Health and Human Services, 110
National Vaccine Program Office, 126
Office of Minority Health and Health Disparities, 2, 30, 149, 152
Department of Justice, 6, 16, 149, 186
Department of Veterans Affairs (VA), 2, 28, 30, 94, 130, 171, 172
Detroit, 121
Discrimination. *See* Stigmatization and discrimination
Drug treatment programs and facilities. *See also* Illicit-drug users
educational programs on viral hepatitis, 8, 88-89, 95-96, 100, 176

funding, 176
integrated approach, 14, 149, 179
prevention of seroconversion, 177, 178
screening and testing, 176
staff knowledge of hepatitis, 85, 88, 96
vaccination opportunities, 121, 124, 129
Drug users. *See* Illicit-drug users

E

Economic issues. *See also* Funding; Insurance coverage
screening and testing, 27, 161-162, 163
vaccination, 54, 57-58, 117-119, 124, 137-138
Educational programs. *See also* Knowledge and awareness of chronic hepatitis
advocacy efforts, 153-154
for alternative-medicine professionals, 86, 87, 89
for at-risk populations, 4, 14, 85-86, 92-93, 95-96, 97, 98-100, 153-154
CDC initiatives, 4, 8-9, 86, 87, 96, 97
contacts, 97, 98
content, 86-87
continuing medical education, 87
educational programs, 4, 8-9, 86, 87, 96, 97
evaluation of, 97
funding, 99, 152
for general population, 4, 96, 97, 98, 99, 153
goals, 9, 97
for health-care and social service workers, 4, 8-9, 58, 82, 84-88
integration into other programs, 9, 92, 95-96, 98
linguistically and culturally appropriate, 9, 87, 90, 92, 93, 97, 98-99, 101, 153, 183
outreach component, 96, 97, 98-99, 100
peer education, 95, 100
in perinatal facilities, 99-101
recommendations, 4, 8-9, 85-89, 96-101
safety precautions and procedures, 88
on screening and testing, 9, 58, 98
vaccination, 8, 9, 97, 101
Electronic medical records, 7, 50, 51, 60, 65, 68, 69, 70
Egyptian immigrants, 24, 159

Emerging Infections Program, 43, 58, 59
Employee Retirement Security Act, 134
End-stage renal disease patients, 113, 131, 152
Epidemiologic Surveillance Project, 60
Epidemiology and Laboratory Capacity for Infectious Diseases program, 59
Exposure routes
knowledge and awareness, 95
sexual, 1, 23, 44, 72, 84, 119-120
unsafe vaccine injections, 24

F

Federal Employees Health Benefits Program, 5, 13, 130, 148, 172
Florida Hepatitis Prevention Program, 186-187
Food and Drug Administration, 109
Foreign-born populations. *See also* Asians and Pacific Islanders; Hispanics
access to care, 56
culturally appropriate programs, 13, 56, 173-174, 183-184
educational outreach to, 9, 90, 91-92, 97, 98-99, 101, 174-175
exposure routes, 120
geographic regions of endemicity, 81-82
HBV, 1-2, 8, 13, 14, 23, 27, 81-82, 89-90, 91-92
health disparity, 27
incidence and prevalence of HBV, 8, 27, 79, 86, 93
knowledge and awareness of risks to, 13, 79, 81-82, 86, 87, 89-90, 173-174
liver cancer and cirrhosis, 29
recommendations, 14, 175
screening and testing, 5, 13, 14, 90, 91, 148, 153-154, 155, 156, 161-162, 173
vaccination, 5, 10, 13, 14, 90, 91, 92-93, 116, 117-118, 120, 132, 148, 157, 161-162
viral hepatitis services for, 5, 13-14, 148, 173-175
Funding
education, 99, 152
surveillance, 3, 7, 42, 57, 58-59, 63, 65, 66, 67, 71, 129
vaccination, 57, 118, 120, 129, 134

INDEX

G

General population
    education program, 4, 96, 97, 98, 99
    knowledge and awareness of chronic hepatitis, 3, 4, 9, 17, 33, 34, 79, 98
    recommendations, 13
    screening and testing, 13
    viral hepatitis services, 13, 170-173
Guillain-Barré syndrome, 32

H

Health Disparities Collaborative, 188
Health Resources and Services Administration (HRSA), 6, 16, 127, 148-149, 151-152, 187, 188-189, 192
Health-care providers and workers
    APIs, 82
    educational programs, 4, 8-9, 58, 82, 84-88
    guidelines for, 80
    immunization, 124
    knowledge and awareness of hepatitis, 3, 4, 8, 17, 33, 34, 79, 80-89, 154-155, 171, 182-183
    outreach to, 97
    safety precautions and procedures, 88
    vaccination, 88, 93, 113, 117, 118, 124, 125
Healthcare Effectiveness Data and Information Set (HEDIS), 126
Healthcare Systems Bureau, 152
Hemodialysis, 21, 22, 24, 44, 93, 113, 156, 158, 162
Hepatitis A, 30, 48, 49, 50, 57, 58, 137, 150-151, 189, 190
Hepatitis B. *See also* Vaccination for Hepatitis B; *specific populations and services*
    acute infection, 1, 19, 23, 27, 34, 48, 50, 59, 70-71, 99, 117, 118, 119, 120, 121, 125, 161, 189
    adults, 27, 47, 117-125, 132
    at-risk populations, 1-2, 21-22, 27, 81-82, 120-125
    case definition, 48, 50, 51, 52
    causative agent, 19, 21
    children, 23, 25, 30, 47, 116-117, 128-132

chronic infection, 19, 22, 23, 34, 48, 51, 52, 59-60, 64
community knowledge and awareness, 89-93
contact screening, 48, 82, 86
deaths, 20, 23, 26, 34, 83
economic issues, 25, 26, 128-135
education programs, 83, 90, 92-93
exposure routes, 1, 21, 23, 26, 44, 90
geographic differences, 27, 81
HBsAg determinant of infection, 10, 21, 22, 46, 48, 51, 52, 54, 55, 56, 69, 82-83, 99, 100-101, 109, 110, 111, 112, 113, 114, 115, 124, 156, 157, 159, 160, 161, 162, 166, 174, 181, 182, 183
health-care provider knowledge, 81-83
health-care use trends, 30
health-care workers, 91, 124
HIV-infected people, 29, 124
immunization, *see* Vaccines and vaccination
incidence and prevalence, 1-2, 21, 23, 26-27, 29, 83, 118, 119
infants, 1, 25
institutionalized developmentally disabled people, 124
insurance coverage, 5, 128-134
knowledge and awareness of, 81-83, 89-93, 127-128
liver cancer and liver disease from, 29-30
medical management, 82, 90, 166-167
men who have sex with men, 91
mistrust of vaccination, 127-128
progression of infection and clinical outcomes, 22, 23, 25, 29, 46; *see also* Liver cancer and liver cirrhosis
public vaccine programs and insurance, 128-132
racial/ethnic differences, 27, 29
reactivation, 162
registries of immunization, 126-127
risk factors, 27
screening and testing, 5, 8, 13, 14, 23, 27, 47, 48-49, 51, 81, 82-83, 86, 90, 91, 124-125, 152, 156-157, 160-162
stigma/discrimination, 23, 91-92
surveillance, 44, 46, 47, 48, 50, 51, 52, 59-60, 61, 64, 71

Hepatitis B immune globulin (HBIG), 4, 9-10, 55, 69, 110, 111, 112-113, 114, 115, 182, 183-184
Hepatitis B Initiative, 92
Hepatitis C. *See also specific populations and services*
   acute infection, 19, 28, 29, 34, 47, 49, 51, 71, 136, 137, 163, 165
   adults, 51
   at-risk populations, 21-22, 28, 93-101, 158
   case definition, 49, 50, 53, 68
   causative agent, 19, 21, 137
   children, 51
   chronic infection, 17, 22, 34, 51-52, 59, 64, 136-138
   economic issues, 25, 26, 137-138
   education programs, 84-85, 95-96
   exposure routes, 2, 5, 21, 24, 26, 28, 44, 84
   health-care provider knowledge, 83-85
   in HIV-infected people, 30
   knowledge and awareness, 83-85, 93-96
   medical management, 167-169
   mortality, 20, 23, 26, 34, 45
   prevalence and incidence, 21, 22-23, 24, 26, 28-29, 137, 138
   prevention, 5, 24, 79, 136-138, 196-187
   progression of infection and clinical outcomes, 22, 24, 29-30, 47, 84; *see also* Liver cancer and liver cirrhosis
   racial/ethnic differences, 29-30, 168-169
   risk factors, 29-30, 84
   screening and testing, 5, 8, 28, 51-52, 53-54, 62, 68, 84, 85, 86, 93-94, 152, 157-159, 162-165
   spontaneous resolution, 51, 136
   stigma/discrimination, 24, 85, 94-95
   surveillance, 28, 44, 45, 47, 49, 51-52, 53-54, 59-60, 61, 62, 63, 64, 71
   vaccine development, 2, 5, 24, 136-138
Hepatitis C Continuity Program, 185-186
Hepatitis D, 30
Hepatitis E, 30
Hepatocellular carcinoma. *See* Liver cancer and liver cirrhosis
High-risk populations. *See* At-risk populations
Hispanics, 2, 10, 27, 30, 93, 116, 121, 159, 168-169, 184-185

HIV/AIDS, 124
   burden of disease, 25, 26
   coinfection, 23, 29, 72, 81-82, 190
   funding for activities, 45, 150-151
   HBV vaccination, 93, 113, 120, 124, 129
   mortality, 20, 45
   partner services, 63, 72
   Prevention for Positives initiatives, 95
   public awareness campaign, 98
   screening and testing, 120, 156, 162
   surveillance, 59, 61, 62, 63, 64, 66, 67, 72
HIV/AIDS Bureau, 152
Homeless people, 56, 62, 71, 152, 154-155, 187, 188, 191

I

Illicit-drug users, injection drug users. *See also* Drug treatment programs and facilities
   access to health services, 2, 24, 29, 56, 85, 176
   acute infections, 120, 137, 189
   contact notification, 63, 72, 86
   education programs, 95-96, 97, 154, 179
   gaps in services for, 175-181
   HBV, 1, 14, 23, 61-62, 82, 83, 120-121, 122-123, 176
   HCV, 2, 5, 8, 14-15, 24, 28-29, 61, 62, 83, 84, 86, 93-94, 95-96, 136-137, 148, 158, 175-176
   health-care use, 14, 176
   high-risk period, 14-15
   knowledge and awareness of risks to, 82, 83, 86, 94, 95-96
   needle-exchange/safe injection programs, 5, 9, 14, 28, 80, 88-89, 94, 97, 100, 120-121, 148, 155, 166, 177, 180
   prevalence and incidence of infection, 14, 27, 61-62, 82, 96, 120, 176
   recommendations, 15, 179-181
   referral for medical management, 148
   screening, testing, and counseling, 14, 62, 83, 85, 86, 94, 148, 156-157, 158, 162, 163, 179
   stigmatization and discrimination, 24, 85

surveillance, 2, 56, 61-62, 63
transmission of hepatitis, 1, 14, 24
vaccination, 14, 93, 120-121, 122-123, 124, 129, 157
viral hepatitis services, 5, 14-15, 63, 148-149, 175-181
Illicit-drug users, non-injection drug users, 9, 14, 96, 97, 122-123, 175-176
Immigrant services, 8. *See also* Foreign-born populations
Immunization. *See also* Vaccines and vaccination
HBIG adjuvant, 4, 9-10, 55, 69, 110, 111, 112-113, 114, 115, 182, 183-184
Immunoglobulin M (IgM) antibody, 48, 49, 50, 51, 52, 160, 161
Immunosuppresive therapy, 162
Incarcerated populations
acute infections, 121
education programs, 5, 8, 9, 99-100
HBV, 16, 27, 62, 83, 90-91, 121-124, 184
HCV, 8, 16, 28, 62, 83, 86, 100, 184
knowledge and awareness of risks to, 83, 86, 90-91
prevalence and incidence of infection, 121, 184
racial/ethnic differences, 184-185
recommendations, 186
screening and testing, 16, 156-157, 185
size of, 62, 99
surveillance, 62
vaccination, 121-124, 157, 185
viral health services, 6, 16, 149, 184-186
Incidence of hepatitis. *See* Prevalence and incidence of hepatitis
Infants. *See also* Perinatal infections
antiviral therapy, 183-184
followup, 56
HBV case definition, 55
HBV infection, 4, 9-10, 25, 54-55, 75, 93, 100, 110, 111-116, 173, 182
immunization, 4, 9-10, 25, 54-55, 75, 93, 100, 110, 111-116, 173, 182
incidence and prevalence of hepatitis, 100, 111, 112, 182
potential for and progression to chronic infection, 22, 46, 51, 82, 113, 156
preterm, 111, 112, 114, 115
screening/testing, 54, 162
surveillance, 182

Infectious Diseases Society of America, 159
Inflammatory bowel disease, 162
Influenza, 20, 27, 110
Information systems, 5, 11, 72, 126-127
Initiative on Immunization Registries, 126
Institute of Medicine, 127-128
Institutionalized developmentally disabled people, 62, 93, 113, 124, 156-157
Insurance coverage
gaps and barriers, 11, 134-135, 170
private plans, 11, 12, 132-134
public plans, 11-12, 128-132, 172-173; *see also specific programs*
recommendations, 11-12, 172-173
screening and testing, 13, 148
vaccination, 5, 11-12, 128-132, 135
International Symposium on Viral Hepatitis and Liver Disease, 82, 83
Injection-drug users. *See* Illicit-drug users
Iowa, 95
Italy, 163

J

Jade Ribbon Campaign, 92, 153-154

K

Knowledge and awareness of chronic hepatitis. *See also* Educational programs
age and, 93
asymptomatic infected individuals, 1, 3, 24, 26, 27, 50, 51, 90
at-risk populations, 3, 4, 8, 9, 13, 34, 82, 89-91, 93-96, 173
of clinical outcomes, 80, 83, 89
community, 89-101
contact notification and screening, 9, 84
correctional facilities, 88-89, 99-100
and discrimination and stigma, 8, 9, 85, 91-92, 94-95
drug-treatment facilities and needle-exchange programs, 5, 8, 9, 100
exposure routes, 95
general public, 3, 4, 9, 17, 33, 34, 79, 98
HBV, 81-83, 89-93, 127-128
HCV, 83-85, 93-96

health-care and social-service providers, 3, 4, 8, 17, 33, 34, 79, 88-89, 154-155, 171, 182-183
mistrust of vaccination, 8, 127-128
perinatal facilities, 82-83, 100-101
policy-makers, 3, 17, 98
of prevalence and incidence, 8, 79, 80, 81, 83, 89, 153-154
of prevention approaches, 80, 89
race/ethnicity and, 93
recommendations, 4, 8-9, 85-89, 96-101
or risk factors and high-risk population characteristics, 80, 81-84, 89
of screening, testing, and management methods, 5, 8, 9, 79, 80, 82-83, 84, 90
surveillance and, 45
Korean Americans, 90

L

Lamivudine prophylaxis, 162, 170, 183
Lao People's Democratic Republic, 115-116
Liver cancer and liver cirrhosis
  age and, 79
  deaths, 1, 23, 24, 25, 29
  incidence and prevalence, 22-23, 79, 154
  prevention, 1, 19, 109
  progression of infection to, 46-47
  racial/ethnic differences, 29-30, 153-154, 169
  risk factors, 29-30, 169
  surveillance, 67, 72
  survival rate, 23
Liver transplants, 25, 67, 110, 169

M

Maryland, 27 n.1, 116, 173
Massachusetts, 63, 69, 186
Measles, 20, 116 n.1, 136
Medicaid, 13, 128-129, 132, 148, 152, 168, 172
  Early Periodic Screening, Diagnosis, and Treatment, 11, 130-131, 134
Medical management of hepatitis, 3, 5, 166-170
  access to, 56, 79, 130, 183
  antiviral therapy, 6, 15, 24, 79, 86, 149, 184
  coinfections, 23
  components of, 155
  costs and cost-effectiveness, 163, 169-170
  disparities, 169
  education on, 86
  goals, 166
  guidelines, 30, 32, 80, 155, 166-168
  insurance coverage, 130, 170
  interferon-alpha-based treatment, 30, 170
  provider knowledge, 82, 86
  racial/ethnic disparities, 168-169
  referral for, 5, 6, 14, 15, 31, 56, 62-63, 70, 72, 83, 120-121, 148, 149, 153, 166, 170, 171, 177, 181, 182, 183, 189
Medicare, 5, 13, 128, 130, 132, 134, 148, 152, 168, 172
Men who have sex with men, 21, 27, 44, 71, 81, 82, 91, 97, 113, 156, 162, 191
Metabolic syndrome, 30
Minnesota, 58, 172
Mobile health units, 6, 13, 16-17, 120-121, 122, 149, 189, 191-192
Montana, 116
Multiple sclerosis, 32

N

National Alliance of State and Territorial AIDS Directors (NASTAD), 42-43, 58, 59, 60, 61, 63, 189
National Center for HIV/AIDS, Viral Hepatitis, Sexually Transmitted Diseases, and Tuberculosis Prevention, 26, 45, 150-151
National Center for Immunization and Respiratory Diseases, 15, 126, 181-182
National Electronic Disease Surveillance System (NEDSS), 61
National Electronic Telecommunications System for Surveillance (NETSS), 60-61, 64
National Health and Nutrition Examination Survey, 62
National HIV Behavioral Surveillance System, 62, 72

INDEX

National Immunization Program, 126
National Immunization Surveys, 111-112, 126, 128
National Institutes of Health, 6, 15, 30, 149, 184
National Vaccine Advisory Committee (NVAC), 126, 127
National Viral Hepatitis Roundtable, 2, 30
Needle-stick injuries, 1, 21, 88, 158
New Haven, 120, 122-123
New Jersey Academy of Family Physicians, 82, 83
New York City, 28, 58, 85, 90, 92, 120-121, 122, 173, 186, 190
New York state, 58, 185-186
Nosocomial infections, 24, 67, 87, 88

O

Occupational Safety and Health Administration, 88
Office of Management and Budget, 129
Omnibus Budget Reconciliation Act of 1993, 128-129
Optic neuritis, 32
Oregon, 58
Outbreak
　detection and control, 48, 67, 70
　prevention, 88

P

Partner services
　CDC guidelines, 63
　contact notification, 9, 15, 63
　cost-effectiveness, 63
　funding, 72
　screening and testing, 48, 82, 86, 98, 100, 154, 162
　surveillance, 48, 62-63, 68, 72
　vaccination, 54, 57-58, 62, 93, 113, 117, 119-120
Perinatal hepatitis B coordinators, 15, 54, 152
Perinatal infections. *See also* Pregnant women
　educational programs on, 99-101
　HBV, 46, 111-116, 152
　immunization, 9, 54-55, 111-116
　knowledge and awareness, 82-83, 100-101
　prevention, 5-6, 15, 54, 183-184
　progression of, 46
　screening and testing, 54-56
　surveillance, 54-56
Peripartum antiviral therapy, 6, 15, 149, 184
Policy-makers
　knowledge and awareness of chronic hepatitis, 3, 17, 98
Polio, 20, 110, 116 n.1
Pregnant women. *See also* Perinatal infections
　antiviral therapy, 6, 15, 149, 184
　case management, 70, 149, 182
　education, 97, 100-101
　educational programs on viral hepatitis, 9, 99-100
　foreign-born women, 23, 182-183
　HBV, 6, 15, 23, 25, 82-84, 90, 149, 182-183
　HCV, 83-84
　household contacts and sexual partners, 54, 182
　knowledge and awareness of risks to, 82-84
　lamivudine prophylaxis, 162, 170, 183
　medical management, 6, 15, 149, 182-183
　recommendations, 15-16, 184
　screening and testing, 15, 25, 54-56, 69, 82-83, 84, 111, 120, 149, 162, 181-182
　surveillance, 54, 69, 70, 182
　vaccination, 4, 10, 54, 111-116, 129, 131, 132, 182
　viral hepatitis services, 15, 149, 181-184
Prevalence and incidence of hepatitis
　accuracy of estimates, 50-51, 56, 57, 66, 70-71
　acute infections, 1, 50, 70-71, 99, 118, 119, 120, 121, 125
　APIs, 1-2, 23, 27, 29, 81-82, 83, 93, 117-118, 153-154, 161, 183, 184-185
　at-risk populations, 62, 81
　CDC estimates, 25, 26, 27, 62, 120, 182, 189
　chronic infections, 1, 34, 121
　definitions, 7 n.1
　immigration and, 2
　knowledge and awareness of, 8, 79, 80, 81, 83, 89, 153-154

monitoring and reporting, 71; *see also* Surveillance
U.S., 1, 2, 25-29, 86
worldwide, 22-24
Prevention and control of hepatitis. *See also* Counseling; Educational programs; Medical management of hepatitis; Screening and testing; Vaccines and vaccination; Viral hepatitis services
barriers to, 2-3
CDC recommendation, 30
charge to committee, 31
education on, 80, 87
funding, 44, 54
harm reduction, 155, 166
knowledge and awareness of methods, 84, 86
needle-exchange/safe injection programs, 5, 9, 14, 28, 80, 88-89, 94, 97, 100, 120-121, 148, 155, 166, 180
perinatal transmission, 25, 183-184
research recommendations, 15
state plans, 152-153
strategies, 25, 31, 84, 177-179
Prevention for Positives initiatives, 95
Public Health Information Network (PHIN), 7, 61, 64, 65, 70

R

Race/ethnicity
and knowledge and awareness of hepatitis, 93
vaccination disparities, 10, 116-117, 121
Racial and Ethnic Approaches to Community Health (REACH) 2010, 93
Recommendations
at-risk populations, 14, 15, 16-17, 175, 179-181, 184, 186
committee approach, 32
community health centers, 188-189
education programs, 4, 8-9, 85-89, 96-101
insurance coverage, 11-12, 172-173
integrated services, 192
outcomes of implementing, 17, 34
screening and testing, 4, 6, 13, 16, 148
vaccination, 4-5, 9-12, 93, 114, 117, 125, 127, 135, 136, 138

Referral for additional services, 5, 6, 14, 15, 31, 56, 62-63, 70, 72, 83, 120-121, 148, 149, 153, 166, 170, 171, 177, 181, 182, 183, 189
Reporting systems and requirements, 59-61, 68
Resource allocation, 45
barriers to, 3
CDC, 5-6, 14, 15, 16-17, 26, 42, 54, 126-127, 148-150, 151, 152, 153, 175, 183, 186, 192
Respiratory syncytial virus, 20
Rheumatoid arthritis, 162
Rhode Island, 90
Risk factors for hepatitis
APIs, 90
CDC, 156, 157-158, 159
knowledge and awareness of, 80, 81-84, 89
screening for, 3, 5, 8, 11, 13, 16, 85, 86, 124-125, 148, 153, 155, 156-159, 162
Ryan White CARE Act and program, 33, 152, 170

S

Safety precautions and procedures, 88
San Diego, 134, 170, 189-190
San Francisco, 58, 81, 120, 121, 122-123, 173, 174, 182
Schistosomiasis-eradication campaign, 24
Scotland, 122-123
Screening and testing
access to, 3
acute infections, 47-51, 160, 161, 163, 165
antigens and antibodies used for, 160, 161
at-risk populations, 3, 4, 5, 6, 9, 11, 13-14, 16, 27, 71-72, 91-92, 97, 120, 124-125, 148, 152, 153-154, 156-157, 158-159, 161-162, 173
barriers to, 124-125
CDC recommendations, 82-83, 84, 156-157, 159, 183
community-based programs, 5, 13
confirmatory tests, 162-163
contacts/partners, 48, 82, 86, 98, 100, 154, 162

cost-effectiveness, 27, 161-162, 163
cultural aversion to, 91-92, 98
education on, 9, 58, 98
electronic laboratory reporting, 7, 60, 65, 68-69, 70
enzyme immunoassay, 51, 53, 54, 162-163, 164-165
followup/repeat, 48-49, 80
general population, 13
goals, 154-155
guidelines, 80, 86
HBV, 5, 8, 13, 14, 23, 27, 48-49, 51, 81, 82-83, 86, 90, 91, 124-125, 152, 156-157, 160-162
HCV, 5, 8, 28, 51-52, 53-54, 62, 68, 84, 85, 86, 93-94, 152, 157-159, 162-165
importance, 23
insurance coverage, 13, 148, 171
interpretation of results, 94, 160-161, 162, 164-165
knowledge and awareness of methods, 5, 8, 9, 79, 80, 82-83, 84, 90
laws, 83
nucleic acid testing, 49, 53-54, 68, 159, 163, 164-165
pregnant women, 15, 25, 54-56, 69, 82-83, 84, 111, 120, 149, 162
recombinant immunoblot assay, 49, 53, 163, 164-165
recommendations, 4, 6, 13, 16, 148
referral for medical management, 5, 6, 14, 15, 31, 56, 62-63, 70, 72, 83, 120-121, 148, 149, 153, 166, 170, 171, 177, 181, 182, 183, 189
reporting test results, 4, 6, 7, 41-56, 58, 59-61, 65, 66, 67, 68-69
resource allocation, 3, 17, 45
resources available for, 49, 54, 56, 57-58
risk-factor, 3, 5, 8, 11, 13, 16, 85, 86, 91, 124-125, 148, 153, 155, 156-159, 162
serologic, 4, 5, 6, 7, 13, 47, 51, 53-54, 120, 148, 156, 159-165
VA program, 28, 158
Section 317 Immunization Grant program, 11, 126, 129, 130, 132, 134, 135, 153
Services. See Viral hepatitis services
Sexual exposure to hepatitis, 1, 23, 44, 72, 84, 113, 119-120

Sexually transmitted diseases (STDs)
  clinic services for hepatitis, 6, 13, 14, 16-17, 54, 86, 87, 119-120, 124, 125, 129, 134, 149, 151, 170, 171, 176, 189-190, 191, 192
  disease intervention specialists, 63
  funding for services, 45, 151
  integrating services for STD and hepatitis, 189-190
  partner notification, 63
  surveillance, 59, 61, 63
Shelter-based programs, 6, 13, 16-17, 149, 189, 191, 192
Social and peer support, 3, 95, 100, 155
Social-service providers. See also Substance-abuse services and providers
  educational programs, 88-89
  knowledge and awareness of hepatitis, 80-89
Society of General Internal Medicine, 82
South Dakota, 116
Southeast Asian immigrants, 24, 79, 82, 183
Standardization of data, 69
State and territorial health departments
  case followup, 55
  cooperative agreements with CDC, 4, 7, 42, 54, 57, 64-66, 67
  funding, 152
  surveillance role, 4, 6, 7
STD/HIV clinics, 87, 189-190
Stigmatization and discrimination, 8, 9, 23, 24, 56, 85, 87, 89, 91-92, 94-95, 97, 98, 170, 174
Study to Reduce Intravenous Exposures (STRIVE), 95
Sub-Saharan African immigrants, 23, 79, 82, 90
Substance Abuse and Mental Health Services Administration (SAMHSA), 149, 152
Substance-abuse services and providers. See Drug treatment programs and facilities
Surveillance
  acute infections, 29, 44, 47-51, 59, 64, 67, 71
  analyzing, reporting, and disseminating findings, 67, 70-71
  applications of data from, 41, 42, 43-46
  at-risk populations, 2, 4, 6, 7, 32, 61-62, 67, 68, 71-72

automated data collection, 7, 51, 56, 60, 65, 68-70
AVHPC surveys, 42-43, 54, 55, 57, 58, 59, 61, 64, 70
case definitions, 7, 48, 49, 50, 51, 52, 53, 54, 55, 65, 68, 69
case management uses, 43, 45-46, 57-58, 62-63, 65, 68, 70, 72
CDC initiatives, 4, 6, 7-8, 42-43, 44, 45, 50, 57, 58, 59-61, 63, 64, 65-66, 67, 68, 69, 70-71, 150
challenges, 29, 47-54, 56, 60
chronic infections, 25, 44, 51-54, 59, 64, 67, 71
committee charge and approach, 31-32, 41-42
confidentiality safeguards, 43-44, 65
core activities, 4, 6, 7, 43, 66, 67, 68
current system, 3, 25, 34, 41-42
design of programs, 6, 59
disease-specific issues, 46-56
electronic medical records, 7, 50, 51, 60, 65, 68, 69, 70
enhanced projects, 58, 62, 71-72
evaluation of systems, 63-64, 66, 69, 70
funding, 3, 7, 42, 57, 58-59, 63, 65, 66, 67, 71, 129
identifying infections, 4, 6, 41-56, 69
infrastructure and process-specific issues, 57-66, 67, 70
jurisdictional issues, 56, 57, 60, 65-66
and knowledge and awareness of hepatitis, 45
liver cancer and cirrhosis, 67, 72
model programs, 43, 65, 66-72
outbreak detection and control uses, 44, 48, 67, 70
partners of infected people, 48, 62-63, 68, 72
perinatal infections, 54-56
PHIN-compliant systems, 7, 61, 64, 65, 70
pregnant women, 54, 69, 70, 182
programmatic design and evaluation uses, 3, 41, 45, 57, 67
quality of data, 50, 57, 64, 66, 67, 71, 79, 94
recommendations, 4, 6-7, 43, 63-66
reporting systems and requirements, 7, 48, 51, 58, 59-61, 65, 66, 67, 68-69
resource allocation uses, 3, 17, 45

serologic testing, 4, 6, 7, 47, 51, 53-54, 68, 71, 159-165
standardization issues, 6, 7, 41, 56, 61, 64, 65, 66-67, 68, 69, 70
state-CDC cooperative agreements, 4, 7, 42, 54, 57, 64-66, 67
targeted, 43, 66, 71-72
underreporting/misclassification of infections, 3, 27, 34, 47, 50, 60, 62, 70-71
vaccinations, 59, 72, 111

T

Tattooing and piercing, 99, 158-159
Transverse myelitis, 32
Travelers, 22, 93, 113, 117, 156
Tuberculosis, 20, 26, 45, 61, 150, 151, 186

U

United Kingdom, 162
US Preventive Services Task Force, 82-83, 159, 181
US Public Health Service, 132, 150, 159, 190

V

Vaccines and vaccination, HBV
  accessibility, 120-121, 124, 128, 129, 134, 135
  ACIP recommendations, 4, 9-10, 11, 55, 83, 88, 93, 100, 110-115, 116, 125, 127, 132, 133, 134, 181
  adults, 11, 32, 93, 110, 111, 113, 116, 117-125, 126, 127, 128, 129, 132, 134
  at-risk populations, 4, 9, 10-11, 27, 81, 93, 113, 117-125
  barriers to, 8, 10, 11-12, 118, 120, 124-125, 127-136
  CDC recommendations and programs, 12, 110-111, 124-125, 126, 128-129, 134, 136, 153, 157
  children and adolescents, 4, 9, 10, 25, 30, 93, 97, 110, 111, 112, 116-117, 126, 127, 128-132, 134
  cost-effectiveness, 54, 57-58, 117-119, 124, 137-138, 162

INDEX

coverage data, 111-112, 114-115, 116, 117, 118, 120, 121, 126, 132
education programs, 8, 9, 97, 101
efficacy, 110
evaluation of programs, 45
foreign-born people, 5, 10, 13, 14, 90, 91, 92-93, 116, 117-118, 120, 132, 148, 152, 161-162
formulations, 109-110, 136
funding for, 57, 118, 120, 129, 134, 152
geographic variability, 116
HBIG adjunct, 110, 114
health-care and social-service workers, 88, 93, 113, 117, 118, 124, 125
HIV-infected people, 93, 113, 120, 124, 129
identifying at-risk adults for, 124-125
illicit-drug users, 14, 93, 120-121, 122-123, 124, 129
immunization-information systems, 5, 11, 72, 126-127
incarcerated people, 11, 113, 121-124, 125
incentives, 121
infants, 4, 9-10, 25, 54-55, 75, 93, 97, 110, 111-116, 120, 173, 182
institutionalized developmentally disabled people, 93, 124
insurance coverage, 5, 11-12, 128-132, 135
liver cancer prevention, 109
liver transplants and, 110
mandatory, 116-117, 134, 153
mistrust of, 8, 127-128
partners and household members (ring vaccination), 54, 57-58, 62, 93, 117, 119-120, 162
payment for, 57, 128-135, 152, 153
perinatal, 4, 10, 54, 111-116, 129, 131, 132
public programs and insurance, 128-132
racial and ethnic disparities, 10, 116-117, 121
recommendations (committee), 4-5, 9-12, 93, 114, 117, 125, 127, 135, 136, 138
safety issues, 32-33, 127-128
schedules and completion of series, 11, 25, 55, 91, 101, 110, 111, 114, 116 n.1, 120, 121, 125, 127, 157

supply of vaccines, 5, 12, 118, 127, 135-136
surveillance, 59, 72, 111
travelers, 22, 93, 113, 117, 156
WHO guidelines, 30, 114
Vaccines and vaccination, HCV
development, 2, 24, 136-138, 166
feasibility, 136-137
need for, 137
recommendations, 5, 12, 138
therapeutic, 136
Vaccines for Children (VFC) program, 128-129, 130, 131, 134
Veterans, 28, 94, 130-131, 158, 168, 171
Vietnamese Americans, 68, 90, 171
Viral hepatitis services. *See also* Counseling; Educational programs; Medical management of hepatitis; Screening and testing; Vaccines and vaccination
access to, 2, 3, 34, 56, 79, 151, 169, 170
adult viral-hepatitis prevention coordinators, 42-43, 57, 59, 61, 64, 70, 152-153
adults, 3, 5, 6, 13, 16-17, 56, 79, 149, 189-192
case management, 45-46, 57-58, 62-63, 70, 72, 149, 170
CDC allocations for, 5-6, 14, 15, 16-17, 26, 42, 54, 126-127, 148-150, 151, 152, 153, 175, 183, 186, 192
community-based approaches, 5, 6, 13, 14, 16, 148, 149, 174-175, 186-188
core components, 5, 12, 13, 148, 153, 154-157
current status, 148-154
design and evaluation of programs, 3, 41, 45, 57, 67
foreign-born people, 5, 12, 13-14, 16, 92, 148, 173-175
funding (public), 148-149, 150-152, 171, 172-173
gaps in, 12-17, 170-192
general population, 12, 13, 148, 170-173
HBV, 5-6, 14, 15, 148, 149, 153, 182-183
HCV, 5, 14, 148-149, 153
identifying infected persons, *see* Screening and testing
illicit-drug users, 2, 5, 12, 14-15, 148-149, 175-181

incarcerated populations, 6, 13, 16, 149, 184-186
integrated approach, 14, 16-17, 149, 171-172, 179, 180-181, 189-192
knowledge and awareness of, 91
mobile health units, 6, 13, 16-17, 120-121, 122, 149, 189, 191-192
model programs, 33, 152, 157, 170, 171-172
nongovernmental organizations, 153-154
pregnant women, 5-6, 13, 15, 54, 70, 149, 181-184
prevention, 3, 5, 12, 15, 166, 177-179, 183-184; *see also* Vaccines and vaccination
program venues for high-risk groups, 13, 176-177
recommendations, 5-6, 12-17, 148-149, 172-173, 179-181, 192

shelter-based programs, 6, 13, 16-17, 149, 189, 191, 192
social support, 3
at STD/HIV clinics, 6, 13, 14, 16-17, 54, 86, 87, 119-120, 124, 125, 129, 134, 149, 151, 170, 171, 176, 189-190, 191, 192
Viral Hepatitis Surveillance Emerging Infections Program, 58
Vitamin K prophylaxis, 115

W

Washington State Basic Health Insurance Plan, 171
Whites, 2, 10, 27, 30, 33, 81, 116, 168, 169, 184-185
World Health Organization, 23, 30, 115
  Collaborating Center for Reference and Research on Viral Hepatitis, 151